NEOPLASIA OF HEAD AND NECK

Proceedings of the Annual Clinical Conferences on Cancer
sponsored by The University of Texas System Cancer Center
M. D. Anderson Hospital and Tumor Institute,
and published by Year Book Medical Publishers, Inc.

TUMORS OF THE SKIN
TUMORS OF BONE AND SOFT TISSUE
RECENT ADVANCES IN THE DIAGNOSIS OF CANCER
CANCER OF THE GASTROINTESTINAL TRACT
CANCER OF THE UTERUS AND OVARY
NEOPLASIA IN CHILDHOOD
BREAST CANCER: EARLY AND LATE
LEUKEMIA-LYMPHOMA
REHABILITATION OF THE CANCER PATIENT
ENDOCRINE AND NONENDOCRINE
HORMONE-PRODUCING TUMORS
NEOPLASIA OF HEAD AND NECK

NEOPLASIA OF HEAD AND NECK

A Collection of Papers Presented at the
Seventeenth Annual Clinical Conference on Cancer, 1972,
at The University of Texas System Cancer Center
M. D. Anderson Hospital and Tumor Institute,
Houston, Texas

YEAR BOOK MEDICAL PUBLISHERS, INC.
35 East Wacker Drive, Chicago

Library of Congress Catalog Card Number: 74-78368
International Standard Book Number: 0-8151-0210-0

Acknowledgments

FOR THEIR SUPPORT in making possible both the Seventeenth Annual Clinical Conference and the publication of this monograph, the staff of M. D. Anderson Hospital and Tumor Institute of The University of Texas System Cancer Center gratefully acknowledges the assistance of the Texas Division of the American Cancer Society, American Cancer Society, Inc., and the Division of Continuing Education of The University of Texas Health Science Center at Houston.

The program was arranged and organized by a committee composed of the following staff members of M. D. Anderson Hospital: Richard H. Jesse, chairman; Robert D. Lindberg, co-chairman; and members A. J. Ballantyne, James M. Bowen, Sebron C. Dale, Joe B. Drane, Robert C. Hickey, Renilda Hilkemeyer, Mario A. Luna, and Edna P. Wagner.

This volume was prepared for publication by the following members of the M. D. Anderson Hospital Department of Publications: R. W. Cumley, Joan E. McCay, Dorothy M. Beane, Susan Birkel Freitag, Walter J. Pagel, Carol A. Flynn, Susan L. Huey, D. Ruth SoRelle, Jane E. Parker, and Larry W. Dybala. The secretarial efforts of Mrs. Connie Fox and Mrs. Alice Rojas of the Department of Publications and Miss Nancy Jordan of the Section of Head and Neck, Department of Surgery, are greatly appreciated.

Many of the illustrations in this volume were prepared by members of the M. D. Anderson Hospital Department of Medical Communications.

Contents

Introduction

R. LEE CLARK, M.D., M.Sc., D.Sc. (Hon.)

*President, The University of Texas System Cancer Center; and Professor
of Surgery, The University of Texas M. D. Anderson
Hospital and Tumor Institute, Houston, Texas*

EACH YEAR we consider it a privilege and a welcome responsibility to share with physicians of the area the knowledge that we have acquired in treating the patients they have referred to us. This mutual sharing of problems and knowledge fulfills the assigned mission of The University of Texas M. D. Anderson Hospital, as envisioned by the State Legislature and the Board of Regents of The University of Texas back in 1941, when legislation was passed to establish a state cancer hospital and research institute.

This Seventeenth Annual Clinical Conference on Neoplasia of Head and Neck is a singularly timely one, as it exemplifies all the aspects that are emphasized in the new cancer research and demonstration program being designed and activated by this country.

In the past, the National Cancer Institute has interpreted its role as primarily that of fostering cancer research in the United States and has not considered clinical application within its purview. During the conferences convened to draft recommendations for new legislation to expand the national effort to reduce cancer mortality in this country, it became obvious that little progress would be made if mechanisms were not designed to translate the knowledge, acquired through research, to widespread application at the bedside and in the outpatient clinics.

Consequently, there is a new emphasis on establishing additional comprehensive cancer research and demonstration centers that conduct multidisciplinary programs of research, education, and patient care; sustain active information exchange with other cancer institutions, national and international; and are actively involved in community programs to rehabilitate disabled cancer patients and return them to their communities prepared for a quality existence and productive activities.

There are few anatomic areas attacked by cancer which demonstrate such a dramatic need of multidisciplinary teamwork for adequate medical and rehabilitative management as the head and neck. Often the initial diagnosis is made by a dentist alert to the possibilities of neoplastic changes in the oral cavity, or by a dermatologist, an internist, or an eye, ear, nose, and throat specialist. Other members of the team may be the diagnostic radiologist, the pathologist, the endocrinologist, the head and neck surgeon, the dental surgeon, the neurosurgeon, the radiotherapist, the chemotherapist, the plastic surgeon, the maxillofacial prosthodontist, the nutritionist, and the specialists in the various rehabilitative programs; for example, speech therapists, occupational therapists, etc.

Each of these individuals has a clearly defined role in the total treatment plan and each plays a vital part in coordinating his particular contribution with the sequential events so essential for comprehensive therapy.

This cooperative environment is an ideal one for educational purposes. The student seldom observes such teamwork in the average general teaching hospital. He is able to acquire a much more comprehensive view of how the bench scientist, the kinetic engineer, the clinical scientist, and the medical and paramedical specialists all contribute to high-quality care of an individual cancer patient. In such an environment, there is no competition for patients or for financial remuneration, and all those involved have the common bond of educating the young in addition to the goal of improved cancer treatment.

As cancer treatment has significantly improved, through the concept of multidisciplinary teamwork involving persons especially trained in oncology, more and more of the specialty boards have realized a real need for an oncology subspecialty within each of the specialty training programs.

The recognition of such a need for training is exemplified by a meeting held October 15, 1972. Representatives from the Society of Head and Neck Surgeons, the American Society of Head and Neck Surgery, and the American Boards of General Surgery, Otolaryngology, and Plastic Surgery recommended that, following certification by respective boards, a certificate of proficiency in oncological head and neck surgery should be awarded by each Society and/or Board after completion of one year in an approved program. This recommendation is to be submitted for approval of the membership of each society and board.

In 1950, The University of Texas Dental Branch and M. D. Anderson Hospital and Tumor Institute entered into a cooperative program designed to correct deformities of patients subjected to surgical treatment for cancer of the head and neck. Prosthetic devices are designed and constructed for those individuals whose deformities cannot be corrected by plastic surgery, or those who will need a cosmetic device during the interim between widely spaced surgical procedures. In 1966, this program was expanded and became the Regional Maxillofacial Restorative Center, serving not only the cancer patients of Texas but those of the four surrounding states as well. The Center receives additional support from the Social Rehabilitation Service and, until September of 1972, the Regional Medical Program of Texas.

This rehabilitation program is only part of a total program soon to be housed in the nation's first hospital organized totally for the rehabilitation of cancer patients and known as the Rehabilitation and Extended Care Annex of The University of Texas M. D. Anderson Hospital and Tumor Institute. This hospital has four floors and will provide space for 110 inpatients, the majority of whom will be ambulatory and capable of self-care while receiving physical, psychological, or vocational rehabilitation following their treatment for cancer. An adjacent facility already houses 19 indigent ambulatory patients. M. D. Anderson Hospital owns and will operate this rehabilitation facility as an integral part of its total program and will be responsible for the major supportive services for the hospital.

We wish to thank the American Cancer Society, both the national organization and the Texas Division, and the Division of Continuing Education of The University of Texas Graduate School of Biomedical Sciences for their assistance in making this Conference possible. And, once again, we express our appreciation to the Board of Regents of The University of Texas for their never-failing support as we strive to carry out our mission for the citizens of Texas.

The Heath Memorial Awards

ROBERT C. HICKEY, M.D.

Director, The University of Texas System Cancer Center,
M. D. Anderson Hospital and Tumor Institute,
Houston, Texas

THE HEATH MEMORIAL AWARD is made possible again this year through the generosity and concern of the late William Womack Heath and his lovely wife, Mavis Barnett Heath. Mr. and Mrs. Heath established the award seven years ago; it honors the memory of Mr. Heath's three brothers, Guy H., Dan C., and Gilford G. Heath, and acknowledges an individual who has made "outstanding contributions to the better care of the cancer patient by the clinical application of basic cancer knowledge."

It is a privilege to present the Heath Award to two men this year—men who are long-standing associates and friends. Both are on the staff of The University of Texas System Cancer Center, M. D. Anderson Hospital and Tumor Institute. The Award Committee and others reflected on the propriety of an award to staff members, since all previous awardees have been from other institutions and organizations. Upon reflection, however, the Committee members were overwhelmed by the impropriety of omission. One cannot sum up in five minutes the accomplishments of one man, not to mention those of two, but I shall give some very brief background information. Both awardees are educators and clinical scientists. In 1952, when Dr. William S. MacComb came to M. D. Anderson Hospital from Memorial Hospital in New York, he and Dr. Gilbert H. Fletcher combined the modalities of surgery and radiotherapy to create a better treatment program for some types of cancer of the head and neck.

In addition to his many contributions to the improvement of surgical techniques in his specialty, Dr. William Spencer MacComb is Professor of Surgery of the Head and Neck Service of M. D. Anderson Hospital and has trained more than 150 Surgical Fellows on that service. (My first surgical thyroidectomy was done under the tutelage of this man.)

He was a founder and first President of the James Ewing Society. He is the only person to serve as President of three well-known societies—the James Ewing Society, the American Radium Society, and the Society of Head and Neck Surgeons—and to be honored by all three with their respective awards. He is presently the Surgical Director of the Regional Maxillofacial Restorative Center which is dedicated to the rehabilitation of cancer patients who have undergone extensive operations on the head and neck region and who require prostheses or plastic or oral surgery to repair the residual disabling defects of curative surgical procedures.

Dr. Gilbert Hungerford Fletcher is Professor of Radiotherapy and has been Head of the Department of Radiotherapy (originally known as the Radiotherapy Section) since his affiliation with M. D. Anderson Hospital in 1948. In addition to the M.D. degree, Dr. Fletcher also has degrees in civil engineering, physics, and mathematics.

He has been honored by the Countries of Peru, Italy, and Great Britain. As a Fellow of the American College of Radiology, he serves as a consultant to the Surgeon General of the United States and is a member of the Cancer Program Committee of the National Institutes of Health.

Dr. Fletcher and the late Dr. Leonard Grimmett designed and developed the prototype of the first 1,000-curie cobalt teletherapy unit approved by the Atomic Energy Commission in 1950 for use in the treatment of patients. It became a working reality in 1954, and modifications of this unit are being used in hospitals throughout the world.

Both Dr. Fletcher and Dr. MacComb have written chapters on surgery and radiotherapy of head and neck cancer for textbooks, and in 1967 they published a book entitled *Cancer of the Head and Neck*. Each is responsible for numerous other publications.

The procedures established by these two men have been adopted widely by teams of cancer therapists and are undoubtedly responsible in great measure for making a more superior, comprehensive therapeutic management of disease available for patients with cancer of the head and neck.

It is my privilege to introduce first Dr. William S. MacComb, whose presentation is "A Review of Cancer Treatment for Neoplasms of the Head and Neck," and then Dr. Gilbert H. Fletcher, who shares with us his extensive knowledge in a presentation on "Radiation Therapy and Subclinical Cancer."

HEATH MEMORIAL AWARD LECTURE
Head and Neck Cancer: Reminiscences and Comments

WILLIAM S. MacCOMB, M.D.

Professor of Surgery and Emeritus Chief of the Head and Neck Section, The University of Texas System Cancer Center, M. D. Anderson Hospital and Tumor Institute, and Surgical Director, Regional Maxillofacial Restorative Center, Houston, Texas

To HAVE BEEN DESIGNATED CORECIPIENT of the Heath Award is a great honor. Since I first entered medical school nearly 50 years ago, the diagnosis and treatment of cancer of the head and neck areas have undergone progressive changes, not entirely commensurate, however, with discoveries and advancements in other fields of medicine.

Until the early 1920's, little was attempted for patients with cancer of the head and neck, except for those with laryngeal lesions. If, as rarely happened, the diagnosis was made early, partial laryngectomies were performed with some success. Only an occasional patient who underwent total laryngectomy survived. Presumably, this operation was performed only in advanced stages of the disease, and the mortality rate was high. Few laryngologists had sufficient experience and courage to attempt a total laryngectomy.

Aside from laryngeal cancer, few reports on treatment of cancer of the head and neck are to be found in those early years. In H. T. Butlin's book on the tongue published in 1885, only one short chapter was devoted to cancer. Mortality for operations of tongue lesions was high and the end results were most discouraging.

In 1906, Dr. George Crile, Sr., reported that some patients afflicted with cancer of the head and neck (chiefly those with intraoral lesions) could be benefited by "block dissection of the neck," later known as the radical neck dissection. Dr. Crile's contentions were based on his observations and a review of autopsies in which death had resulted from intraoral cancer. Approximately 25 per cent of these patients had died of uncontrolled regional metastases and not from the primary disease itself. Dr. Crile's report was at first received with skepticism, but it did create interest in these patients, even though more than 15 years were to elapse before the operation was generally recognized for its intrinsic value. Delay in acceptance of the operation as an essential part of the treatment of the head and neck cancer patient was the result of the initially high operative mortality rate, caused in a large part by the use of general anesthesia. When local block and infiltration anesthesia came into vogue, the mortality rate immediately dropped to a quite acceptable level.

When Dr. Robert Greenough of Boston and the others on his committee of the American College of Surgeons met in 1930 to draw up the minimum requirements for the diagnosis of cancer and for cancer clinics, they discussed the probability of medical society censure. They suggested that treatment for cancer should require a group of physicians to achieve a correct diagnosis; namely a surgeon, a pathologist, a radiologist and an internist, and that treatment should not be attempted by an individual physician without this backup. Prior to 1926 the need for a positive biopsy specimen from a suspected lesion was not believed necessary before the institution of treatment. Instead, the concept of John Mackenzie, who in 1900 stated that "the removal of a piece of [for] microscopical examination too often means the beginning of the end," was generally accepted. This idea gradually changed, however, to that expressed by S. C. Thomson and L. Colledge of London in their book devoted to cancer of the larynx and published in 1930, which stated with regard to reports on biopsy specimens:

"Many mistakes have arisen from reports based on inadequate or badly collected specimens. The tragic course followed by the illness of the Emperor Frederic is a familiar example, and numerous errors of this kind have been reported. Consequently, reports must be accepted with reserve, and, in our opinion, the surgeon himself should be able to verify and confirm the report of the pathologist. We have not fallen into error by resorting to this diagnostic aid, but this is only because we have at times declined to accept the pathological report and relied on our own clinical observations."

These authors advised that only those expert in this field should attempt to obtain tissue from the larynx for a biopsy specimen by indirect laryngoscopy, and suggested instead the direct method following the invention by

Dr. Chevalier Jackson, Sr., of the anterior commissure laryngoscope and tissue forceps.

During my years in medical college, little time and effort was expended on teaching about cancer. Near the Medical School at the University of Buffalo, there existed an institution called the Gratwick Laboratory, founded in 1898 by Dr. Roswell Park. This institution, organized for cancer research, in 1911 became the New York State Institute for the Study of Malignant Disease and later the now-famous Roswell Park Memorial Institute. While I was in medical school, the director of that institute, Dr. Burton Simpson, lectured to the junior and senior classes once each year. I am afraid these lectures of one hour each made very little impression upon the students, and certainly not much upon me.

In the years of internship and residency, my attention however, was drawn to the frequency of cancer in general, and particularly to cancer in abdominal sites. These patients were usually in an advanced stage of carcinomatosis and the surgeon's comment invariably was, "Refer patient to the radiologist." What ultimately happened to the patient was, of course, "death from uncontrolled cancer." I cannot now remember a single instance of cancer in the head and neck regions being seen during those years. Why? I cannot say, but I strongly suspect that they either were unrecognized or were not being treated. Of course, it may be that they were being referred to more distant cancer centers.

Certainly, in the late 1920's few patients with head and neck cancer were treated by physicians other than the general surgeons. The otolaryngologists were adverse to any involvement in what was to them a most distressing and uncontrollable problem. Plastic surgeons were just beginning to consider treatment for lesions arising in skin. Dermatologists were treating early skin cancers by curettage and electrodesiccation, frequently without first establishing the diagnosis microscopically. Thus, not infrequently patients later developed parotid or cervical node involvement following treatment for what had been clinically believed to be basal cell epithelioma.

In 1930, I was on the private service at St. Luke's Hospital in New York, where I was fortunate to observe the work of Dr. William MacFee, a dour Scotsman and an expert and meticulous surgeon with a special interest in cancer of the head and neck, who had been trained by W. K. Simpson. Also at St. Luke's, I first met Dr. Maurice Lenz, who was treating head and neck cancer patients by radium packs externally applied and intraoral cancer with radium needle implants. At the same institution, Dr. Francis Carter Wood and Dr. Leila Knox, though both primarily pathologists, had established a department of radiotherapy.

At the close of 1930, through the interest of Dr. Lenz I was referred to Dr. James Ewing, Dr. Douglas Quick, and the director of Memorial Hospital, Dr. Burton J. Lee. So, on January 1, 1931, I began my career at that institution, first as an intern for six months; then, through the persuasion of Dr. George Pack, I continued further training for a period of three and one-half years.

Among the dedicated people at Memorial Hospital in those years were some who became my devoted and life-long friends and were to play such important roles in my future. Among these were Dr. Lloyd Craver, Dr. Edith Quimby, Dr. Gioacchino Failla, and finally Dr. Hayes Martin, whose offer in January 1931 resulted in my appointment to a position on his head and neck service where I was to remain for 17 years. Dr. Martin, though trained in general surgery, had been attached to the head and neck service at Memorial Hospital since 1928, and in 1934 had been appointed Chief of the Department.

Coutard's publication in 1932 on the use of external radiation for treatment of laryngeal cancer attracted Dr. Martin's attention. His scientific interest was aroused and with his customary zeal and energy he initiated a program for treatment of patients with cancer of the larynx by means of external radiation therapy. All of this now is ancient history, but many of us then in training at Memorial became embued with the enthusiasm of Dr. Martin and, under the aegis of Dr. Ewing who had already become a vigorous proponent of the use of radiation therapy in the treatment of cancer, pursued similar professional courses. Dr. Ewing himself was an ardent antagonist to the use of surgical procedures in cancer therapy.

In the early 1930's, Dr. Martin became a leader in the field of radiotherapy in the treatment for head and neck cancer. He invented the cylinders for circular fields as well as the peroral cone for treatment for intraoral cancers.

During the period of my fellowship training, I first saw patients treated for laryngeal and pharyngeal cancer by the Coutard method of 3,000 r (skin dose) delivered by 198 kv to either side of the neck over a period of three weeks. In reviewing this period of therapy today, I can well understand how few of these patients tolerated what are now known to be excessive doses of radiation, given too rapidly and, in the beginning, over unnecessarily large fields. External treatment to both primary and regional sites was supplemented when necessary by gold radon seeds inserted interstitially. The method of preparing gold seeds was an invention of Dr. Failla at the behest of Dr. Henry Harrington Janeway, who had been treated for a tumor of the upper jaw with the old glass, unfiltered, radon tubes and who found the pain resulting from this type of radiation unbearable.

Dr. Martin, with many of the resident training staff, published the end results of treatment by radiation therapy for cancer of various anatomical sites in the head and neck area. The results may not seem impressive today, but at that time they were better than any previously obtained by any therapeutic approach.

However, the ill effects resulting from complications of the radiation therapy, often resulting in mortality, could not be ignored. Unfortunately, at that time, the staging of cancer had not been considered. In retrospect, many of those patients probably should not have been treated by radiation because of advanced disease; others undoubtedly could have been treated with smaller fields of radiation. Age and poor general condition were not considered deterrents to active therapy, nor was the alcoholic individual ever excluded. As a consequence, morbidity and mortality were higher than would now be considered acceptable.

During the war years, Dr. Martin and his staff gradually replaced the radiotherapeutic approach with the surgical approach. Since Dr. Martin and his staff were trained primarily as general surgeons, and since residents at Memorial Hospital were accepted only after primary training in general surgery, the gradual transition to the surgical approach was logical.

Surgical procedures were mostly limited to radical neck dissections, performed under block and local infiltration anesthesia, and heavy sedation. These procedures were often carried out on patients who had previously received irradiation and who presented with uncontrolled cervical metastatic tumors. These metastatic masses were often ulcerated from radiation and accompanying infection. Such situations were, of course, most undesirable for performing a major surgical procedure, and it is hardly necessary to say that it was usually only the younger physicians who had the temerity to undertake these difficult procedures. These operations were not only hard on the patient, but also were arduous for the surgeon, especially during the summer months before the days of air conditioning.

Other surgical procedures were more limited. Tracheostomies were performed frequently, especially at the end of the course of radiothrapy. Gastrostomies, usually the Janeway type (since none were considered temporary) were frequently necessary. Primary intraoral cancers, except for those of the tongue and lip, were rarely treated by surgical procedures. Tongue lesions were often managed by an overdosage of gold radon seeds followed in approximately 48 hours by cautery removal. Only extensive cancer of the lip was primarily treated surgically; early lesions were treated by radium molds.

Hemorrhage from ulcerating tumors caused by radiation, residual disease, infection, or combinations of these conditions, was not infrequent. It was often necessary to ligate the external carotid artery or its branches; again, such ligations were always done under local infiltration anesthesia.

At first, only early lesions were selected for surgical removal. Following early successes, the surgical approach was broadened to include more advanced primary tumors, often with regional involvement.

Antibiotics were not available in those days to the civilian population. Anesthesia was induced by the same routine methods formerly employed, except that sodium pentothal, which had become available by the late 1930's, was increasingly utilized. The need for intratracheal intubation was also then recognized. Blood transfusions, formerly given by the multiple syringe direct method only, were replaced by blood banks in the early war years.

By the end of the war, there were no borders beyond which the surgeon would not venture in the treatment for head and neck cancer. Consequently, some patients, though possibly cured temporarily of cancer, found themselves unable either to return to their former occupation or to undertake any activity requiring contact with the public. In fact, eating and talking were functions often to be undertaken alone or in the immediate confines of their homes. By the late 1940's and early 1950's, the limits of surgical removal of cancerous tissues were reached, and with this realization a need for a modified approach became evident.

Meanwhile, radiotherapists also had made tremendous advances in the treatment of patients with head and neck cancer. Not only new instruments but also new techniques had produced better results than had been obtained in prewar years. Still, the therapists were also learning that there was a limit to what could be effected in cures for these tumors.

Thus, it was natural that the surgeon and the radiotherapist should each turn to the other discipline for help in treating patients with the more advanced cancers. Such cooperation did not develop suddenly. In the beginning, salvage of some patients who presented with residual or recurrent disease after treatment by radiotherapy was obtained by surgical procedures. In these patients, if the surgical approach had been utilized first, it would have been necessary to remove a much large volume of tissue.

However, performing operations in the field of radiation was not without hazards. The upper and safe levels of the tumor dose of radiation therapy were soon recognized after several fatalities resulted from loss of skin flaps, exposure of carotids, and fatal hemorrhages.

From these early experiences developed the planned approach to treatment which is now considered to be the best approach, in general, for the medial and more advanced stages of the disease. The first report Dr. Fletcher and I gave on this approach was presented to the American Radium Society Meeting in 1954 and was entitled "Planned Combination of Surgery and Radiation in Treatment of Advanced Primary Head and Neck Cancers."

With chemotherapy, a new discipline was added to the treatment of patients in the more advanced stages of the disease, as well as to that of those patients in the terminal phases. In the latter case, the use of the chemotherapeutic drugs is sometimes questionable, because frequently the patient's general condition is not improved and the period of his remaining life is not lengthened.

In any discussion of progress in diagnosis of and treatment for head and neck cancer, advances in rehabilitation must be mentioned. In this field, radical progress has been made through the development of the maxillofacial service, an essential discipline in the treatment of many patients with intraoral cancer. The development of new materials has added greatly to the skills of the maxillofacial surgeon. Treatment of the dentulous patient before and after radiotherapy has produced most impressive and excellent effects. Not the least of these improvements is the use of fluoride, which has reduced the incidence of postirradiation caries so that this complication has been almost completely eliminated. Other dental management programs have materially reduced the incidence of osteoradionecrosis.

Diagnostic aids in the field of radiology have also improved. In particular, tomography has brought to laryngology more specific knowledge of the size and outlines of laryngeal tumors. Laryngograms have added more specific information on the extent of these lesions. Tomograms of the paranasal sinuses, as well as of other bony sites, aid materially in defining the amount of tumor involvement. Arteriography has also proved valuable, and lymphangiograms, which have proved useful in other areas of the body, may yet become a comparable aid in determining the presence of cervical node metastases before they are clinically palpable.

One of the greatest aids in advancing the cure rate lies in the now-universal use of frozen sections. It is simply inconceivable today that surgeons could have removed cancers, especially those of the skin, without base and border checks.

In addition to progress in diagnosis of and treatment for cancer of the head and neck, there have been many advances in unraveling the puzzle of the cause of cancer. As the veil of secrecy surrounding the life processes is gradually lifted by the biochemists, the physiologists, the virologists, the geneticists, and others, considerable support is found for Dr. Ewing's prediction that, "If and when the cause of cancer is ever found, it will be due not to any one factor but to more than one, if not to many."

The virus theory which bears great promise does not apply to all types of tumors. In the head and neck areas, neither does the excessive use of alcohol and tobacco account for the origin of all cancer, though undoubtedly it plays a large part, perhaps through the accompanying liver damage resulting from the poor or deficient diets of these patients.

The chronic irritation theory, so popular 30 to 40 years ago, and of which Dr. William B. Coley (but not Dr. Ewing) was a confirmed advocate, is now seldom mentioned. In my own experience, the death of a close relative—so vivid and so personal a tragedy to a boy seven years of age—left a permanent impression upon me that his death from cancer of the head of the pancreas, proven by postmortem examination, could have been the result only of daily trauma incurred over a period of many weeks.

During the early years of my hospital training, other theories intervened. The death of an infant child of close friends resulted from a tumor in the mastoid region. This lesion was found in the child at the age of three months and microscopic examination revealed it to be a very malignant tumor of salivary gland origin. In spite of surgical removal and radiation therapy for the rapid recurrence, death from pulmonary metastases resulted at one year. Did not the presence of this salivary gland tumor in the region of the mastoid lend definitive support to the Cohnheim theory of "misplaced embryonic cells"? In this same family four years later, a boy 12 years old died of acute myelogenous leukemia. And again about 10 years later, another child, not yet born at the time of the death of his brother, also died of leukemia. Finally, the father died in his early seventies of a cancer of the prostate with bizarre metastases, the primary being found only at postmortem examination. Surely heredity and genetics played a large part in the history of this family.

Truly, I believe Dr. Ewing's statement of multiplicity of causes of cancer must be considered seriously and that the answer lies in many factors, more complicated than now realized. The intensive programs now undertaken by the Federal Government give reason to hope that dramatic progress may be imminent. Within a few years perhaps surgical procedures and radiotherapy may become obsolete.

When a "breakthrough" comes, I myself believe it will not be in the field of chemotherapy, but in immunotherapy. The 1972 Nobel Prize awarded to Gerald M. Edelman and Rodney R. Porter for their work on the chemical structure of antibodies may well presage future dramatic developments in the field of immunology in cancer. It would seem that within each individual exists his own form of immunity, and that something, perhaps a latent virus, may at times disturb this balance between the normal and the abnormal cell, thus permitting the cancer cell to multiply without restraint. An example is the patient who presented originally with an epiglottic lesion with bilateral node involvement. After a total laryngectomy and a bilateral neck dissection, this man, after 10 years and 3 months with no evidence of disease, suddenly developed a local area of recurrence over the hyoid cartilage. The disease repeatedly recurred in spite of surgical excisions, radiation therapy, and chemotherapy. Yet, the areas of recurrence always lay within the cervical region. For the last 10 months he existed with slowly progressing disease, under constant sedation, and unaware of his surroundings. Death occurred only recently. Why did not this patient develop pulmonary or generalized metastases? Who can say? Somewhere within his body tissues lay the answer to an unexplained mystery, apparently connected with immunity now locally lost.

The history of this patient also demonstrates the fallacy of the term "five-" or "ten-year cure" of cancer. As the years have passed, this fact has become more clearly evident. Once a patient has developed a cancer in any organ or tissue, he is clearly more susceptible to the development of another, should he be cured of the first. This has been demonstrated with increasing frequency in the cancers of the head and neck region. Should a cancer be controlled for several years, the patient, as he grows older, enters an age group where he becomes increasingly susceptible to the development of another cancer. With advancing age, changes in immunity, perhaps associated with endocrine changes, are probably linked with the development of late recurrences or of new tumors.

Finally, what does the future hold for the diagnosis of and treatment for head and neck cancer? Is there any evidence or prospect of improvement? Having no prescient qualities, I can only pretend a simulated clairvoyance tempered by an assumed hopefulness. At present, the final answer to improved results in the treatment for cancer must still lie in early diagnoses. True, some cancers develop without symptoms and are well advanced before their presence is even suspected; but too many patients are first seen in the last stages of their disease. Delay may be the result of lack of adequate education on the part of the patient (including the inability to face the truth as to the most likely diagnosis), or the fault may lie with the physician or dentist who, for lack of education, sees the patient with his initial complaint but postpones positive action.

It is at this point, in my opinion, that the greatest advance can be made in the cancer field. Education of the laity probably has progressed as far as possible with aid of the press, radio, and television. In the past half century however, education in the professional field, including the medical schools, has been negligent. With cancer occupying its present place as a major cause of death, more emphasis should be placed on teaching diagnosis of and treatment for this disease throughout medical school and in the postgraduate years.

The time now allotted for training on the Head and Neck Service in most cancer centers is not comparable to that of 25 years ago. As a result, many residents enter practice adept in the surgical procedures or radiotherapy but too often not completely trained in the proper approach to the diagnosis of head and neck cancer or, still more important, not sufficiently experienced in selecting the best approach to treatment.

A broader educational base as well as a longer period of time for training are required to attain the best experience for the individual who proposes to devote his professional life primarily to this specialty.

Over the years, it has been my privilege to be associated with many residents during their training period, and I wish to pay tribute to all of them. In their practice in cities throughout the United States and in some foreign countries, many have become international leaders in the field of cancer. Though I may have played some small part in stimulating their interest in this particular phase of cancer, and perhaps was able to contribute to their actual training, I undoubtedly acquired as much if not more knowledge from them as they from me.

Each new generation of residents appears to have attained a broader base of professional knowledge and greater experience in the practice of medicine, except in that relating to the treatment of patients with cancer of the head and neck. In these areas, their education and training have been deficient. However, the future appears somewhat brighter, since many otolaryngologists now recognize the need for a better training program in this field. In only a few geographical areas, however, has the need of training residents in the value of the proper use of surgical procedures combined with radiation therapy been recognized.

There is a great need for continuing education for the medical, dental, and nursing professions, such as is demonstrated in state programs like MIST (Medical Information Service via Telephone) or the Dial Access system now functioning at M. D. Anderson Hospital.

Because of the recently nominated Cancer Commission, the attention of the public and of the medical profession is now concentrated on this disease. It is to be hoped that, though the greatest emphasis must remain on continued research and investigation of new forms of treatment for the patient with head and neck cancer, professional education should not and must not be relegated to the inferior position it has previously held in this troika of the cancer program. The cure rate of cancer in most anatomical sites appears to have leveled off in the past decade. Therefore, perhaps in the immediate future a greater effort should be made to establish the cause or causes of cancer.

Is the future of cancer therapy still to be retained within cancer centers? Hopefully, it may and should. The tendency, however, seems to be for this function to be taken over by the university centers. In any case, wherever the emphasis and the responsibility may eventually lie, it is to be hoped that, as the walls of brick become higher and the ivory towers more remote, it may not be forgotten that the basic problem is the treatment of the cancer patient.

REFERENCES

Butlin, H. T.: *Diseases of Tongue*. Philadelphia, Pennsylvania, Lea Brothers and Company, 1885.

Coutard, H.: Roentgen therapy of epitheliomas of the tonsillar region, hypopharynx, and larynx from 1920 to 1926. *American Journal of Roentgenology*, 28: 313-331, September 1932.

Crile, G., Sr.: Excision of cancer of the head and neck. *Journal of the American Medical Association*, 47:1780-1786, 1906.

MacComb, W. S. and Fletcher, G. H.: Planned combination of surgery and radiation in treatment of advanced primary head and neck cancers. *American Journal of Roentgenology, Radium Therapy and Nuclear Medicine*, 77:397-414, March 1957.

Mackenzie, J. N.: Cancer of the larynx. *Transactions of the American Laryngological Association*, 22:56-65, 1900.

Ogura, J. H.: Surgical pathology of cancer of the larynx. *Laryngoscope*, 65:867-926, October 1955.

Thomson, S. C., and Colledge, L.: Diagnosis and prognosis. In *Cancer of the Larynx*. London, England, Kegan Paul, Trench, Trubner & Co., Ltd., 1930, pp. 50-68.

Radiation Therapy and Subclinical Disease

GILBERT H. FLETCHER, M.D.

Head, Department of Radiotherapy, The University of Texas System Cancer Center, M. D. Anderson Hospital and Tumor Institute, Houston, Texas

Original Concept of Cancerocidal Dose

RADIOTHERAPY has, until recently, operated under two concepts:

1. The concept of an all-or-none cancerocidal dose.

2. The concept of intrinsic radiosensitivity, *i.e.* the belief that a particular histological type of cancer cannot be eradicated unless a dose specific for that cancer is given.

Radiotherapists have ignored the significance of the size of the tumor to be treated. For example, Paterson, in the 1949 edition of his textbook and in his 1952 study of optimal dosage, using the external beam, selected 5,000 roentgens in three weeks or 5,500 roentgens in five weeks as optimal for squamous cell carcinomas, irrespective of the size of the lesion. As an exception, Baclesse (1953) had the concept that cancer at the site of origin was more radioresistant than at the periphery of the tumor. He designed the shrinking-field technique which delivers higher doses to the central mass. Clinically uninvolved areas of the neck were given significantly lower doses when treated electively.

The emphasis in radiotherapy has been primarily directed to controlling gross masses. Little attention, if any, has been given to the amount of irradiation necessary to control occult or subclinical deposits of cancer cells.

Subclinical Disease

INCIDENCE

The incidence of subclinical disease has been well established for various lymphatic areas. The term "subclinical disease" refers to microscopic disease as well as to aggregates of cancer cells not of sufficient size to be palpated.

In several series of patients with squamous cell carcinomas of the mobile tongue who had an elective radical neck dissection, the incidence of occult deposits in the neck has ranged from 40 to 60 per cent (Kremen, 1956; Lyall and Schetlin, 1958; Roux-Berger, Baud, and Courtial, 1949; Southwick, Slaughter, and Trevino, 1960). It has been established from many series that almost 40 per cent of breast cancer patients with clinically negative axillae have positive nodes in the surgical specimen of the axillary dissection (Cutler and Connelly, 1969). The incidence of supraclavicular disease appearing later in patients with adenocarcinomas of the breast, treated by radical mastectomy, with positive nodes in the axillary specimen has been found to be 20 to 25 per cent if no postoperative irradiation is given (Jackson, 1966; Robbins, Lucas, Fracchia, Farrow, and Chu, 1966).

CONTROL BY IRRADIATION

At M. D. Anderson Hospital, most patients with squamous cell carcinomas of the nasopharynx, faucial arch, tonsillar fossa, and base of the tongue are treated by irradiation (Fletcher, 1972b, 1973). The upper neck, to the level of the superior border of the thyroid cartilage, is treated with the area of the primary lesion through parallel opposed portals. The lower neck is treated with an anterior portal and the larynx is shielded. The dose to the upper neck nodes is never less than 5,000 rads and is often 6,000 rads. The given dose to the lower neck is 5,000 rads. The dose to the midjugular nodes may be as low as 4,500 rads. The nodes in the supraclavicular fossa and posterior cervical triangle, located immediately under the skin, receive 5,000 rads.

Early in the megavoltage irradiation program at M. D. Anderson Hospital, all patients with base of tongue and tonsillar fossa lesions did not receive treatment to the lower neck. A variable approach was used in the treatment of faucial arch lesions. Irradiation might be given to the ipsilateral or bilateral subdigastric areas only. Table 1 compares the appearance of neck disease in two groups of patients, those receiving partial neck irradiation and those receiving whole neck irradiation (Berger, Fletcher,

TABLE 1.—Control of Subclinical Disease in Squamous Cell Carcinomas of the Nasopharynx, Tonsillar Fossa, Base of Tongue, and Faucial Arch: Primary Lesion and Initial Neck Disease Controlled[*]

New Disease in Areas of Neck Initially Clinically Negative	
Partial Neck Irradiation	Whole Neck Irradiation
185 pts. (12 N_3[†])	284 pts. (100 N_3[†])
	4,500–5,000 rads/5 weeks to initially uninvolved areas
12.0% (22/185)	1.7% (5/284)

[*]All treatments 1,000 rads per week, 5 days a week.
[†]Either fixed node(s) (N_{3A}) or bilateral clinically positive node(s) (N_{3B}) in the upper portion of the neck.
(Courtesy of Berger, Fletcher, Lindberg, and Jesse, 1971.)

Lindberg, and Jesse, 1971). New neck disease appeared in 12 per cent of the patients whose necks were only partially irradiated. These patients had a low risk of occult disease since less than 10 per cent were initially staged as N_3. In contradistinction, new disease appeared in only 1.7 per cent of the patients whose entire necks were irradiated. These patients generally had cancers of the nasopharynx, tonsil, or base of the tongue, with more than 33 per cent initially staged N_3 and, therefore, having a high risk of occult disease. The lower incidence of new disease in the higher risk groups attests to the value of elective radiotherapy (Berger, Fletcher, Lindberg, and Jesse, 1971; Million, Fletcher, and Jesse, 1963).

Table 2 is a composite of results of various studies (Jesse, Barkley, Lindberg, and Fletcher, 1970; Lindberg, Barkley, Jesse, and Fletcher, 1971; Northrop, Fletcher, Jesse, and Lindberg, 1972). The appearance of new disease in the contralateral neck is low in patients with lesions of the floor of the mouth, oral tongue, faucial arch, supraglottic larynx, or pyriform sinus who received various amounts of external irradiation to the first lymphatic levels with a significant contribution to the equivalent contralateral lymphatics. Only 3 per cent (6 of 187) developed new disease compared with 24.5 per cent (46 of 187) in patients who had only an ipsilateral radical neck dissection.

In comparison with the nonirradiated patients, contralateral disease is diminished 60 to 70 per cent in patients receiving 3,000 rads in three weeks to 4,000 rads in four weeks to the opposite submaxillary and subdigastric areas. No patient in our series who had a faucial arch lesion developed contralateral neck disease when the opposite subdigastric nodes were given 5,000 rads in five weeks. Postoperative radiotherapy (6,000

TABLE 2.—CONTROL OF SUBCLINICAL DISEASE IN SQUAMOUS CELL CARCINOMAS OF THE FLOOR OF MOUTH, ORAL TONGUE, FAUCIAL ARCH, SUPRAGLOTTIC LARYNX, AND PYRIFORM SINUS: PRIMARY LESION AND INITIAL NECK DISEASE CONTROLLED*

	NEW DISEASE IN OPPOSITE SIDE OF THE NECK INITIALLY CLINICALLY NEGATIVE		
	Without Irradiation	With Irradiation	
Floor of Mouth (N_1 & N_2)†	47.5% (9/19)	10.5% (3/28)	3,000 rads/3 wks to 4,000 rads/4 wks {to opposite subdigastric & submaxillary triangle nodes
Oral Tongue (N_1 & N_2)†	27.0% (8/30)	9.0% (2/22)	
Faucial Arch (N_1 & N_2)†	30.0% (3/10)	0% (0/72)	
			5,000 rads/5 wks {to opposite subdigastric nodes
Supraglottic Larynx and Pyriform Sinus†	20.0% (26/128)	1.5% (1/65)	6,000 rads/6 wks upper neck 5,000 rads/5 wks given dose to lower neck
Total	24.5% (46/187)	3.0% (6/187)	

*All treatments 1,000 rads per week, 5 days a week.
†N_1—Single clinically positive node $\leq$ 3 cm.
N_2—Single clinically positive node > 3 cm. not fixed or multiple clinically positive ipsilateral nodes.
(Courtesy of Fletcher, In Press.)

TABLE 3.—EVOLUTION OF NECK DISEASE IN N₀* PATIENTS WITH SQUAMOUS
CELL CARCINOMA OF THE SUPRAGLOTTIC LARYNX WITH PRIMARY
CONTROLLED ACCORDING TO METHOD OF TREATMENT
JANUARY 1948 THROUGH DECEMBER 1967
(MINIMUM TWO-YEAR FOLLOW-UP)

SITE	NO. OF PTS. BY INITIAL TREATMENT OF PRIMARY	NO. OF PTS. DEVELOPING NECK NODES
Suprahyoid	2 Surg.	0
Epiglottis	14 XRT	0
	1 Preop.	0
Infrahyoid	20 Surg.	8
Epiglottis	6 XRT	0
	1 Postop.	0
False Cords	16 Surg.	4
	12 XRT	1†
Arytenoids	1 Surg.	1
	4 XRT	0
Aryepiglottic	4 Surg.	1
Folds	8 XRT	0
Total	43 Surg.	14
	44 XRT	1
	1 Postop.	0
	1 Preop.	0

Abbreviations: Surg., Surgery; XRT, Irradiation; Preop., Preoperative; Postop., Postoperative.
*Clinically negative neck.
†5 × 5 cm. portal, a node developed above the treatment field in the high jugular area.
(Courtesy of Fletcher, 1972a.)

TABLE 4.—CERVICAL LYMPH NODE METASTASES UNKNOWN PRIMARY CANCER:
CLINICAL MANIFESTATION OF SUBCLINICAL DISEASE WITH OR
WITHOUT IRRADIATION IN 184 PATIENTS*
(THREE YEARS TO UNLIMITED FOLLOW-UP)

	SURGERY		COMPREHENSIVE IRRADIATION†		COMBINATION‡	
Appearance of nodes in the contralateral side of neck in 164 patients	16%	(16/97)	0%	(0/39)	0%	(0/28)
Primary lesions appearing posttreatment in the head and neck area	20%	(21/104)‖	6%	(3/52)§	14%	(4/28)

*20 patients had initial bilateral neck disease.
‖16 patients—nasopharynx, oropharynx, and hypopharynx.
†Comprehensive irradiation includes nasopharynx, tonsillar fossa, base of tongue, upper part of supraglottic larynx and hypopharynx, and the whole neck.
§2 patients developed a lesion in the oral cavity and 1 in the hypopharynx.
‡Irradiation limited to neck.

TABLE 5.—Supraclavicular Node Metastases after Radical Mastectomy When Axillary Nodes Are Positive in the Surgical Specimen

Christie Hospital[*] Manchester, England Memorial Center Hospital[†] New York, New York	M. D. Anderson Hospital Houston, Texas	
Without Postoperative Irradiation	With Postoperative Irradiation 250 Kv $\leq$ 3,500 rads node dose/4 wks.	
		7% (6/89)
20–25%	^{137}Cs, ^{60}Co, Electron Beam 5,000–5,500 rads GD/4 wks.	
		1.3% (4/273)
	With Preoperative Irradiation ^{60}Co 4,000 rads GD/4 wks.	
		3% (4/121)

[*]Jackson, 1966.
[†]Robbins, *et al.*, 1966.
GD, given dose.
(Courtesy of Fletcher, 1972a.)

rads to the opposite upper neck and 4,500 or 5,000 rads to the lower neck) eliminates more than 90 per cent of contralateral metastases in patients with supraglottic or pyriform sinus lesions.

Table 3 shows that, with a minimum of 5,000 rads to the high and mid-jugular nodes, no patients with squamous cell carcinoma of the supraglottic larynx developed neck disease if the neck nodes were initially clinically negative. Table 4 shows that, with 5,000 rads given in five weeks to the nasopharynx, oropharynx, and whole neck in patients treated for cervical lymph node metastases with an unknown primary cancer, contralateral neck metastases and new primaries are eliminated in the irradiated structures.

Similar results have been obtained in the elective irradiation of the supraclavicular area in patients with breast cancer and positive axillary nodes in the surgical specimen (Table 5).

Clinical Dose-Response Curve for Subclinical Disease

Table 6 shows that control rates are increased as the dose levels are increased. The 90-plus per cent control point is firm both for squamous cell carcinomas of the upper respiratory and digestive tract and for adenocarcinomas of the breast. The other control points are ranges because of variations in dose. Using Cohen's mathematical model (1968), a curve

TABLE 6.—Per Cent of Control of Subclinical Disease
as a Function of Dose*

Adenocarcinoma of the Breast		Squamous Cell Carcinoma of the Upper Respiratory and Digestive Tracts	
3,000–3,500 rads		3,000–4,000 rads	
(89 patients)	60–70%	(50 patients)	60–70%
4,000 rads		5,000 rads	
(121 patients)	80–90%	(356 patients)	>90%
5,000 rads		6,000 rads	
(273 patients)	>90%	(65 patients)	>90%

*1,000 rads per week, 5 days a week.
(Courtesy of Fletcher, In Press.)

Fig. 1.—Probability of cure versus dose per fraction for a model epidermoid tumor with M cells. For a 10^6 (1 mm.^{3}) cell aggregate, the probability of cure drops from 99 per cent with 4,400 rads to 52 per cent with 3,600 rads and to less than 5 per cent with 3,200 rads (approximately equivalent to 2,000 rads in five consecutive days). (Adapted from Herring and Compton, 1970.)

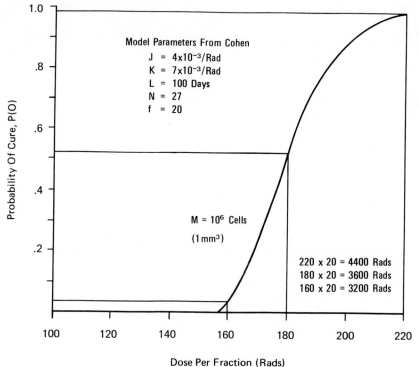

Model Parameters From Cohen
$J = 4 \times 10^{-3}$/Rad
$K = 7 \times 10^{-3}$/Rad
$L = 100$ Days
$N = 27$
$f = 20$

$M = 10^6$ Cells
(1 mm^3)

220 x 20 = 4400 Rads
180 x 20 = 3600 Rads
160 x 20 = 3200 Rads

Probability Of Cure, P(O)

Dose Per Fraction (Rads)

can be constructed in agreement with our clinical data. The slope of the dose-response curve is very steep, showing a drastic decrease in effectiveness with smaller doses (Herring and Compton, 1970) (Fig. 1). The steepness of the curve and the low doses employed suggest that the tumor cell aggregates in the undisturbed lymphatics are oxic.

Tumor Control

Tumor control dose is a better term than is cancerocidal dose since any amount of irradiation will be lethal to a percentage of the total cancer cell population. The curves of clonogenic ability (Puck and Marcus, 1956) and the oxygen effect (Gray, 1961) have shown that the total number of cells and the percentage of those cells in an anoxic stage are paramount factors in determining the dose required to eradicate a cancer. Control of the disease is essentially a function of tumor size and tumor bed. A smaller radiation dose should be required to eradicate small aggregates of cancer cells (microscopic or not clinically detectable) than the dose required to eradicate a palpable mass because of fewer cells and a smaller, if any, anoxic compartment. Anoxic cells, even a limited number, exert a powerful influence on the tumor lethal response. A mathematical model of the influence of cell numbers and the proportion of anoxic cells in determining the single dose needed to eradicate a mammalian cell population is shown in Table 7.

It also should be possible to establish a correlation between tumor size and tumor control dose. Table 8 provides data on control of subclinical disease and gross cancer showing clearly that, in order to obtain equiva-

---

TABLE 7.—INFLUENCE OF CELL NUMBER AND PROPORTION OF ANOXIC CELLS ON SINGLE DOSE NECESSARY FOR ERADICATION OF A MAMMALIAN CELL POPULATION (HELA CELLS)

OXIC CELLS
 A single dose of 380 rads kills 90% of the cell population
ANOXIC CELLS
 A single dose of $380 \times 2.5 = 950$ rads kills 90% of the cell population
 All Cells Oxic
  10^9 cells (3 cm. dia.) 380 rads kill 90% of $10^9 \rightarrow 10^8$ surviving cells
  10^2 (100) cells 380 rads kill 90% of $10^2 \rightarrow 10^1$ surviving cells
  10^9 cells $380 \times 9 = 3{,}160$ rads to zero surviving cells

 1/1000 Cells Anoxic
  Oxic cells $10^9 \rightarrow 10^6 = 380 \times 3 = 1{,}140$ rads
  Anoxic cells $10^6 = 950 \times 6 = 5{,}900$ rads
                           $\overline{7{,}040}$ rads to zero surviving cells

TABLE 8.—Dose-Tumor Volume Relationships* for Approximately 90 Per Cent Control in Squamous Cell Carcinomas of the Upper Respiratory and Digestive Tracts

Subclinical Disease in Lymphatics of the Neck (All Anatomical Sites)	Gross Disease Supraglottic Larynx and Tonsillar Fossa			
	< 2 cm.	2–4 cm.	4–6 cm.	(Massive) > 6 cm.
≤ 1,575 rets	1,800 rets	1,900 rets	2,000 rets	2,100 rets
	6,090 rads/	6,800 rads/	7,310 rads/	7,890 rads/
(5,000 rads/5 wks.)	30 tx/6 wks.	35 tx/7 wks.	37 tx/7½ wks.	40 tx/8 wks.

*The number of rads and weeks are for 1,000 rads per week which, on the main, have been the dose-time schedules used in the material analyzed. Longer treatment times are used in the supraglottic larynx lesions than in those of the tonsillar fossa.
Abbreviations: tx, treatments; wks., weeks.

lent control rates, higher doses are needed for the larger tumors. The higher total doses have usually been given in longer treatment times.

Histological Varieties of Epithelial Tumors

The radiosensitivity of squamous cell carcinomas versus adenocarcinomas has long been argued. The concept that radiosensitivity depends upon the degree of cellular differentiation has also been argued. Present clinical

TABLE 9.—Carcinoma in Salivary Glands: Local Failures* by Histology in Patients Irradiated after Surgical Excision for Definite† or Probable Subclinical Disease, January 1948 through December 1968, Analysis March 1972

Histology	Number of Patients	Number of Recurrences
Malignant mixed tumor	3	1‡
Mucoepidermoid carcinoma (high grade)	4	0
Adenoidcystic carcinoma	9	1‡
Adenocarcinoma	4	0
Squamous cell carcinoma	7	0
Undifferentiated carcinoma	1	0
Unclassified neoplasm	2	0
Total	30‖	2 (6.5%)§

*Patients who died from intercurrent disease or distant metastases in less than 3 years NED locally are excluded.
†Approximately half of the patients had definite residual disease left after the surgical excision.
‡At 7 and 31 months.
‖2 submaxillary glands.
§(Beahrs, 1960)   Moderately malignant tumors of the parotid gland 37.5%.
   Recurrences < 3 years   Highly malignant tumors of the parotid gland 72.5%.
NED, no evidence of disease.
(Courtesy of Fletcher, 1973.)

data show that all epithelial malignant tumors are equally radiosensitive. As an example, in a recent review (King and Fletcher, 1971), no difference is seen in control by irradiation of subclinical disease between the various histological types of malignant epithelial tumors of the major salivary glands (Table 9).

Applications of the Concept of Control of Subclinical Disease by Modest Doses of Irradiation

HEAD AND NECK TUMOR

There are two basic clinical applications:
1. Elective irradiation of clinically uninvolved lymphatic areas.
2. Combination of irradiation and surgery, pre- or postoperatively.

ELECTIVE IRRADIATION.—In the highly metastasizing lesions of the naso-pharynx, tonsillar fossa, base of tongue, and hypopharynx, elective irradiation of potentially involved cervical nodes is mandatory. In tumors of the supraglottic larynx in N_0 patients, the subdigastric and upper midjugular nodes are included in the treatment of the primary lesions. This proximal relay of lymphatics, the first to be involved, should be treated electively in the N_0 patients because of the potential for neck disease to appear later unless the primary lesion is small (Table 10). The opposite lymphatic levels should be irradiated in those patients who have a high risk of contra-lateral metastases; for example, those with lesions of the floor of the mouth or of the oral tongue and clinically positive nodes in the neck.

COMBINATIONS OF IRRADIATION AND SURGERY.—Surgery and irradiation have been combined since the early days of this century. The irradiation

TABLE 10.—PERCENTAGE OF PATIENTS WITH SQUAMOUS CELL CARCINOMA INITIALLY N_0 DEVELOPING NECK DISEASE BY T STAGING

		ORAL CAVITY		FAUCIAL ARCH	
Primary Stage	No. of Pts.	Pts. Developing Neck Metastases	Pts. Having Had Partial Neck Treatment*	⅔ of the Patients Have Had Area I or Areas I and II Irradiated	Pts. Developing Neck Metastases
T_1	169	23% (39/169)	5% (9/169)	Usually angle node only, occasionally	16% (7/43)
T_2	200	26% (52/200)	24% (48/200)	all subdigastric nodes irradiated	18.5% (12/65)
T_3	110	29% (32/110)	52% (57/110)	All subdigastric nodes usually	10% (4/39)
T_4	42	26% (11/42)	69% (29/42)	irradiated	16.5% (2/12)

*Irradiation limited to the subdigastric and submaxillary triangle nodes.
(Courtesy of Fletcher and Jesse, 1971.)

has been given either before or after the surgical procedure. The effectiveness of this combined treatment has been evaluated cyclically both positively and negatively.

In 1954, at the American Radium Society Meeting at the Homestead in Virginia, Doctor MacComb and I presented a paper on "Planned Combination of Surgery and Radiation in the Treatment of Advanced Primary Head and Neck Cancers," (MacComb and Fletcher, 1957). The rationale was that "the peripheral extensions of advanced squamous cell carcinoma are fairly radiosensitive. The central areas, which represent the point of origin of the tumor, are poorly vascularized and often difficult to control by irradiation. Recurrences or reactivation of cancer cells commonly occur at such central points."

Recurrence of cancer at the primary site after surgical excision is the result of microscopic disease extending along the fascial planes, nerve sheaths, periosteum, or bone beyond the limits of resection. The surgeon is often unaware that microscopic disease is at the line of resection.

Conversely, irradiation easily eradicates cancer at the periphery of the lesion where the amount of cancer is small and the cells are well oxygenated. Irradiation fails in the center of large masses, either primary or metastatic, which contain hypoxic areas. The rationale of combining both disciplines is to make use of their complementary effectiveness in those situations where:

1. Cancer has spread beyond possible resection (extensive primary lesions).

2. The lesion is too diffuse for en bloc removal (radical neck dissection is ineffective when multiple nodes are positive).

3. Both primary and potential nodal involvement make success doubtful with surgical excision alone (disease is located close to vital structures).

The goals of preoperative irradiation and postoperative irradiation are essentially the same.

1. To eradicate subclinical disease, usually microscopic beyond the margins of surgical resection.

2. To decrease the incidence of recurrences in the surgical field by decreasing the number of viable cells in the operative field or by destroying residual foci of cells.

3. To eradicate new disease in adjacent areas by sterilizing microscopic foci of cancer (contralateral neck, *etc.*).

In order to accomplish these goals, at least 5,000 rads should be given to the primary lesion or tumor bed area and to the entire neck. The sequence of treatment is determined primarily by the type of surgical procedure required. The healing problem after 5,000 rads are given to the

TABLE 11.—Disease Control*: Immediate Postoperative Irradiation versus Irradiation for Gross Recurrence

	IMMEDIATE POSTOPERATIVE IRRADIATION†	IRRADIATION FOR GROSS RECURRENCES
Patients treated	19	147
Patients NED	8	16
Per cent NED	42%‡	11%‡

*Follow-up of 1 to 6 years.
†Lack of clearance in surgical specimen.
‡p < .001.
NED, no evidence of disease.
(Adapted from Fletcher and Evers, 1970.)

primary cancer and the entire neck is increased drastically by the extensiveness of the surgical procedure.

The oral, pharyngeal, and laryngeal mucosa often have multifocal areas of cancer some distance from the main tumor, and the contralateral neck may also contain metastatic deposits. The surgeon, therefore, must either remove only the gross cancer and rely on radiation treatment of areas of microscopic disease, or perform a superradical procedure designed to remove all possible microscopic spread. The latter procedure involves the risk of both prolonged healing and delay in initiating radiation therapy.

The surgical procedure must permit rapid primary healing so that irradiation will not be delayed, since gross recurrent disease is infrequently eradicated (Table 11). Most patients should begin radiotherapy within three weeks of their operation. The surgical procedure must not remove so much tissue that irradiation is technically impossible. For example, a laryngopharyngectomy with bilateral radical neck dissection leaves only the skin over the vertebral bodies and the enclosed spinal cord (Fig. 2), presenting a technical challenge to irradiation making it almost impossible. A better procedure would be to remove the gross disease in the neck by modified or partial neck dissection, leaving sufficient tissue for postoperative radiation therapy (Fig. 3).

The opposite side of the neck as well as the surgically disturbed area must be irradiated in order to prevent the appearance of new disease. Radical surgical procedures interfere somewhat with the blood supply to the center of the operative field and the subclinical cancer deposits lie in tissues which may be slightly less than euoxic but not anoxic. Therefore, a slightly lowered radiosensitivity may be present. The site of the resected primary and the upper portion of the neck are irradiated with 6,000 rads

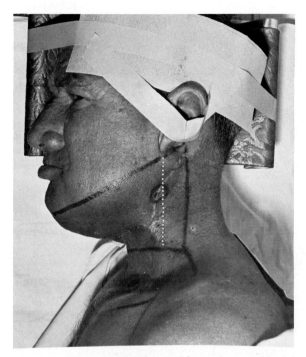

Fig. 2.—Patient seen on May 1, 1968 with a marble-sized mass in the left submaxillary region. On the laryngeal surface of the epiglottis a raised ulcerated lesion was seen extending to the left false and true cords. In the right midjugular chain, there was a node 3 cm. in diameter and in the left one a 4 to 5 cm. node. Biopsy: Grade IV squamous cell carcinoma.

On May 7, 1968 a laryngectomy and a bilateral neck dissection were done. There were positive nodes in both sides of the neck. Irradiation was delayed for two months because of slow wound healing. A midline dose of 6,000 rads was given to the upper neck; after 4,500 rads, the posterior margin of the parallel opposing portals was moved forward to exclude the spinal cord. Additional therapy with the 9 Mev electron beam was used to supplement the dose to 6,000 rads. The lower neck received 5,000 rads given dose in five weeks with an anterior portal, the stoma being shielded.

Even with the availability of an electron beam, adequate irradiation of the surgical area, which extended to the mastoid was difficult.

The patient developed a recurrence in the right neck in August, 1969, and died in November, 1969. (Courtesy of Fletcher, Lindberg, and Jesse, 1970.)

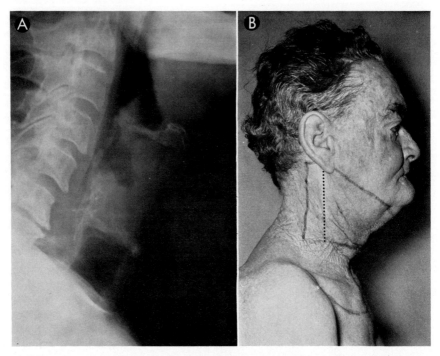

FIG. 3.—Patient seen in November, 1970, with an ulcerated lesion of the infrahyoid epiglottis. Clinical examination and lateral soft tissue film showed involvement of the pre-epiglottic space and of the valleculum. A 1.3 cm. node was palpable in the left subdigastric area and two 3.0 cm. subdigastric nodes were present in the right subdigastric area. Biopsy: Squamous cell carcinoma.

The plan of treatment was total wide-field laryngectomy with bilateral modified radical neck dissection and postoperative irradiation therapy.

A wide-field laryngectomy (including larynx, strap muscles, and a generous portion of the base of the tongue) was done. The sternomastoid muscle was not removed on either side. Of 13 nodes recovered during the right modified neck dissection, three were positive by microscopic examination. On the left side, one node, attached to the jugular vein, was resected. Of 17 nodes removed, two were positive. Pathological diagnosis was squamous carcinoma, Grade II, involving the epiglottis with perforation of the epiglottic cartilage to the pre-epiglottic space, with extension to the right and left aryepiglottic folds, right and left false cords, and right and left arytenoid regions (margins of surgical excision were free of tumor). The wound was closed primarily and the patient was ready for postoperative irradiation 12 days after the surgical procedure.

A, lateral soft tissue film showing an extensive tumor of the infrahyoid epiglottis.

B, lateral portal covering upper neck. A midline dose of 6,000 rads was given in six weeks to the upper neck. The posterior margins of the parallel opposing portals were moved forward at 4,500 rads without need of a supplemental dose because the scar was limited.

A given dose of 5,000 rads in five weeks was delivered to the lower neck with an anterior portal, shielding the stoma of the tracheostomy.

The patient died in September, 1971, from distant metastases with no evidence of disease in the neck. (Courtesy of Fletcher, 1973.)

TABLE 12.—Squamous Cell Carcinoma of Tonsillar Fossa, Base of Tongue, Supraglottic Larynx, and Hypopharynx[*]: Failures in Ipsilateral Side of Neck
(Primary Controlled When Neck Disease Becomes Manifest)
Patients Have Survived at Least 24 Months

TREATMENT	No Neck Treatment			N_1	N_{2A}	N_{2B}	N_{3A}	N_{3B}	TOTAL
	None	Partial	Complete						
Radiation	–	13/85	1/50	8/52	6/22	7/27	8/21	11/35	18.5% (54/292)
Surgery	16/29	8/23	2/28	5/47	1/13	7/30	5/12	7/17	25.6% (51/199)
Combined	–	1/5	0/6	0/21	0/17	0/28	3/13	5/15	8.6% (9/105)

[*]1948 through 1967.
(Courtesy of Barkley, Fletcher, Jesse, and Lindberg, 1972.)

in six weeks without producing significant sequelae. The lower portion of the neck receives 5,000 rads in five weeks.

A marked diminution in recurrences in radically dissected necks is obtained by either pre- or postoperative irradiation (Table 12). Squamous cell carcinomas of the tonsillar fossa and base of the tongue have been given preoperative irradiation, whereas carcinomas of the supraglottic larynx and hypopharynx have been treated with postoperative irradiation.

Subclinical disease can be treated by the association of conservative surgery and comprehensive irradiation. Not only can pre- or postoperative irradiation be used with some modifications of the routine surgical procedures of radical neck dissection, laryngectomy, or composite operation, but in well-selected situations one can go a step further. For example, to manage disease in the neck when the primary lesions are in the tonsillar fossa or base of the tongue, the whole neck is treated in conjunction with the primary treatment followed by a limited neck dissection. This method of management may be very effective for parotid gland tumors when the facial nerve is not grossly involved, permitting preservation of the nerve if postoperative irradiation is given. Facial paralysis is then avoided.

APPLICATIONS OUTSIDE THE AREA OF HEAD AND NECK CANCERS

Head and neck cancers offer an excellent testing ground for any clinical approach since such cancers provide the best opportunity for the clinician to follow the evolution of disease at the primary site and in the regional lymphatics.

The concept of management of subclinical disease with modest doses of irradiation associated with conservative surgical procedures can be extended to areas other than malignant tumors of the head and neck. This approach is very effective in the management of locally advanced breast cancer where simple mastectomy and sometimes dissection of enlarged axillary nodes followed by irradiation of approximately 5,000 rads to the entire area produces very high local and regional control rates (Table 13) (Brown, Horiot, and Fletcher, in press). The control rates are lower with irradiation alone and the very high doses (9,000 to 10,000 rads to the primary tumor) which are required produce severe late fibrosis.

For gynecological malignant diseases, there are multiple applications of the combination of conservative surgery with irradiation. The use of a conservative extrafascial hysterectomy after slightly less radical irradiation diminishes the incidence of central failures in large, bulky central tumors, primarily the barrel-shaped endocervical cancers. The use of postoperative irradiation to the whole abdomen is effective for ovarian cancers only after removal of all palpable disease (Delclos and Quinlan, 1969).

For embryonal carcinoma of the testes, retroperitoneal lymphadenectomy combined with irradiation considerably increases the probability that this dissected area will remain free of disease (Castro, 1969).

This approach is applicable to other than epithelial tumors. For example, in soft tissue sarcomas, simple surgical excision is fraught with an incidence of local recurrences as high as 70 per cent in some series (Atkin-

TABLE 13.—LOCAL CONTROL IN PATIENTS WITH LATE STAGE III (UICC) CANCER OF THE BREAST TECHNICALLY SUITABLE FOR RADICAL MASTECTOMY*

	WITH SIMPLE MASTECTOMY		WITHOUT SIMPLE MASTECTOMY
	Jan. 1955–Dec. 1963 103	Jan. 1964–Dec. 1967 32	Jan. 1955–Dec. 1967 229
Chest Wall†‡	88% (91/103)	97% (31/32)	78% (179/229)
Axilla†‖	88% (91/103)	100% (32/32)	89.5% (205/229)
Supraclavicular†§	93% (96/103)	100% (32/32)	98% (224/229)
Parasternal†	99% (102/103)	100% (32/32)	– –

Survival rates: (Modified life table method)		
	With Simple Mastectomy	5 yrs.—45.5% 10 yrs.—21.5%
	Without Simple Mastectomy (Irradiation alone)	5 yrs.—30.0% 10 yrs.—12.5%

*January 1955 through December 1967, Analysis as of January 1972. By 36 months, 90 per cent of recurrences have developed.
†A patient may have a recurrence in more than one location.
‡Patients treated from January 1955 through December 1963 had 4,000 to 4,500 rads to the chest wall and from 1964 on, 5,000 rads minimum.
‖Axilla: January 1955 through December 1963, 4,400 to 5,000 rads usually with no boost. Since 1964 after 5,000 rads, 1,000 to 2,000 rads boost to palpable nodes.
§Two of the seven supraclavicular failures were in the four patients with initial supraclavicular nodes.
(Courtesy of Fletcher, 1973.)

TABLE 14.—Soft Tissue Sarcomas of Extremities (All Histologies):
1954 through 1969 with a Minimum Follow-up of 24 Months

	RADIOTHERAPY ALONE		EXCISION + RADIOTHERAPY	
SITE	Total Cases	Local Recurrence°	Total Cases	Local Recurrence†
Head & Neck plus Trunk	25	16 (65%)	29	12 (40%)
Extremities	10	7 (70%)	48	7‡ (14.5%)

°96 per cent recurrence by 2 years.
†84.5 per cent recurrence by 2 years.
‡2 recurred in arm, 3 in thigh and 2 in leg.
(Adapted from Lindberg, 1973.)

son, Garvan, and Newton, 1963). It is still 30 per cent with a radical compartmental dissection, short of ablative surgery for the extremities (Brennhovd, 1966; Cantin, McNeer, Chu, and Booher, 1968; Martin, Butler, and Albores-Saavedra, 1963).

The alleged radioresistance of the soft tissue sarcomas is probably the result of the enormous mass of cancer which cannot be eradicated even with very high doses. After simple excision, subclinical disease can be easily controlled, as shown in Table 14. It is of interest that failures are essentially in the upper arm, thigh, and leg. When the lesion becomes obvious to the patient, it is usually large and has already grown deeply into the fascial planes. In these thick parts, even after excision, there still may be a considerable amount of disease left. Conversely, in the areas beyond the elbow, around the knee, and the ankle, disease is recognized early and almost 100 per cent control is obtained by shelling out the mass and giving postoperative irradiation.

For cancer of the rectosigmoid, thought should be given to carrying out an anterior resection and, depending upon the surgical findings, giving postoperative radiotherapy. The lymphatic drainage areas must be encompassed generously since their involvement worsens the prognosis when even an abdominoperineal resection only is done. Pelvic recurrences are quite high with abdominoperineal resection when disease has penetrated through the wall of the bowel (Gilbertsen, 1960). Not only could the incidence of pelvic recurrences be diminished but the patients would be spared a colostomy, the psychological effects of which are very significant.

Quality of Life

To live is not merely to exist. The goal of cancer treatment, whether surgical, radiotherapeutic, or a combination of both, must be not only to eradicate disease and keep the patient alive, but also to maintain a desirable quality of life for the patient. Sequelae, even though neither fatal nor crippling, may still diminish normal functions and create cosmetic blemishes which are incompatible with a normal life.

In the present evolution of cancer management, Carlisle's maxim might be appropriate to meditate upon, "Our main purpose is not to see what lies dimly at a distance but to do what lies clearly at hand."

One could take exception to this maxim, which reflects the excessive intellectual dryness of the age of reason. However, it is unfair to the patient with cancer not to make the best use of information available today and, instead, give overwhelming attention to the possibilities of a cure lying dimly at a distance. Some of the existing solutions will not only preserve the patient's life but also will insure normal function and cosmesis.

Acknowledgments

This investigation was supported by Public Health Service Research Grants CA-06294 and CA-05654 from the National Cancer Institute.

REFERENCES

Atkinson, L., Garvan, J. M., and Newton, N. C.: Behavior and management of soft connective tissue sarcomas. *Cancer,* 16:1552-1562, December 1963.

Baclesse, F.: L'etalement ou le "fractionnement" dans le roentgentherapie seule des epitheliomas du pharynx et du larynx, de l'uterus et du vagin, du sein (étude del. 449 cas). *Acta Unio internationalis contra cancrum,* 9:29-33, 1953.

Barkley, H. T., Jr., Fletcher, G. H., Jesse, R. H., and Lindberg, R. D.: Management of cervical lymph node metastases in squamous cell carcinomas of the tonsillar fossa, base of tongue, supraglottic larynx, and hypopharynx. *American Journal of Surgery,* 124:462-467, 1972.

Beahrs, O. H., Woolner, L. B., Carveth, S. W., and Devine, K. D.: Surgical management of parotid lesions. *Archives of Surgery,* 80:890-904, June 1960.

Berger, D. S., Fletcher, G. H., Lindberg, R. D., and Jesse, R. H., Jr.: Elective irradiation of the neck lymphatics for squamous cell carcinomas of the nasopharynx and oropharynx. *American Journal of Roentgenology, Radium Therapy and Nuclear Medicine,* 11:66-72, January 1971.

Brennhovd, I. O.: The treatment of soft tissue sarcomas—a plea for a more urgent and aggressive approach. *Acta chirurgica scandinavica,* 131:438-442, May 1966.

Brown, G. R., Horiot, J-C., Fletcher, G. H., White, E. C., and Ange, D. W.: Simple mastectomy and irradiation therapy for locally advanced breast cancers technically suitable for radical mastectomy. *American Journal of Roentgenology, Radium Therapy and Nuclear Medicine.* (In press.)

Cantin, J., McNeer, G. P., Chu, F. C., and Booher, R. J.: The problem of local recurrence after treatment of soft tissue sarcoma. *Annals of Surgery,* 168:47-53, July 1968.

Castro, J. R.: Lymphadenectomy and radiation therapy in malignant tumors of the testicle other than pure seminoma. *Cancer,* 24:87-91, July 1969.

Cohen, L.: Theoretical iso-survival formulae for fractionated radiation therapy. *British Journal of Radiology,* 41:522-528, July 1968.

Cutler, S. J., and Connelly, R. R.: Mammary cancer trends. *Cancer,* 23:767-771, April 1969.

Delclos, L., and Quinlan, E. J.: Malignant tumors of the ovary treated with megavoltage postoperative irradiation. *Radiology,* 93:659-663, September 1969.

Fletcher, G. H.: Local results of irradiation in the primary management of localized breast cancer. *Cancer,* 29:545-551, March 1972a.

————: Elective irradiation of subclinical disease in cancers of the head and neck. *Cancer,* 29:1450-1454, June 1972b.

————: Dose response curve of subclinical aggregates of epithelial cells and its practical application in the management of human cancers. In *Biological and Clinical Basis of Radiosensitivity,* A collection of papers presented at an International Conference at the Instituto Regina Elena, Rome, Italy, October, 1971. Milton Friedman, Ed. (In press.)

————: *Textbook of Radiotherapy,* 2nd Ed. Philadelphia, Pennsylvania, Lea and Febiger, 1973, pp. 121-151.

Fletcher, G. H., and Evers, W. T.: Radiotherapeutic management of surgical recurrences and postoperative residuals in tumors of the head and neck. *Radiology,* 95:185-188, April 1970.

Fletcher, G. H., and Jesse, R. H.: Interaction of surgery and irradiation in head and neck cancers. *Current Problems in Radiology,* R. D. Moseley, Ed., Chicago, Year Book Medical Publishers, Inc., 1:3-37, July-August 1971.

Fletcher, G. H., Lindberg, R. D., and Jesse, R. H.: The combination of radiation and surgery in oropharynx and laryngopharynx squamous cell carcinoma. In Saegesser, F., and Pettavel, J., Eds.: *Surgical Oncology.* Bern, Switzerland: Hans Huber Publishers, 1970, pp. 347-366.

Gilbertsen, V. A.: Adenocarcinoma of the rectum: Incidence of locations of recurrent tumor following present-day operations performed for cure. *Annals of Surgery,* 151:340-348, March 1960.

Gray, L. H.: Radiobiologic basis of oxygen as a modifying factor in radiation therapy. *American Journal of Roentgenology, Radium Therapy and Nuclear Medicine,* 85:803-815, May 1961.

Herring, D. F., and Compton, D. M. J.: *The Degree of Precision Required in the Radiation Dose Delivered in Cancer Radiotherapy.* Report #EMI-216 from Enviro-Med. Inc., La Jolla, California, July 10, 1970.

Jackson, S. M.: Carcinoma of the breast—the significance of supraclavicular lymph node metastases. *Clinical Radiology,* 17:107-114, April 1966.

Jesse, R. H., Barkley, H. T., Lindberg, R. D., and Fletcher, G. H.: Cancer of the oral cavity. Is elective neck dissection beneficial? *American Journal of Surgery,* 120:505-508, October 1970.

King, J. J., and Fletcher, G. H.: Malignant tumors of the major salivary glands. *Radiology,* 100:381-384, August 1971.

Kremen, A. J.: Results of surgical treatment of cancer of the tongue. *Surgery,* 39: 49-53, 1956.

Lindberg, R. D.: The role of radiation therapy in the treatment of soft tissue sarcoma in adults. In *Seventh National Cancer Conference Proceedings,* Philadelphia, Pennsylvania, J. B. Lippincott Co., 1973, pp. 883-888.

Lindberg, R. D., Barkley, H. G., Jr., Jesse, R. H., and Fletcher, G. H.: Evolution of the clinically negative neck in patients with squamous cell carcinoma of the faucial arch. *American Journal of Roentgenology, Radium Therapy and Nuclear Medicine,* 111:60-65, January 1971.

Lyall, D., and Schetlin, D. F.: Cancer of the tongue. *Annals of Surgery,* 134:313, 1958.

MacComb, W. S., and Fletcher, G. H.: Planned combination of surgery and radiation in treatment of advanced primary head and neck cancers. *American Journal of Roentgenology, Radium Therapy and Nuclear Medicine,* 77:397-414, March 1957.

Martin, R. G., Butler, J. J., and Albores-Saavedra, J.: Soft tissue tumors: Surgical treatment and results. In *Tumors of Bone and Soft Tissue,* Chicago, Year Book Medical Publishers, Inc., 1963, pp. 333-347.

Million, R. R., Fletcher, G. H., and Jesse, R. H.: Evaluation of elective irradiation of the neck for squamous cell carcinoma of the nasopharynx, tonsillar fossa, and base of tongue. *Radiology,* 80:973-988, June 1963.

Northrop, M. F., Fletcher, G. H., Jesse, R. H., and Lindberg, R. D.: Evolution of neck disease in patients with primary squamous cell carcinoma of the oral tonque, floor of mouth, and palatine arch and clinically positive neck nodes neither fixed nor bilateral. *Cancer,* 29:23-30, January 1972.

Paterson, R.: *The Treatment of Malignant Disease by Radium and X-ray: Being a Practice of Radiotherapy,* Baltimore, Maryland, Williams and Wilkins Company, 1949.

————: Studies in optimum dosage. *British Journal of Radiology,* 25:505-516, 1952.

Puck, T. T., and Marcus, P. I.: Action of x-rays on mammalian cells. *Journal of Experimental Medicine,* 103:653-666, 1956.

Robbins, G. F., Lucas, J. C., Fracchia, A. A., Farrow, J. H., and Chu, F. G. H.: An evaluation of postoperative prophylactic radiation therapy in breast cancer. *Surgery, Gynecology and Obstetrics,* 122:979-982, May 1966.

Roux-Berger, J. L., Baud, M., and Courtial, J.: Cancer de la partie mobile de la langue. Le curage ganglionaire prophlactique est-il justifie? Statistique de la Foundation Curie, *Memorias de l'Academie de chirurgie,* 75:120-126, January 26-February 2, 1949.

Southwick, H. W., Slaughter, D. P., and Trevino, E. T.: Elective neck dissection for intraoral cancer. *Archives of Surgery,* 80:905-909, June 1960.

Evaluation of Patients with Head and Neck Cancer

KENT C. WESTBROOK, M.D.

Department of Surgery, University of Arkansas Medical Center,
Little Rock, Arkansas

CANCER OF THE HEAD AND NECK threatens the patient, his family, and his physician. The patient faces possible loss of sensory organs, decreased physiologic function, altered personal appearance, and death. The patient's family is threatened by the loss of their relative plus the serious problems associated with a prolonged illness. The physician is confronted with difficult treatment problems and a high rate of treatment failures.

Yet, these are desperate ills and they demand radical measures to achieve cure or relief of symptoms. The physician's general goals should include relief of symptoms, prolongation of useful life, and assistance with death if it becomes inevitable. He should help the patient and his family to accept the disease, its treatment, and its course. In patients with head and neck cancer, optimal therapy goals include: (1) eradication of the cancer, (2) satisfactory physiological function, and (3) acceptable cosmetic appearance. The correct treatment for any individual patient is that therapeutic approach which most nearly achieves these goals. Selection of correct therapy requires: (1) an accurate, detailed assessment of the patient and his lesion, (2) knowledge of various applicable treatment regimens, and (3) wisdom to choose the optimal therapeutic course for an individual patient.

Most of this conference will concern specific diagnostic and therapeutic procedures, modalities, and regimens. Before this material is presented, we should consider the evaluation of each individual patient. This evaluation is designed to aid in the selection of optimal therapy and involves three groups of variables: (1) tumor factors, (2) patient factors, and (3) physician factors.

39

TABLE 1.—Tumor Factors

1. Anatomical site of primary
2. Extent of primary tumor
3. Stage of cervical nodes
4. Presence or absence of distant metastasis
5. Gross and microscopic tumor pathology

Tumor Factors

Usually, the most important factors in determining the treatment of an individual patient are those related to the tumor. Crucial tumor factors include the anatomical site of the primary, the local extension of the primary, and the presence or absence of metastasis (Table 1).

Anatomical Site of Primary

Anatomical site of origin is significant because of varied clinical courses, different metastatic patterns, and varied surgical or radiotherapeutic accessibility of different sites. Similar histological lesions originating in different portions of the head and neck manifest different clinical courses. For example, squamous cell carcinoma of the lip rarely metastasizes while carcinoma of the tongue frequently does. Very small primaries with cervical node metastases are fairly common in the tonsillar fossa, base of the tongue, pyriform sinus, and nasopharynx. Midline lesions including uvula, floor of the mouth, epiglottis, and nasopharynx tend to produce bilateral metastasis.

The site of early metastasis is closely correlated with the site of origin. For example, tongue lesions usually spread first to submandibular and subdigastric nodes while extrinsic larynx lesions usually go to midjugular and paratracheal nodes.

Certain anatomical sites including the lip, oral tongue, buccal mucosa, and floor of the mouth are relatively accessible and can be handled easily by surgical procedures. Other lesions such as those of the retromolar trigone, faucial arch, pyriform sinus, or oropharynx are more difficult to manage surgically. Nasopharyngeal lesions are essentially inaccessible surgically.

Extent of Primary Tumor

Accurate staging of the primary lesion is important in therapy selection and prognosis. Various staging systems are used for primary tumors of the head and neck, but all include evaluation of the primary tumor and its local extension. Proper primary staging requires an adequate history, physical examination, and laboratory evaluation. Size of the lesion can be determined on physical examination directly by measurement or by comparison with an object of known size. Special roentgenograms help delineate the size of less accessible lesions.

While specific staging criteria are formulated for each anatomical site of origin, a general outline can be used for discussion. Primary lesions of the upper digestive and respiratory tract are staged approximately as follows:

	Size	*Extent*
T_1	Less than 2 cm.	No extension or infiltration, function normal.
T_2	2 to 4 cm.	Minimal extension to adjacent structures and minimal infiltration, slightly decreased function.
T_3	Greater than 4 cm.	Moderate extension to adjacent structures and infiltration, significantly decreased function.
T_4	Massive	Extends outside organ of origin, bone invasion, fixation of structure.

Local extension of head and neck cancers occurs primarily along normal tissue planes formed by mucosa, soft tissues, muscles, nerve sheaths, and vessels. Direct extension into bone or cartilage may occur. Redness of the mucosa at a distance from a primary tumor often indicates mucosal or submucosal spread. Bimanual palpation may delineate tumor growth along soft tissue planes. Cancer infiltration into muscle limits normal movement. For example, pterygoid muscle involvement produces trismus.

Altered sensation from the face usually indicates tumor involvement of the fifth cranial nerve. The mandibular division (V_3) transmits sensation from the chin, floor of the mouth, tongue, and inner cheek via the inferior alveolar, lingual, and buccal nerves. The maxillary nerve (V_2) covers the palate, upper gum, and malar area via the superior alveolar, palatine, and infraorbital branches. The ophthalmic nerve (V_1) supplies the forehead through the supraorbital and supratrochlear nerves. Decreased sensation in these areas is usually the result of tumor infiltrating a nerve.

Nasopharyngeal tumors often spread directly upward toward the cranial cavity involving nerves III to VI. Extraocular movement should be checked in every patient with suspected nasopharyngeal tumor. Retropharyngeal or parapharyngeal node involvement by metastatic lesions of the oropharynx, nasopharynx, and hypopharynx is not rare and can produce a deficit of cranial nerves IX, X, XI, or XII. Involvement of the VII cranial nerve with facial paralysis occurs primarily with malignant parotid tumors and metastatic carcinoma to the parotid nodes.

Referred ear pain is a common symptom in patients with head and neck cancers, and it may develop from several nerve pathways. Lesions of the tongue or floor of the mouth may refer pain along the lingual nerve to the maxillary division of the fifth cranial nerve (V_3) and up the auriculo-temporal nerve to produce pain of the external ear area. Oropharyngeal tumors may refer pain along the glossopharyngeal nerve (IX) to the tympanic nerve producing pain deep in the ear. Hypopharyngeal lesions are supplied by the superior laryngeal nerve, a branch of the vagus (X) nerve which also gives rise to the auricular nerve of Arnold, sensory from deep in the ear. Hence, referred ear pain may occur with varied lesions of the head and neck.

Bone or cartilage involvement may be suggested, on physical examination, by deep fixation. Frequently, however, radiographic techniques including routine studies, angiography, contrast studies, and tomography are essential to delineate the actual extent of a tumor with regard to adjacent soft tissue, cartilage, or bone. Furthermore, bone destruction must be rather extensive before it can even be detected radiographically.

Stage of Cervical Nodes

Most cancers of the head and neck are squamous cell carcinomas and metastasize primarily by the lymphatic system. Therefore, evaluation of the cervical lymphatics is of utmost importance. Tumors of specific anatomical areas have characteristic metastatic patterns. For example, the classical spread of nasopharyngeal lesions is to subdigastric and posterior triangle nodes, that of oral tongue lesions to subdigastric nodes, and that of lip lesions to submental nodes. Various stagings of cervical nodes have been used. The system currently employed at M. D. Anderson Hospital is based on clinical examination, and is as follows:

N_0 —no positive nodes.

N_1 —single positive node less than 3 cm. in diameter.

N_{2a}—single positive node greater than 3 cm. in diameter.

N_{2b}—multiple ipsilateral positive nodes.

N_{3a}—unilateral fixed node.

N_{3b}—bilateral positive nodes, fixed or not fixed.

Nodes are considered fixed when they are clinically attached to the carotid artery, prevertebral muscles, or bony structures of the head and neck.

Positive nodes at multiple levels or in an unusual position (other than first level) usually indicate a more virulent tumor.

OTHER TUMOR FACTORS

Other significant tumor factors include duration of the tumor, gross tumor characteristics, and specific histology of the tumor. Tumors with a long history are usually less aggressive and more amenable to therapy. Exophytic tumors are more easily managed than infiltrative tumors. Most head and neck cancers are squamous cell carcinomas, but other histologic types with special features do occur. For example, adenoid cystic carcinomas frequently spread along nerves and are prone to long-term recurrence. Lymphoepitheliomas produce early lymph node metastases and are very responsive to radiotherapy. The spindle variety of squamous carcinoma seems more virulent than well-differentiated squamous cell carcinoma.

Accurate assessment of the tumor depends upon a history which elicits precipitating factors and determines the exact duration and symptomatology of the lesion. Physical examination includes inspection and palpation of the entire head and neck, with emphasis on the possible routes of spread of the tumor including muscle planes, fascial planes, nerve sheaths, and cervical metastases. Special roentgenograms are indicated in most head and neck lesions. Biopsy is required for definitive histological diagnosis.

Patient Factors

A cancer cannot be considered separate and apart from the patient in whom it occurs. Therefore, patient factors including age, general health, dental health, social habits, socioeconomic factors, previous therapy, and individual desires must be considered in each patient (Table 2). Some patients are not suitable for a major operative procedure with general anesthesia because of severe systemic disease such as recent myocardial infarction or severe cirrhosis. These patients must therefore receive radio-

---

TABLE 2.—PATIENT FACTORS

1. General medical condition
2. Personal habits
3. Socioeconomic factors
4. Dental status
5. Previous treatment
6. Personal desires

---

therapy, chemotherapy or no therapy. Complete dental evaluation and care is necessary before any radiotherapy to the oral cavity. Repair of damaged teeth, extraction of nonsalvageable teeth, smoothing of exostoses, and institution of fluoride prophylaxis should be considered.

Squamous cell carcinoma of the upper respiratory and digestive tracts is frequently associated with heavy drinking and smoking habits. A severe alcoholic is unsuitable for prolonged radiotherapy which requires his daily presence and cooperation. Alcoholism therefore suggests surgical therapy. Heavy smoking increases the complication rate with radiotherapy because of an additive effect on the mucous membranes. Patients must, therefore, stop smoking during radiotherapy. Heavy continued smoking may necessitate splitting radiotherapy or even abandoning it for surgical therapy. Furthermore, the high incidence of second primaries in these patients must be considered in the initial planning of their therapy.

Socioeconomic factors play a definite role in therapy selection. Working patients or patients from long distances frequently can ill afford six to eight weeks for radiotherapy. They are, therefore, treated surgically if both modalities are equal in tumor eradication. Implantation techniques may be utilized in patients best treated with radiotherapy but who object to a prolonged course of external irradiation treatment.

Treatment cannot be administered to a patient against his will, so individual desires must be considered. Some patients refuse surgical therapy because of fear and must be treated by radiotherapy even if such treatment is less than optimal for their problem. Some patients prefer a fairly rapid surgical procedure and recovery rather than a prolonged radiotherapy treatment regimen. A few patients refuse to submit to ablative surgery because of their fear of disfigurement. The desires of the patient must be respected in therapy planning.

Patient factors including the general health of the patient, the habits of the patient, the socioeconomic factors related to the patient, and the desire of the patient may override tumor factors in arriving at a therapy plan.

Physician Factors

The tumor which occurs in a patient must be treated by a doctor or group of doctors. The physician responsible for making therapeutic decisions must be familiar with the various alternative regimens applicable in an individual patient. In any geographical area, surgical skills and radiotherapeutic skills may vary tremendously. Surgical specialties are fairly well represented throughout the United States, though the number of trained head and neck cancer surgeons is limited. The number of radio-

TABLE 3.—Physician Factors

1. Surgical skills
2. Radiotherapy skills
3. Dental skills
4. Rehabilitative skills

therapists skilled in the exacting administration of high-dose therapy to the head and neck is very limited. Therefore, the availability of medical skills must be considered (Table 3).

Furthermore, patients treated with either radiotherapy or surgical therapy of the head and neck often require dental, maxillofacial, or oral surgical care. Radiotherapy to the oral cavity may result in caries, loss of teeth, and osteoradionecrosis unless proper dental hygiene is maintained before, during, and after therapy. Dentists specially trained in this field must be available if radiotherapy is to achieve maximal results. Also, certain radiotherapeutic techniques, such as intraoral irradiation, require the manufacture of cones and retracting devices to delineate the field and protect surrounding tissues. This requires a prosthodontist skilled in the production of such appliances. A fair number of patients with cancer of the mouth, oropharynx, or jaws develop trismus and require special exercises and/or appliances to maintain satisfactory function. Ablative procedures within the oral cavity frequently require prosthetic devices. This may be a stabilizing prosthesis, placed at the time of operation, to maintain normal tissue configuration or to secure skin grafts. A temporary prosthesis may be placed in the early postoperative period to facilitate eating or talking. A permanent prosthesis may replace the removed portion of the face or oral cavity to achieve acceptable cosmetic and functional results.

Mandibular resection produces serious problems in which specialized assistance is required. Good occlusion of the remaining teeth must be maintained by mechanical devices, exercises, etc. Replacement of the resected mandible may be feasible in some cases and requires multi-specialty cooperation.

Patients with head and neck cancer have tremendous psychological and sociological problems and hence skilled help consisting of social workers, speech therapists, dieticians, etc., is required in these areas. The implementation of an optimal therapy plan for a patient with cancer of the head and neck often requires specialized surgeons, radiotherapists, dentists, oral surgeons, prosthodontists, social workers, dieticians, rehabilitation specialists, and others. Therefore, the treatment plan of any individual patient must take into account the facilities and help available to the patient.

Summary

Every patient with head and neck cancer is an individual patient with an individual tumor. The ultimate treatment goal is eradication of the cancer with satisfactory functional and cosmetic results. Selection of the optimal treatment requires accurate diagnosis, knowledge of treatment modalities, and wisdom to integrate these into a suitable therapeutic regimen. Careful evaluation of tumor factors, patient factors, and physician factors form the foundation for this decision.

Radiotherapy—Before or After Surgery?

ROBERT D. LINDBERG, M.D.,
RICHARD H. JESSE, M.D., AND
GILBERT H. FLETCHER, M.D.

*Departments of Radiotherapy and Surgery, The University of Texas
System Cancer Center, M. D. Anderson Hospital and
Tumor Institute, Houston, Texas*

IN RECENT YEARS, the survival rates for surgical treatment of head and neck cancer have assumed a gradual plateau. This indicates that the surgical techniques have nearly reached the limits of their effectiveness. There have been attempts to increase the surgical cure rates by more radical procedures, but in general, the gains are too small to justify the ensuant morbidity, dysfunction, and disfigurement. With an increased understanding of tumor biology and a better understanding of the patterns of spread, most surgeons have realized that frequently their results depend upon the biological behavior of the particular tumor rather than the technical refinements of the surgical procedures. Therefore, during the past 20 years, surgeons have sought suitable surgical adjuvants to circumvent the biological behavior of tumors.

The combination of surgery and radiotherapy in treatment for malignant tumors was reported by Symonds (1913-1914). Before 1950, there were conflicting reports in the literature on the benefits of a combined approach. With the advent of megavoltage radiotherapy in the 1950's, however, there was renewed interest in the combined approach. In 1957, a report by MacComb and Fletcher advocated radiation therapy and surgery in the treatment for selected advanced head and neck lesions. In recent years, there has been more widespread interest in combining the two modalities of treatment (Fletcher and Jesse, 1962).

47

The purpose of this presentation is to discuss the rationale and the pros and cons of pre- and postoperative radiation therapy. The discussion will be limited to the epithelial cancers of head and neck origin.

Rationale

The cause of local and regional failures cannot be dissociated. Recurrence of cancer at the primary site after surgery results from: (1) microscopic extensions of disease beyond the limits of resection, (2) seeding of the wound at the time of surgery, and/or (3) not removing all the gross disease. Recurrences in the radically dissected neck are usually because the disease, diffusely spread through lymphatic channels, cannot be totally removed. Thus, radiation therapy is needed to eradicate cancer at the periphery of the primary site and in the heavily infested neck.

PREOPERATIVE IRRADIATION

The first purpose of preoperative radiation therapy is to render inoperable lesions operable. Primary or metastatic lesions may be so large that they are technically inoperable and/or attached to structures such as the carotid artery which should not be removed. Radiation therapy, at the 5,000 to 6,000 rad level, may provide sufficient shrinkage of the tumor so that a surgical freeing may be possible.

The second purpose of preoperative radiation therapy is to decrease the incidence of local and regional recurrences. Animal experiments, reported by Perez and Powers (1967), have shown that the number of viable tumor cells is markedly decreased with moderate doses of irradiation, and thus fewer cells will be present to reseed the surgical area. Preoperative irradiation eradicates subclinical disease which might have spread beyond the margins of the surgical resection. In fact, 4,500 to 5,000 rads in five weeks eradicate at least 90 per cent of well-oxygenated subclinical disease, and 3,000 rads in three weeks to 4,000 rads in four weeks may eradicate 60 to 70 per cent (Fletcher, 1972).

The third and perhaps the most important potential benefit of preoperative irradiation is to decrease the frequency of distant metastases. Since preoperative irradiation decreases the number of viable cancer cells, theoretically there should be less chance of distant metastasis caused by a surgical manipulation of the tumor. This theoretical concept is difficult to prove or disprove.

PREOPERATIVE IRRADIATION—LOW DOSE VERSUS HIGH DOSE

Among the advocates of preoperative irradiation there is considerable argument regarding the most effective dose which is well tolerated. There are numerous conflicting and confusing reports in the literature.

Biller and Ogura (1970) reported on 292 patients presenting with pharyngeal and laryngopharyngeal cancers treated with and without preoperative irradiation. In their series, the patients received 1,500 to 3,000 rads in two to three weeks with ^{60}Co teletherapy, covering the primary lesion and the ipsilateral neck. Surgery was performed three to four weeks following radiation therapy. An incontinuity neck dissection was performed regardless of whether clinically metastatic nodes were palpable. Of the 189 patients with lesions arising in the supraglottic larynx, glottis, lingual surface of epiglottis, vallecula, or base of tongue, 79 received preoperative irradiation. The remaining 110 patients were treated by surgery alone. There were no statistically significant differences between the two groups in local or neck recurrence, or survival. Next they compared lesions of the pyriform sinus. Of 103 patients, 41 received preoperative irradiation. The three-year survival rate with preoperative irradiation was 60 per cent (25 of 41), whereas the group treated by surgery alone was 41 per cent (26 of 62). The results were statistically significant, with a χ^2 of .0007. The neck recurrences were not influenced by preoperative irradiation.

Strong (1969) reported a statistically significant decreased incidence of node recurrence in the radically dissected neck with 2,000 rads in five fractions to the entire neck preoperatively. The survival rates, however, were unchanged. A pilot study (unpublished data, 1970) at M. D. Anderson Hospital showed that 2,000 rads given dose in 96 hours was ineffective when the primary lesions were large or when the neck nodes were fixed.

Galante, Benak, and Buschke (1970) reported on a series of patients with oral cavity lesions treated with 5,000 to 6,500 rads tumor dose in six to seven weeks followed by surgery. The two-year determinate survival was 55 per cent (16 of 29).

Hendrickson (1970) reported on a series of 71 patients with advanced laryngeal carcinomas treated by preoperative radiation therapy who were randomly assigned to receive either 2,000 rads in two weeks or 5,000 rads in four weeks (29 and 42 patients, respectively). The four-year NED (no evidence of disease) rate was 58 per cent (17 of 29) for low dose versus 50 per cent (21 of 42) for high dose.

Silverstone, Goldman, and Ryan (1970) reported on 53 patients with advanced squamous cell carcinoma of the laryngopharynx treated with 5,500 rads over five weeks followed by radical surgery in three to six weeks. The two-year survival was 90 per cent (44 of 49) absolute and 96 per cent (44 of 46) determinate. The five-year absolute survival rate was 67 per cent (18 of 27), and determinate rate was 86 per cent (18 of 21). The effectiveness of local eradication of the tumor within the head and neck area was 90 per cent (48 of 53). No one has been able to duplicate these results.

On reviewing the literature, no practical information was found regarding the proper dose of preoperative irradiation.

POSTOPERATIVE IRRADIATION

The rationale for postoperative irradiation is similar to that for preoperative irradiation: to increase the local and regional control rate by eradicating (1) the microscopic extensions beyond the margins of the surgical resection, and (2) the cancer cells in the operated area which cause seeding.

Pros and Cons

PREOPERATIVE IRRADIATION

The main argument in favor of preoperative irradiation is that no interference with the blood supply has occurred. It is argued that tumor cells shed into the surgical wound must be hypoxic; therefore, radiation therapy is more effective if given preoperatively. Although surgical precedures do interfere with the blood supply, the tissues are not anoxic. In addition, subclinical nests of cancer cells at the periphery are relatively unaffected and remain oxygenated.

Postoperatively, because of the possibility that the tumor cells remaining in the bed are slightly hypoxic with perhaps 10 to 15 per cent decreased radiosensitivity, the dose is increased to 6,000 rads in six weeks. The necessity of the additional 1,000 rads in postoperative radiation therapy is a matter of conjecture. Comparison of pre- and postoperative radiation therapy in the treatment of primary lesions of the paranasal sinus (Table 1) and of neck nodes (Table 2) shows no difference in failure rates. Pre- and postoperative irradiation are equally effective in controlling local and regional node disease, *i.e.*, 5,000 rads tumor dose in five weeks compared to 6,000 rads tumor dose in six weeks, respectively (Table 2).

A second argument for preoperative irradiation is that after 5,000 rads in five weeks, the margin of surrounding normal tissue may be less than if

TABLE 1.—SQUAMOUS CELL CARCINOMA
PARANASAL SINUS (1952 TO 1961)

	PREOPERATIVE IRRADIATION	POSTOPERATIVE IRRADIATION
Total Cases		
Treated for Cure	22	18
Three-Year Survival	10 (45.5%)	7 (39%)
Local Recurrence	8 (36.5%)	6 (33%)
Distant Metastasis	2 (9.0%)	1 (5.5%)

Adapted from Jesse, 1965.

radiation therapy were not used. The same reasoning can be used for a limited surgical procedure and postoperative irradiation.

The third and probably most potent argument for preoperative irradiation is the potential decrease in the incidence of distant metastasis. Biller and Ogura (1970) reported on 292 patients presenting with pharyngeal and laryngopharyngeal cancers treated with and without preoperative irradiation (3,000 rads in three weeks). The incidence of distant metastasis was essentially the same in both groups (Table 3) (Ogura, 1972). Whether high-dose preoperative irradiation (5,000 rads tumor dose in five weeks) will diminish the incidence of distant metastases remains to be seen.

The arguments against preoperative radiation therapy are: First, there is an increased patient morbidity and mortality, *i.e.*, delayed healing, increased fistula formation, and increased incidence of carotid artery rupture. Numerous authors (Hendrickson, 1970; Silverstone, Goldman, and Ryan, 1970; Rush, Mooney, Jewell, and Greenlaw, 1971), however, report that the complication rate is not increased significantly even after high-

TABLE 2.—FAILURE OF INITIAL TREATMENT IN IPSILATERAL SIDE OF NECK[*]
SQUAMOUS CELL CARCINOMA 1948 THROUGH 1967,
ANALYSIS OF JANUARY 1972

TREATMENT	N1	N2A	N2B	N3A	N3B	TOTAL
Preoperative Irradiation						
Tonsillar Fossa & Base of Tongue	0/4	0/9	0/14	1/3	1/7	2/37 (5.4%)
Postoperative Irradiation						
Supraglottic Larynx & Hypopharynx	0/17	0/8	0/14	2/10	3/8	5/57 (8.8%)

[*]Failures/total patients.
Adapted from Barkley, Fletcher, Jesse, and Lindberg, 1972.

TABLE 3.—LARYNGOPHARYNX AND PHARYNX, SQUAMOUS CELL
CARCINOMA: INCIDENCE OF DISTANT METASTASIS

SITE	SURGERY ALONE		PRE-OP XRT[*]	
Supraglottic Larynx	4/52	(7.6%)	6/35	(17%)
Glottic	2/43	(4.6%)	2/30	(6.6%)
Lingual Surface of Epiglottic and Base of Tongue	1/15	(6.6%)	2/14	(14%)
Pyriform Sinus	1/62	(1.6%)	4/41	(9.7%)
Total	8/172	(4.7%)	14/120	(11.6%)

[*]1,500 to 3,000 rads in one to three weeks.
Ogura, Personal Communication, 1972.

dose preoperative irradiation, *i.e.*, 5,000 rads tumor dose in five weeks or more. The field sizes used by these investigators are often smaller than would be used if the pateints were treated by radiotherapy alone. The speed of healing depends upon the radiation dose, the size of the portals, the extent of the surgical procedure, and the nutritional status of the patient at the time of surgery. Any kind of surgical procedure may be done after doses of 2,000 rads in two weeks to 3,000 rads in three weeks. After 4,000 rads in four weeks, surgery can usually be performed two to three weeks after completion of therapy. After 5,000 rads in five weeks to 6,000 rads in six weeks, slow healing on mucosal suture lines can be expected, and the patient must be carefully evaluated to be sure that he is in positive nitrogen balance. This may require five to six weeks postradiation. After 6,000 rads in six weeks, bilateral neck dissection must be staged. When contemplating extensive surgical procedures, the surgeon should ask the therapist to modify treatment portals to spare possible donor areas for skin flaps. Alterations of the portals should not, however, spare areas where there may be cancer or reasonable risk of infestation. Often a compromise must be made by using a more limited surgical procedure for the heavily irradiated patient than would ordinarily be used in the nonirradiated patient.

The second objection to preoperative irradiation is more theoretical than practical. Some surgeons argue that because of tumor regression they can no longer decide the normal tissue margin. The surgical procedure must be planned before initiation of therapy; the limits of the resection are dependent upon the original extent of the lesion rather than the amount of tumor regression. All areas of original gross tumor must be removed. However, wide margins of grossly normal tissue are not necessary after high-dose preoperative radiation therapy. The extent of the resection can be tattooed prior to the radiation therapy. More important is the realization that frozen section checks of the surgical margin cannot be relied on, especially after irradiation.

Third, the patient's age is important. Rarely will a patient over 70 tolerate high-dose radiation therapy followed by extensive surgery. Younger patients (50 or 60 years old) in good physical condition and positive nitrogen balance tolerate the treatment well.

POSTOPERATIVE IRRADIATION

Postoperative radiation therapy has fallen into such disrepute that even some radiation therapists have categorically stated that if postoperative radiation therapy is indicated, preoperative radiation therapy should have been given. Such a statement cannot be defended, since many times the indications for radiotherapy are not clinically apparent and are appreciated only at the time of surgery. Most data on which these assumptions are based come from the well-known inability of radiation to eradicate grossly recurrent disease. If radiation therapy is delayed until there is a gross recurrence, the effectiveness of the treatment is very limited. Immediate postoperative radiation therapy, however, is effective in eliminating subclinical disease at the surgical margin, and when given electively to the undissected neck, prevents further manifestation of disease (Fletcher, 1972; Barkley, Fletcher, Jesse, and Lindberg, 1972; Berger, Fletcher, Lindberg, and Jesse, 1971).

The surgeon must decide either to remove the gross cancer and leave areas of in situ or microscopic disease to be treated by radiation, or to do a superradical procedure which removes all the possible areas of microscopic spread. The latter procedure causes prolonged healing time and delayed postoperative radiation therapy. The surgical procedure must be designed to remove the gross disease and still obtain the fastest possible healing. Immediate rather than delayed reconstruction is advisable, so that radiotherapy can be started as soon as possible.

In addition to radiation therapy as a planned procedure after surgery, it is also used in selected patients when: (1) there is a question as to the adequacy of the surgical margin, (2) the primary disease was more extensive than suspected, and (3) there are multiple foci of microscopic invasion and/or carcinoma in situ.

Discussion

No blanket statement is possible regarding combined surgery and radiation therapy in the treatment for head and neck cancer. Patients who will benefit from combined treatment are those in whom the cancer, primary lesion and/or nodal metastasis, is advanced with a significant probability of local and/or regional failure if treated by a single modality. In the treatment plan, one cannot dissociate the primary lesion from the cervical metastasis. When combined therapy is indicated, the sequence of modalities depends on the location and extent of the primary lesion and the nodal metastasis.

ORAL CAVITY, FAUCIAL ARCH, AND OROPHARYNX

Planned combined surgical and radiation therapy procedures are used in patients with T_4 lesions. Selected T_3 lesions of the anterior two thirds of tongue, floor of mouth, and retromolar trigone are also treated by combined treatment. We prefer initial resection with immediate closure followed by postoperative radiation therapy. Closure of these wounds can be by primary suture, split skin grafts, or undelayed pedicle. The closure is designed so that within three weeks the primary site and the lower neck can be treated postoperatively to 6,000 and 5,000 rads, respectively, at 1,000 rads per week.

Patients with nodes fixed to the carotid artery should never have primary radical neck dissection, since the chance of eradicating the cancer is slight. Proper treatment is to administer 5,000 rads or more preoperatively, which will often render the neck mass resectable. Radical or modified neck dissection is then performed.

GLOTTIC

Patients with fixed cord lesions confined to the larynx without positive nodes are treated by surgery alone. Postoperative radiation therapy would not benefit these patients since there is not extension outside the larynx. Patients with vocal cord lesions extending beyond the larynx, *i.e.*, through the thyroid cartilage and/or subglottically into the trachea, or those with positive neck nodes are treated surgically with postoperative radiation therapy covering the entire neck.

SUPRAGLOTTIC LARYNX

T_3 and T_4 lesions of the infrahyoid epiglottis, false cords, and aryepiglottic folds are best treated by initial laryngectomy. Since most false cord lesions can be removed with a good surgical margin, postoperative irradiation is not given unless lymph node metastases are found. In contrast, the

TABLE 4.—Supraglottic Larynx, NED at
Two Years: 1948 through 1965

Margin (Suprahyoid Epiglottis and Aryepiglottic Folds)

Stage	Surgery	Radiation	Combined Surgery and Radiation
T_1	–	9/12	–
T_2	5/5	16/22	–
T_3	1/11	7/13	5/9
T_4	2/9	12/20	5/5

Vestibule (Infrahyoid Epiglottis and False Cords)

T_1	–	4/7	2/2
T_2	13/20	12/18	8/9
T_3	24/34	3/7	3/10
T_4	9/22	3/11*	9/11

*Six patients—N_3.
Adapted from Fletcher, Jesse, Lindberg, and Koons, 1970.

surgical clearance in advanced lesions of the supraglottic margin, *i.e.*, suprahyoid epiglottis and aryepiglottic folds, and the infrahyoid epiglottis is narrow. The addition of postoperative radiation therapy decreases the incidence of local recurrences only when the tumor extends to the pharyngeal wall, preepiglottic space, or base of tongue (Tables 4 and 5). Thus, by surgical determination of the extent of the lesion, radiation therapy may be avoided in some patients.

Postoperative irradiation is given when: (1) The surgical margin is narrow, (2) disease has spread outside the larynx, and/or (3) multiple metastatic nodes are found at surgery. The primary site and upper portions of the neck are irradiated to 6,000 rads tumor dose in six weeks and the lower part of the neck receives 5,000 rads given dose in five weeks.

TABLE 5.—Patients with Advanced Tumors of the Epiglottic and
Aryepiglottic Folds or N_2–N_3 Neck Disease, NED at Two
Years: February 1948 through December 1965

	Surgery Alone	Surgery + Postop. Irrad.
T_3–T_4 Suprahyoid Epiglottis and Aryepiglottic Folds	3/20 (15.0%)	10/14 (71.5%)
T_4 Infrahyoid Epiglottis	8/17 (47.0%)	8/10 (80.0%)
N_2–N_3	13/34 (38.0%)	15/21 (71.0%)

Courtesy of Fletcher and Jesse, 1971.

Fixed nodes associated with supraglottic cancers are given preoperative radiation therapy to a dose of 5,000 rads or more followed by partial or radical neck dissection and laryngectomy.

PYRIFORM SINUS

From 1954 through 1961, 35 patients were treated by laryngectomy, partial pharyngectomy, and radical neck dissection, and 21 patients had surgery and postoperative irradiation. Although the local recurrence rate was decreased with combined treatment, the survival rates were similar (Table 6). In an attempt to increase the survival rate, 57 patients from 1962 through 1965 had a more extended surgical procedure including laryngectomy, circumferential pharyngectomy, radical neck dissection, and retropharyngeal node dissection. The local control rate above the clavicle was not significantly improved by the extended surgical procedure and the survival rates were unchanged due to the increase in distant metastasis and death from intercurrent disease. The addition of postoperative radiation therapy diminishes the incidence of failures above the clavicle. In order to be effective the treated volume must include the primary (6,000 rads in six weeks), the lower neck bilaterally (5,000 rads in five weeks), and the retropharyngeal nodes (5,000 rads in five weeks).

NECK

Postoperative radiation therapy is indicated after radical neck dissection irrespective of the site of the primary lesion for the following findings in the surgical specimen: (1) connective tissue disease, (2) multiple levels of involvement, and/or (3) a high percentage of nodes involved.

TABLE 6.—PYRIFORM SINUS[e]

	RECURRENCE ABOVE CLAVICLE	5-YEAR ABSOLUTE SURVIVAL
1954 through 1961		
Surgery Alone	20/35 (57%)	8/35 (23%)
Surgery + Megavoltage Irradiation	6/21 (28.5%)	5/21 (24%)
1962 through 1965		
Superradical Surgery	28/57 (48%)	11/44[†] (25%)

[e]The T and N distribution is the same in the three groups.
[†]Number of patients with 5-year follow-up.
Courtesy of Fletcher, 1973.

Summary

1. Combined surgery and radiation is beneficial only when there is a high incidence of local and/or regional failures by either modality alone.

2. The sequence of the two modalities depends on the anatomical site and stage of the primary lesion and the neck disease.

3. The effectiveness of preoperative or postoperative radiation therapy in controlling local and regional disease is equal.

4. When preoperative irradiation is used, the dose should be 5,000 rads in five weeks since that dose will control more than 90 per cent of the subclinical disease.

5. When postoperative irradiation is used, the entire surgical area must be irradiated as soon as possible. The recommended dose is 6,000 rads in six weeks in the scar area.

Acknowledgments

This investigation was supported by Public Health Service Grants CA-06294, CA-05654, and CA-05099 from the National Cancer Institute.

REFERENCES

Barkley, H. T., Jr., Fletcher, G. H., Jesse, R. H., and Lindberg, R. D.: Management of cervical lymph node and metastases in squamous cell carcinomas of the tonsillar fossa, base of tongue, supraglottic larynx, and hypopharynx. *The American Journal of Surgery*, 124:462-467, October 1972.

Berger, D. S., Fletcher, G. H., Lindberg, R. D., and Jesse, R. H.: Elective irradiation of the neck lymphatics for squamous cell carcinoma of the nasopharynx and oropharynx. *The American Journal of Roentgenology, Radium Therapy and Nuclear Medicine*, 111:66-72, January 1971.

Biller, H. F., and Ogura, J. H.: Planned preoperative irradiation for laryngeal and laryngopharyngeal carcinoma. *Frontiers of Radiation Therapy and Oncology*, 5:100-105, 1970.

Fletcher, G. H.: Elective irradiation of subclinical disease in cancers of the head and neck. *Cancer*, 29:1450-1454, June 1972.

———: *Textbook of Radiotherapy*. 2nd edition. Philadelphia, Pennsylvania, Lea and Febiger, 1973, pp. 122-123.

Fletcher, G. H., and Jesse, R. H.: The contribution of supervoltage roentgenotherapy to the integration of radiation and surgery in head and neck squamous cell carcinomas. *Cancer*, 15:566-577, May-June 1962.

———: Interaction of surgery and irradiation in head and neck cancers. *Current Problems in Radiology*, 1:3-37, July-August 1971.

Fletcher, G. H., Jesse, R. H., Lindberg, R. D., and Koons, C. R.: The place of radiotherapy in the management of the squamous cell carcinoma of the supraglottic larynx. *The American Journal of Roentgenology, Radium Therapy and Nuclear Medicine*, 108:19-26, January 1970.

Galante, M., Benak, S., Jr., and Buschke, F.: Radical preoperative radiation therapy in primarily inoperable advanced cancers of the oral cavity. *Frontiers of Radiation Therapy and Oncology*, 5:93-99, 1970.

Hendrickson, F. R.: The results of low dose preoperative radiotherapy for advanced carcinoma of the larynx. *Frontiers of Radiation Therapy and Oncology*, 5:123-129, 1970.

Jesse, R. H.: Preoperative versus postoperative radiation in the treatment of squamous carcinoma of the paranasal sinuses. *The American Journal of Surgery*, 110:552-556, October 1965.

Lindberg, R. D.: Unpublished data. 1970.

MacComb, W. S., and Fletcher, G. H.: Planned combination of surgery and radiation in treatment of advanced primary head and neck cancers. *The American Journal of Roentgenology, Radium Therapy and Nuclear Medicine*, 77:397-414, March 1957.

Ogura, J. H.: Personal communication. September 1972.

Perez, C. A., and Powers, W. E.: Studies on optimal dose of preoperative irradiation and time for surgery in the cure of a mouse lymphosarcoma. *Radiology*, 89:116-122, July 1967.

Rush, B. F., Jr., Mooney, C., Jewell, W. R., and Greenlaw, R.: Integrated radiation and operation in the treatment of carcinoma of the head and neck: Experience in 101 patients. *Journal of Surgical Oncology*, 3(2):151-156, 1971.

Silverstone, S. M., Goldman, J. L., and Ryan, J. R.: Combined high dose radiation therapy and surgery of advanced cancer of the laryngopharynx. *Frontiers of Radiation Therapy and Oncology*, 5:106-122, 1970.

Strong, E. W.: Preoperative radiation and radical neck dissection. *Surgical Clinics of North America*, 49:271-276, April 1969.

Symonds, C. J.: Cancer of the rectum: Excision after application of radium. *Proceedings of the Royal Society of Medicine*, Clinical Section 7:152, 1913-1914.

The Role of High LET Radiotherapy in the Management of Head and Neck Cancer

DAVID H. HUSSEY, M.D.

*Department of Radiotherapy, The University of Texas System
Cancer Center, M. D. Anderson Hospital and Tumor
Institute, Houston, Texas*

IN THE PAST TWO DECADES, advances in the field of radiotherapy have resulted in a substantial improvement in local control, while the incidence of normal tissue complications has declined. Nevertheless, a significant number of tumors continues to be locally incurable at doses within tissue tolerance. In an effort to improve the local control rate and decrease the incidence of complications and bothersome sequelae, a variety of new forms of radiotherapy have been proposed. These include irradiation with fast neutrons, heavy ions, and negative pi mesons. These new forms of radiotherapy will be described, their rationale discussed, and their potential role in the management of head and neck cancer outlined.

Scope of the Problem

The American Cancer Society has estimated that 10,000 patients in the United States die of head and neck cancer each year. Based on consultation with head and neck surgeons, Suit (1970) has estimated that 40 per cent, or 4,000 of these, die as a result of uncontrolled local disease. Additional patients who might benefit from an improved form of local management include: (1) those patients dying of distant metastasis with local cancer requiring palliation, and (2) those patients presently cured with surgical therapy or conventional radiotherapy who might be spared the functional and cosmetic impairment of current treatment methods.

Fast Neutrons

Fast neutrons are uncharged heavy particles of approximately the same mass as protons and greater than 500 KeV energy. They produce biological changes mainly by interaction with the nuclei of H, C, O, and N. Recoil protons from hydrogen and inelastic scatter account for most of the neutron energy transfer. These secondary particles are referred to as having a "high" linear energy transfer (LET*); that is, they deposit a large amount of energy per unit path length traveled. By way of contrast, photons from ^{60}Co or x-rays give rise to electrons, secondary particles of low linear energy transfer.

RATIONALE

There are several reasons why fast neutrons may be more effective in the treatment of massive local disease than conventional radiotherapy:

1. Decreased oxygen dependence.—Numerous radiobiological studies

FIG. 1.—Typical cell survival curves for fast neutrons and x-rays under anoxic and well-oxygenated conditions. (RBE, OER, and gain factors are calculated for a level of 0.1 per cent cell survival.)

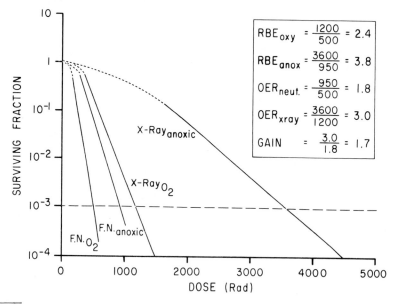

$$RBE_{oxy} = \frac{1200}{500} = 2.4$$

$$RBE_{anox} = \frac{3600}{950} = 3.8$$

$$OER_{neut.} = \frac{950}{500} = 1.8$$

$$OER_{xray} = \frac{3600}{1200} = 3.0$$

$$GAIN = \frac{3.0}{1.8} = 1.7$$

*The term linear energy transfer (LET) refers to the energy deposited per unit track length (units of KeV/micron) by an ionizing particle as it traverses through matter.

have shown that hypoxic cells are 2.5 to 3.0 times (OER†) more resistant to the effects of conventional x- and gamma irradiation than are well-oxygenated cells. While the cells in most normal tissues are well oxygenated, most solid tumors have hypoxic regions which have outgrown their vascular supply. It has been postulated that these cells remain viable and provide a focus for local recurrence. With high LET radiation, radiosensitivity is less dependent upon the state of oxygenation (Fig. 1). Consequently, fast neutrons may be more efficient in the radiotherapy of bulky tumors than x- or gamma radiation.

2. Decreased cell cycle dependence.—Another possible advantage of high LET radiation relates to the variation in radiosensitivity with the mitotic cell cycle. With conventional x- and gamma radiation, radiosensitivity can fluctuate by a factor of 2.5 among the various stages. It is possible that local tumor recurrences occasionally result from regrowth of noncycling cells or cells in a more resistant phase of the cell cycle. Sinclair (1970), using fission neutrons, and Bird and Burki (1971), using heavy ions, have reported that there is less cell cycle variation in radiosensitivity with high LET radiation. If this is confirmed, it would represent another mechanism for improved results with high LET radiotherapy.

GAIN FACTOR

Alper and Moore (1967) originated the term "gain factor" (G), to express the potential advantage of fast neutron irradiation over conventional radiotherapy in hypoxic situations. It is defined as the ratio of the OER for x-rays to the OER for neutrons, and represents the gain in effectiveness against the anoxic compartment. For equal damage to oxygenated tissues, fast neutrons increase the injury to anoxic cells as if the dose to these cells only has been increased by the ratio OER x-rays ÷ OER neutrons. With single fractions, gain factors of 1.6 to 2.0 have been measured.

In practice, the "effective gain factor" is smaller than maximum because (1) not all cells in tumors are anoxic, and (2) reoxygenation occurs during intervals between fractions, diminishing the influence of hypoxic cells. Using a mouse rhabdomyosarcoma system, Barendsen (1971) determined that the "effective gain factor" decreased from 1.9 for 800 rad fractions to 1.2 for 100 rad fractions of 14 MeV neutrons.

An "effective gain factor" as low as 1.2 might still lead to a significant improvement in local control. A dose of fast neutrons equivalent to 6,500

---

†The term oxygen enhancement ratio (OER) refers to the ratio of the radiation dose required to produce a specified biological effect under anoxic conditions to the dose required to produce the same effect under well-oxygenated conditions.

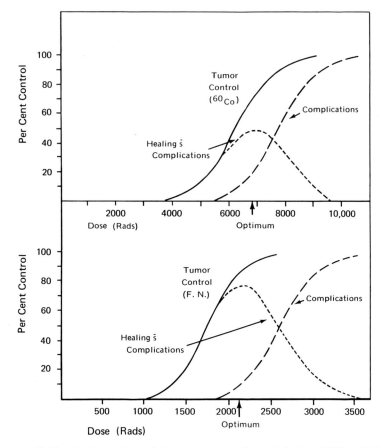

Predicted local control rates for fast neutrons assuming a gain factor at 1.2 (hypothetical).

FIG. 2.—Hypothetical tumor control and complication frequency curves for ⁶⁰Co and fast neutrons, assuming an "effective gain factor" for fast neutrons of only 1.2. For the same frequency of complications, the local control rate is considerably improved (the scales on the abscissa are normalized by an RBE of 3.0 for fast neutrons relative to ⁶⁰Co).

rads with ⁶⁰Co in six and a half weeks (relative to the normal tissues) would be equivalent to 7,800 rads in tumor control (Fig. 2).

OTHER FACTORS

The two machines showing potential for fast neutron radiotherapy are the large cyclotrons and the deuterium on tritium neutron generators (Table 1). With the large cyclotrons, fast neutrons are produced by bom-

TABLE 1.—COMPARISON OF FAST NEUTRON
THERAPY SOURCES

D-T GENERATORS	VARIABLE ENERGY CYCLOTRONS (TAMVEC[*])
Disadvantages:	Advantages:
Poor output	Good output
Short target life	Long target life
Large target size	Small target size
Difficult collimation	"Easier" collimation
Fixed depth dose	Variable depth dose
Satisfactory depth dose	Excellent depth dose
Satisfactory skin sparing	Good skin sparing
Tritium hazard	No tritium hazard
Advantages:	Disadvantages:
Low cost	Expensive
Small, mobile	Large, poor mobility

[*]Texas A & M Variable Energy Cyclotron.

barding a beryllium target with deuterons ($Be^9(d,n)B^{10} + 4.36$ MeV). This results in a spectrum of neutron energies ranging from zero to the deuteron energy plus 4 MeV. Since most of the neutron energy is derived from the deuterons, penetration can be varied by altering the incident deuteron energy. The D-T generator uses the nuclear reaction ($t(d,n)He^4 + 17.5$ MeV) to produce a fixed, nearly monoenergetic, 14 MeV neutron beam. The penetration is similar to that of the ^{60}Co (Fig. 3).

The principal advantage of fast neutron therapy over other forms of high LET radiation is that a relatively low cost source for fast neutron radiotherapy is feasible. The D-T generators of the future will never match the skin sparing or the excellent and variable depth doses which can be obtained with cyclotrons, and it is unlikely that they will ever duplicate their output. Nevertheless, the D-T generators are much less expensive. McFarlin (personal communication) has estimated that a 35 MeV fixed energy cyclotron would cost $2.1 million to construct and house, with an additional $350,000 per year required for operations and maintenance. A D-T generator could be built for $250,000.

The main disadvantages of fast neutron therapy, as compared to conventional radiotherapy sources and other high LET radiation methods, are collimation and field shaping. A finite target size, transmission through the collimator, and scatter within the patient result in a poorly defined beam edge. The low-dose region at the edge of the beam is accentuated biologi-

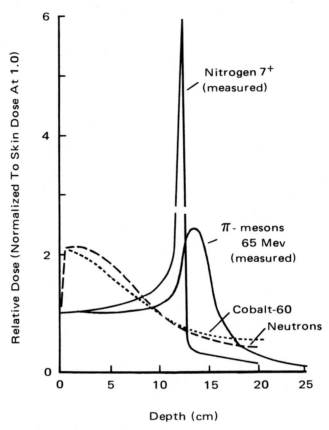

Fig. 3.—Depth dose curves for 278 MeV nucleon nitrogen—14 ions, 65 MeV negative pi mesons, ^{60}Co gamma rays, and 14 MeV neutrons (D-T generator), all normalized to skin entrance dose. (Courtesy of Tobias, C. A., *et al.*, 1971.)

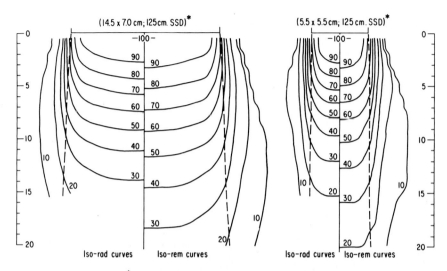

Based on Field's RBE variation with fraction size for skin and a tumor dose of 155 rads at 10.0 cm. (n+γ).

Fig. 4.—Physical and biological isodose distributions for fast neutrons produced by bombarding beryllium with 16 MeV deuterons (TAMVEC). Fast neutrons of this energy range produce depth dose distributions similar to kilovoltage x-rays. Higher energy neutrons produce better depth doses, but retain the poorly defined beam edge. This is accentuated biologically since the RBE is higher in low dose regions. (Adapted from Field and Hornsey, 1971.)

cally since the relative biological effectiveness (RBE*) is higher with low doses (Fig. 4).

CLINICAL STUDIES

In 1938, six years after Chadwick's discovery of the neutron, Stone (1948) performed the first clinical trial of fast neutron therapy, treating 250 patients deemed incurable by conventional means. Although the cancer was locally controlled in a number of cases, the study was terminated in 1943 because of a high incidence of late skin and subcutaneous damage. In retrospect, this was the result of inadequate knowledge of the physics and radiobiology of the fast neutron beam leading to an overdosage.

In 1966, the Medical Research Council Cyclotron Unit at Hammersmith Hospital in London, England, initiated a second clinical trial of fast neu-

*For the purposes of this paper, the term relative biological effectiveness (RBE) refers to the ratio of the dose of ^{60}Co gamma rays required to produce a specified biological effect to the dose of high LET radiation required to produce the same biological effect.

TABLE 2.—Fast Neutron Therapy: Preliminary Hammersmith
Results*, November 1969 through July 1972,
107 Evaluable Patients†

Total Number	Recurrences	Alive with Tumor Regressing < 6 mo.	> 6 Mo.	N.E.D. > 1 Yr.	> 2 Yrs.
107	18	37	52	40	14

*Catterall, M., 1972.
†An additional 94 patients died too soon to evaluate local control.

tron therapy. This trial has benefited from a better understanding of the biological effects of neutrons. Between November 1969 and July 1972, Catterall (1972) treated 201 patients with a wide variety of advanced neoplasms (Table 2). Of these, 94 died too soon to evaluate local control. Of the remaining 107 patients, only 18 have developed recurrent local disease. The preliminary results in oral cavity and salivary gland cancers are particularly promising, but the follow-up period is short. The complication rate is not high, as only five patients have developed necrosis, two of whom had received previous radiotherapy to the neutron-irradiated areas.

The M. D. Anderson-Texas A & M Project

M. D. Anderson Hospital and Tumor Institute has initiated a clinical trial of fast neutron radiotherapy using the cyclotron at Texas A & M University. The Texas A & M Variable Energy Cyclotron (TAMVEC) is capable of accelerating deuterons to energies of 12 to 60 MeV with a high degree of reliability. The energies which are planned for radiotherapy are:

1. 16 MeV deuterons: 7 mean neutron energy (depth dose equivalent to kilovoltage x-rays).

2. 30 MeV deuterons: 13 MeV mean neutron energy (depth dose equivalent to ^{60}Co or a D-T generator).

3. 50 MeV deuterons: 22 MeV mean neutron energy (maximum TAMVEC energy: depth dose equivalent to 18 MeV x-rays).

Following extensive pretherapeutic studies, a pilot study was begun in October 1972 (Fig. 5). Initially, the clinical trial is using neutrons produced by 16 MeV deuterons since there is considerable radiobiological and clinical experience at Hammersmith with this energy beam. Its penetration is similar to kilovoltage x-rays, and skin sparing is limited. Because of the low percentage depth dose, the tumor sites are confined to relatively superficial locations (locally advanced head and neck, skin, and

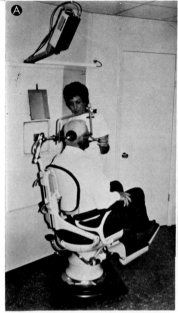

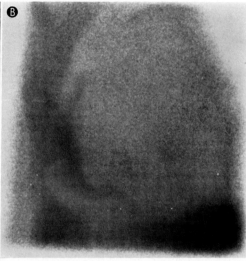

Fig. 5.—*A*, 64-year-old patient with T4N2A squamous carcinoma of the base of tongue in treatment position for fast neutron radiotherapy "boost" following comprehensive ^{60}Co radiotherapy (at TAMVEC). *B*, neutron localization radiograph—same patient.

breast cancer; brain tumors; massive lymphadenopathy; and pulmonary metastases).

A pilot study of deep-seated tumors was started in June 1973, using fast neutrons produced by 50 MeV deuterons. This beam has excellent penetration and skin sparing, and will be suitable for treatment of locally advanced and recurrent gynecological cancer and advanced carcinomas of the prostate and bladder.

Heavy Charged Particles

The heavy charged particles being considered for radiotherapy include protons, alpha particles, and heavy ions such as carbon, nitrogen, neon, and argon. Like x- and gamma rays, heavy charged particles are attenuated by interactions with electrons. These particles lose energy at a rate inversely proportional to their energy, and on entering tissue, deposit a nearly constant amount of radiation along their path. However, as the particle slows to a stop, the amount of radiation deposited increases to a maximum known as the Bragg peak (Fig. 3).

RATIONALE

The rationale for heavy charged particle radiotherapy lies in the physical dose distribution. Conventional x- and gamma rays and fast neutrons are exponentially attenuated as they travel through tissue so that a deep-seated tumor receives less radiation than the superficial normal structures. With heavy ions, the energy of the beam can be adjusted so that the Bragg peak occurs within the tumor, and the intervening normal tissues receive a considerably smaller dose. Unfortunately, the Bragg peak region for heavy ions is quite narrow. To encompass a large tumor, the width must be broadened by varying the energy of the incident beam or by inserting a variable absorber in its path.

OTHER FACTORS

Heavy ions are probably no more effective against the hypoxic compartment than x- and gamma rays. Although the oxygen dependence within the Bragg peak is substantially lower than that of x-rays, the plateau region presents an oxygen effect similar to that of the conventional radiation. When protons or alpha particles are scanned across the tumor, essentially all of the oxygen advantage is lost. The heavier particles, such as nitrogen or neon, have intense Bragg peaks presenting very high LET spectra. Whether the oxygen advantage is lost when these particles are scanned across the tumor remains uncertain.

The principal advantage of heavy ion radiotherapy is that a high dose of radiation can be delivered to a specified tumor volume. A major limitation in the use of heavy particle radiotherapy is the lack of sufficiently accurate means of defining this target volume.

CLINICAL STUDIES

No full-scale clinical trials of heavy ion radiotherapy have been conducted, although some proton radiotherapy has been carried out at Harvard University, and in Sweden and the U.S.S.R.

Negative Pi Mesons

Negative pi mesons have a unit negative charge and a mass 273 times that of an electron (approximately one-seventh the mass of a proton). They are produced when an appropriate target is bombarded by protons of several hundred MeV. Pi mesons interact with tissue in a manner similar to electrons, and on slowing down, their ionization density increases to produce a Bragg peak similar to that of heavy ions. However, at the end of their path, they are captured by an atomic nucleus and decay, releasing a localized burst of secondary particles (protons, alpha particles, heavy ions, and neutrons). This phenomenon is termed "star formation."

RATIONALE

Negative pi mesons show both (1) the oxygen advantage of fast neutrons and (2) the physical dose distribution advantage seen with heavy ions. The area of high dose distribution for pi mesons is broader than the Bragg peak of heavy ions (Fig. 3). For large tumors, the star region can be scanned across the tumor by varying the energy of the incident beam or the interposition of absorbers. Thus, a homogeneous and a high dose of radiation can be delivered to the target volume while the dose to normal tissue outside this region is quite small.

The plateau region of the negative pi meson beam is the result of low LET interactions, and, consequently, shows an oxygen dependence similar to x- and gamma rays (OER of 2.5 to 3.0). However, the star peak is due to secondary radiations of a high average LET. Experiments have indicated that the oxygen enhancement ratio for the peak portion of the curve is in the range of 1.5 to 1.8 (Raju, Amer, Gnanapurani, and Richman, 1970), a value comparable to the OER of fast neutrons. Thus, the oxygen dependence within the target volume is favorable. Because the "star peak" is broad, it can be scanned and still retain the oxygen advantage.

OTHER FACTORS

The principal disadvantage of pi meson radiotherapy is cost. It has been estimated that a pion factory sufficient for radiotherapeutic use would cost $12 million to build and approximately $900,000 per year to maintain and operate.

To make full use of the dose distribution advantage, accurate means of locating the extent of tumors within the body must be developed. Since tissue inhomogeneity (such as bowel gas, or bone) would alter the depth of the "star peak" within the body, methods must be developed to account for these.

CLINICAL STUDIES

To date, there are no machines with a sufficient output of pi mesons to be feasible for radiotherapy. However, a beam satisfactory for radiotherapy is under construction at Los Alamos, New Mexico, and is expected to be available for pretherapeutic studies in early 1973. Other institutions are developing pi meson radiotherapy facilities in Palo Alto, California; Vancouver, British Columbia; and Zurich, Switzerland.

Discussion

Selection of Patients for High LET Radiotherapy

Following preliminary studies to determine normal tissue tolerance, clinical trials to evaluate the effectiveness of high LET radiotherapy should be undertaken. Extensive head and neck carcinomas are among the more suitable tumor populations for such investigations because: (1) The local control rates with conventional radiotherapy are low (Table 3), and the incidence of distant metastasis is less than that for tumors of many sites; (2) they are frequently ulcerated or necrotic, and would be expected to contain a significant hypoxic compartment; (3) they are accessible to clinical examination, facilitating the appraisal of tumor regression and local control; and (4) local recurrences usually occur within two years, allowing an early evaluation of results.

The selection of patients for high LET radiotherapy should not be based strictly on the clinical stage. Each patient should be evaluated on an individual basis, including a consideration of the location, size, and clinical variety (exophytic, infiltrative, or necrotic) of the primary tumor and regional metastases; the functional results of various treatment modalities; and patient factors such as age, general condition, and personal habits.

Most early and moderately advanced cancers of the head and neck are

---

TABLE 3.—Failure to Control the Primary Tumor in Patients Treated by Definitive Radiotherapy (Unlimited Follow-up), January 1948 through December 1968

Site	Favorable			Unfavorable		
Ant. ⅔ tongue	T_{1-2}	20/152	(13%)	T_{3-4}	47/96	(50%)
Lower gingiva	T_{1-2}	5/17	(29%)	T_{3-4}	17/31	(55%)
Floor of mouth	T_{1-3}	24/186	(13%)	T_4	19/24	(79%)
Buccal mucosa	T_{1-3}	13/66	(20%)	T_4	14/29	(48%)
Ant. pillar, R.M.T. and soft palate*	T_{1-3}	37/251	(15%)	T_4	8/20	(40%)
Tonsillar fossa*	T_{1-3}	15/105	(14%)	T_4	8/20	(40%)
Base of tongue*	T_{1-2}	11/64	(17%)	T_{3-4}	28/91	(31%)

*January 1954 through December 1967. Probable new primaries have been excluded.

adequately controlled with surgical therapy, radiotherapy, or a combination of the two, and would not be suitable for study. At the present time, clinical trials of high LET radiotherapy should be reserved for patients with locally infiltrative or bulky cancers, poorly controlled by conventional methods.

OTHER TREATMENT METHODS

There are a number of other ways of circumventing the problem of the hypoxic cell:

1. Ultrafractionation.—If fast neutrons or pi mesons fail to improve upon the results obtained with conventional forms of radiation, it may be that the hypoxic cell problem is already solved through the use of fractionated treatments. Initial treatments kill well-oxygenated cells adjacent to capillaries, bringing the hypoxic cells into closer proximity with the vascular supply. Reoxygenated, these cells are more easily eradicated by subsequent treatments. At M. D. Anderson Hospital and Tumor Institute certain tumors of the head and neck are treated with prolonged fractionation to take full advantage of reoxygenation, as well as to reduce normal tissue reactions.

2. Surgery.—The combination of conservative surgical therapy and moderate doses of conventional radiotherapy is successful in eradicating locally advanced cancer in many clinical situations. This combines the best of both modalities, not only for improved local control rates, but for diminution in the functional and cosmetic losses resulting from more radical surgical procedures and the incidence of complications and sequelae which result from radical irradiation.

3. Modification of the oxygen content of the tumor or the normal tissues.—Here the aim is to increase the radiosensitivity of the tumor by improving the oxygen content of the hypoxic compartment (conventional radiotherapy in hyperbaric oxygen) or to decrease the radiosensitivity of the normal tissues by reducing the oxygen content of the adjacent normal cells (conventional radiotherapy with applied tourniquets). Clinical trials of conventional radiotherapy in hyperbaric oxygen or with applied tourniquets have been under way for a number of years, yet their value is not clearly established.

COMBINATIONS WITH CONVENTIONAL RADIOTHERAPY

Although in some sites it may be used as the sole treatment modality, in the management of many extensive head and neck tumors, high LET radiotherapy will be best employed in combination with conventional irradiation. Even in areas accessible to radium needle implants, such as the tongue and floor of mouth, late-stage disease is treated initially with external conventional radiotherapy to produce tumor shrinkage and eradicate subclinical disease at the regional level. Fletcher (1972) has shown that modest doses of x- or gamma radiation (4,500-5,000 rads/25 fractions/5 weeks) will eradicate subclinical aggregates of epithelial cancer in greater than 90 per cent of cases. Fast neutrons present problems of collimation and field shaping which limit their effectiveness in treating regional disease, and pi mesons and heavy ions are designed to deliver high doses to localized areas.

Combinations with ^{60}Co or x-rays would also reduce the likelihood of subcutaneous fibrosis or other complications which may result from the poor physical dose distributions of fast neutrons (fat absorbs 18 per cent higher dose than other tissues). There would be the added benefit of being able to treat more patients, thus reducing the cost per patient benefited.

Summary

1. Three forms of high LET radiation (fast neutrons, heavy charged particles, and pi mesons) are discussed in terms of the physical and biological properties which have led to their consideration for the radiotherapy of locally advanced cancer.

2. The principal rationale for fast neutron radiotherapy lies in an increased effectiveness in eradicating hypoxic cells which may provide a focus for local recurrence; whereas the main advantage of heavy ion radiotherapy is an improved depth dose distribution, delivering a high dose of radiation to a specified target volume; pi mesons appear to have both an increased effectiveness against the hypoxic compartment and an improved depth dose distribution.

3. The principal advantage of fast neutron therapy over other forms of high LET radiation is that a low cost source for fast neutron therapy (D-T generator) is technologically feasible.

4. Extensive carcinomas of the head and neck are among the more suitable tumor populations to evaluate high LET radiotherapy because of the high local failure rate with conventional radiotherapy alone and the accessibility for clinical follow-up.

5. Patient selection for high LET radiotherapy should be based on an evaluation of the entire clinical picture rather than simply on clinical stage. The combination of conservative surgery and moderate doses of

conventional radiotherapy is often successful in controlling local disease and may be superior to high LET radiotherapy in many clinical situations.

6. In many head and neck cancers, high LET radiotherapy might best be combined with external beam conventional radiotherapy given initially to produce tumor shrinkage and adequate irradiation of areas of subclinical spread.

Acknowledgment

This investigation was supported by Public Health Grant CA-12542 from the National Cancer Institute.

REFERENCES

Alper, T., and Moore, J. L.: The interdependence of oxygen enhancement ratios for 250 kVP X rays and fast neutrons. *The British Journal of Radiology,* 40: 843-848, November 1967.

Barendsen, G. W.: Cellular responses determining the effectiveness of fast neutrons relative to x-rays for effects on experimental tumours. *European Journal of Cancer,* 7:181-190, May 1971.

Bird, R., and Burki, J.: Inactivation of mammalian cells at different stages of the cell cycle as a function of radiation linear energy transfer. In *Biophysical Aspects of Radiation Quality,* IAEA-SM-145/5. Vienna, Austria, International Atomic Energy Agency, 1971, pp. 241-250.

Catterall, M.: The treatment of patients with fast neutrons from the Medical Research Council's cyclotron at Hammersmith Hospital, London. Presented at Particle Accelerators in Radiation Therapy (P.A.R.T.) meeting, Los Alamos, New Mexico, October 1972.

Field, S. B., and Hornsey, S.: RBE values for cyclotron neutrons for effects on normal tissues and tumours as a function of dose and dose fractionation. *European Journal of Cancer,* 7:161-169, May 1971.

Fletcher, G. H.: Elective irradiation of subclinical disease in cancers of the head and neck. *Cancer,* 29:1450-1454, June 1972.

McFarlin, W. E.: Personal communication. 1972.

Raju, M. R., Amer, N. M., Gnanapurani, M., and Richman, C.: The oxygen effect of π mesons in *Vicia faba. Radiation Research,* 41:135-144, January 1970.

Sinclair, W. K.: Dependence of radiosensitivity upon cell age. In *Time and Dose Relationships in Radiation Biology as Applied to Radiotherapy,* BNL 50203 (C-57) (Biology and Medicine-TID-4500). Upton, New York, Brookhaven National Laboratory, 1970, pp. 97-116.

Stone, R. S.: Neutron therapy and specific ionization; Janeway Memorial Lecture. *The American Journal of Roentgenology, Radium Therapy and Nuclear Medicine,* 59:771-785, June 1948.

Suit, H. D.: Introduction. Statement of the problem pertaining to the effect of dose fractionation and total treatment time on response of tissue to x-irradiation. In *Time and Dose Relationships in Radiation Biology as Applied to Radiotherapy*, BNL 50203 (C-57) (Biology and Medicine-TID-4500). Upton, New York, Brookhaven National Laboratory, 1970, pp. VII-X.

Tobias, C. A., Lyman, J. T., Chatterjee, A., Howard, J., Maccabee, H. D., Raju, M. R., Smith, A. R., Sperinde, J. M., and Welch, G. P.: Radiological physics characteristics of the extracted heavy ion beams of the bevatron. *Science*, 174:1131-1134, December 10, 1971.

Surgical Salvage for Radiation Failures

ROBERT M. BYERS, M.D.

*Department of Surgery, The University of Texas System
Cancer Center, M. D. Anderson Hospital and
Tumor Institute, Houston, Texas*

THE INDICATIONS to select one modality of treatment over another in patients with squamous cell carcinoma of the head and neck can be obviously simple or extremely subtle. The selection may be based on tumor factors, patient factors, or often a blending of the two. The extent, size, biological behavior, and cell type are examples of tumor factors. Since these tumors are attached to human beings, all the emotional, psychological, and social factors pertinent to the patient's condition must be kept in sharp focus when the primary means of therapy is selected. The particular modality of therapy chosen may be somewhat less than optimal as far as the tumor is concerned, but may be strategically the best modality when the numerous patient factors operative in the decision are taken into consideration.

If the first method of therapy fails, we must be prepared to offer the patient additional treatment, even if this modality superimposed on the first carries with it an increased risk of complications. Some surgeons are reluctant to operate on patients who have been initially treated with radiation therapy and whose tumors have recurred. This paper examines the effectiveness of surgical treatment in salvaging patients in whom radiation therapy has failed.

Definition

It is hard to distinguish residual disease from recurrent disease, and also recurrent disease from a new primary lesion. Arbitrary definitions must be

75

used so that a worthwhile analysis of the data can be interpreted and compared.

A radiation failure is defined as one in which a tissue diagnosis of recurrent cancer is made at any time during the follow-up period in a patient who was treated originally and solely by radiation. Radiation failures can be grouped into those recurring inside or outside the fields of radiation. Failure of radiation therapy within the fields may be the result of underdosage or a failure of the ionizing radiation to sterilize tumor cells, usually the anoxic ones. Recurrent cancer outside the radiation field may be the result of a geographic miss or a failure on the part of the radiotherapist to appreciate the local extent of the disease.

Methods and Materials

Patients with cancer of the oral cavity, oropharynx, and larynx are included, since 80 per cent of these patients in our series have had radiation therapy selected as the initial form of treatment. We have excluded cancers of the hypopharynx, cervical esophagus, paranasal sinuses, skin, nasopharynx, and salivary glands. Most of these patients are treated surgically or by planned combined methods. Patients with nasopharyngeal cancer are treated exclusively by radiation therapy with little or no hope of salvage by surgery if it fails. The radiotherapist and surgeon agreed upon the selection of radiation therapy as the only modality of treatment and both followed the patients while they were under treatment and during the postradiation period. The minimum follow-up period varied with the various sites—oropharynx and glottic larynx four years, and oral cavity and supraglottic larynx two years. Control of the primary lesion was the only end point since the fate of the patient with regard to cervical metastasis, distant metastasis, and other problems is beyond the scope of this presentation. As long as a patient's primary lesion remained controlled until his demise, he is counted as a local treatment success.

Results

The incidence of radiation failure and surgical salvage are categorized by site.

True Vocal Cord

T_1 and T_2 true cord lesions are treated almost exclusively by radiation therapy at M. D. Anderson Hospital. Anterior commissure involvement

TABLE 1.—VOCAL CORD CARCINOMA*, INCIDENCE OF PRIMARY FAILURE FOLLOWING IRRADIATION (1948 THROUGH 1967)

STAGING	HISTOLOGY	No. of Patients	No. of Failures		No. Failures Controlled by Surgery		Per Cent of Ultimate Failures
T₁							
No visible lesion	Borderline histology	42	4	9.5%	4	100%	0
	Invasive squamous cell carcinoma	27	3	11.0%	3	100%	0
Post-cord stripping	Invasive squamous cell carcinoma	7	1		0		
Visible (one cord)	Invasive squamous cell carcinoma	148	20	13.5%	17/19†	89.5%	2
Bulky lesion	Invasive squamous cell carcinoma	21	2	9.5%	2	100%	0
Anterior commissure involved	Invasive squamous cell carcinoma	36	3	8.5%	3	100%	0
T₂							
Partial mobility, extension beyond cord(s), or anterior commissure involvement outside cord(s)	Borderline histology	4	1		1		0
	Invasive squamous cell carcinoma	109	22	20.0%	14/19‡	73.5%	7.5
Combination of above features	Borderline histology	3	0		...		0
	Invasive squamous cell carcinoma	18	11	61.0%	7/10‖	70.0%	22

*Failures by stage and extensions; borderline histology and invasive squamous cell carcinoma in 415 patients studied from 1948 through 1967 (analysis in June 1971).
†One patient refused treatment.

‡Three patients refused treatment.
‖One patient refused treatment; one patient died following a radical neck dissection 15 months after laryngectomy (no evidence of disease at autopsy).

per se is not a contraindication to radiation therapy unless extensive sub-glottic disease is also present. Our results are illustrated in Table 1. Since 1960, we have done seven limited surgical procedures (cordectomies) for radiation failures. There has been one recurrence following cordectomy with successful treatment by total laryngectomy. The criteria which should be met if a limited surgical procedure for recurrence following radiation therapy is to succeed are:

1. Cancer must have been localized originally.

2. The original extent of the cancer must be circumscribed by the surgical procedure.

3. Regional node metastasis should not be a dominant feature of the disease.

SUPRAGLOTTIC LARYNX

Radiation therapy is usually selected for patients with T_1 and T_2 lesions of any site within the supraglottic larynx. Those having T_3 and T_4 lesions of the supraglottic larynx are usually treated by surgery with postoperative radiation therapy. Table 2 shows the number of radiation failures in patients treated for cancer of the supraglottic larynx. Most of the recurrences appeared within 12 months following completion of radiation therapy. The shortest time was five months; the longest was 52 months. The type of surgical procedure necessary to eradicate the recurrent carcinoma varied. Two patients, including the one with T_1 cancer, were treated with resection of the epiglottis and had no evidence of disease at eight and 11 years respectively. Nine patients required total laryngectomy for ultimate local control of the primary. Surgical salvage occurred mostly in the group of patients with T_2 and T_3 lesions.

TABLE 2.—SUPRAGLOTTIC LARYNX, INCIDENCE OF PRIMARY FAILURE FOLLOWING IRRADIATION (1957 THROUGH 1967)

STAGING	FAILURE BY RADIATION THERAPY		SALVAGE BY SURGERY	ULTIMATE FAILURES	
T_1	1/14	7%	1/1	0/14	0%
T_2	6/27*	22%	4/6	2/27	7%
T_3	5/6	83%	4/5	1/6	16%
T_4	6/32†	18%	2/6	4/32	12%
Total	18/79	23%	11/18	7/79	8%

*One patient refused surgery.
†Three patients refused surgery and one was treated by 5-FU infusion only.

TABLE 3.—ANTERIOR FAUCIAL ARCH AND RETROMOLAR TRIGONE,
INCIDENCE OF PRIMARY FAILURE FOLLOWING
IRRADIATION (1954 THROUGH 1967)

STAGING	FAILURE BY RADIATION THERAPY		SALVAGE BY SURGERY	ULTIMATE FAILURES	
T_1	4/27	15.0%	3/4	1/27	4.0%
T_2	16/87	19.5%	6/16	10/87	11.5%
T_3	13/67	19.5%	9/13	4/67	6.0%
T_4	5/19	26.0%	1/5	4/19	21.0%
Total	38/200	19.0%	19/38	19/200	9.5%

ANTERIOR FAUCIAL ARCH AND RETROMOLAR TRIGONE

Most patients with T_1 and T_2 lesions of the arch and retromolar trigone are treated by radiation therapy. In the past, some patients with T_3 and T_4 lesions were radiated for palliation or because they refused surgery. Radiation therapy would not be selected today for patients with T_3 and T_4 lesions since combined modalities of therapy are now preferred.

Table 3 shows the surgical salvage rate. The surgical procedure necessary to control the disease in many of these patients is limited and can be accomplished intraorally with primary closure. The larger recurrences required a resection of a portion of the mandible with a limited upper neck dissection. Most of these defects could also be closed primarily. The extreme defects were closed by a forehead pedicle since split thickness skin grafts usually do not take in heavily irradiated tissue.

SOFT PALATE

All except the very small lesions of the soft palate are usually treated by radiation therapy because of the rather significant functional defect pro-

TABLE 4.—SOFT PALATE, INCIDENCE OF PRIMARY
FAILURE FOLLOWING IRRADIATION
(1954 THROUGH 1967)

STAGING	FAILURE BY RADIATION THERAPY		SALVAGE BY SURGERY	ULTIMATE FAILURES	
T_1	0/18	0%	0/0	0/18	0%
T_2	0/30	0%	0/0	0/30	0%
T_3	4/22	18%	0/4	4/22	18%
T_4	2/4	50%	1/2	1/4	25%
Total	6/74	8%	1/6	5/74	7%

duced by surgical resection. In addition, the soft palate lesions are often midline, and radiation therapy to both sides of the neck can decrease significantly the appearance of neck metastasis. Localized recurrences can usually be excised intraorally with a minimal defect. Table 4 shows that our results are good in patients with T_1 and T_2 lesions but poor in patients with T_3 and T_4 staging.

TONSILLAR FOSSA

Table 5 shows the results for patients with tonsillar fossa lesions. Radiation therapy does very well with the small localized lesions, but fails significantly as the degree of invasiveness increases. The results of surgical salvage are poor in recurrent T_2, T_3, and T_4 lesions. If the surgeon is going to be effective in controlling the radiation therapy failures in the tonsillar fossa, he must diagnose the recurrence early and must be willing to perform extensive surgery including resection of the palate, pharyngeal wall, and mandible. Many of these patients with this extensive surgical resection will never swallow again, and a laryngectomy may be the only means of preventing repeated episodes of aspiration. Wound healing is definitely impaired if much of the pharyngeal wall is resected. A forehead pedicle flap is often required to repair the surgical defect. If radical neck dissection has been part of the procedure and fistula formation occurs, carotid artery rupture can be an expected sequela.

BASE OF TONGUE

The local failure rate for radiated lesions of the base of the tongue is approximately 25 per cent for the T_2 and T_3 lesions but much higher in the T_4 stage. Table 6 shows that the surgical salvage for all T stages does not exceed 20 per cent. Resecting recurrent disease in the base of the tongue usually requires laryngectomy, and wound healing is generally delayed.

TABLE 5.—TONSILLAR FOSSA, INCIDENCE OF PRIMARY FAILURE FOLLOWING IRRADIATION (1954 THROUGH 1967)

STAGING	FAILURE BY RADIATION THERAPY		SALVAGE BY SURGERY	ULTIMATE FAILURES	
T_1	0/15	0.0%	0/0	0/15	0%
T_2	1/32	3.0%	0/1	1/32	3%
T_3	14/58	24.0%	6/14	8/58	14%
T_4	8/20	40.0%	1/8	7/20	35%
Total	23/125	18.5%	7/23	16/125	13%

TABLE 6.—BASE OF TONGUE, INCIDENCE OF PRIMARY FAILURE
FOLLOWING IRRADIATION (1954 THROUGH 1967)

STAGING	FAILURE BY RADIATION THERAPY		SALVAGE BY SURGERY	ULTIMATE FAILURES	
T_1	2/28	7.0%	2/2	0/28	0.0%
T_2	9/36	25.0%	2/9	7/36	19.5%
T_3	13/58	22.5%	1/13	12/58	20.5%
T_4	15/33	46.0%	2/15	13/33	39.5%
Total	39/155	25.0%	7/39	32/155	20.5%

A medial-based deltopectoral flap can occasionally be used in selected instances for closure. A controlled pharyngeal stoma is a necessity if unwanted fistulas and carotid artery ruptures are to be prevented. Closure of the stoma is done under local anesthesia about three to four weeks later. A midline mandible split-type incision through nonradiated tissue may provide adequate exposure with minimized risk in selected cases.

PHARYNGEAL WALL

Table 7 shows that only five of 52 patients whose pharyngeal wall lesions were treated primarily with radiation therapy have been salvaged surgically. Radiation therapy alone gives good results in patients with T_1 and T_2 lesions. For those with T_3 and T_4 cancers, combined treatment should be planned rather than depending on the surgical salvage of an anticipated radiation failure.

FLOOR OF MOUTH

Radiation therapy is usually selected for most of the T_2 and T_3 tumors and occasionally for the T_4 lesions of the floor of the mouth. If radiation

TABLE 7.—PHARYNGEAL WALLS, INCIDENCE OF PRIMARY FAILURE
FOLLOWING IRRADIATION (1954 THROUGH 1967)

STAGING	FAILURE BY RADIATION THERAPY			SALVAGE BY SURGERY	ULTIMATE FAILURES	
T_1	1/7	(1)	14%	1/1	0/7	0.0%
T_2	6/25	(1)	24%	1/6	5/25	20.0%
T_3	18/41	(3)	44%	3/18	15/41	36.5%
T_4	27/41		66%	0/27	27/41	66.0%
Total	52/114		45.6%	5/52	47/114	41.2%

TABLE 8.—FLOOR OF MOUTH, INCIDENCE OF PRIMARY
FAILURE FOLLOWING IRRADIATION
(1954 THROUGH 1967)

STAGING	FAILURE BY RADIATION THERAPY		SALVAGE BY SURGERY[*]	ULTIMATE FAILURES
T_1	1/49	2.0%	1/1	0.0%
T_2	9/77	11.5%	4/9	6.5%
T_3	14/60	23.0%	11/14	5.0%
T_4	19/24	79.0%	0/19	79.0%
Total	43/210	20.5%	16/43	37.2%

[*]NED at two years after treatment of failure.

fails, the problems for the surgeon are compounded if the recurrence cannot be resected by an intraoral procedure. Table 8 shows that surgical salvage is good if the mandible is not involved (T_4 lesions) (Horiot, Fletcher, Ballantyne, and Lindberg, in press). The problems involved with the reconstruction of the surgical defect are much greater with lesions of the anterior floor of the mouth, particularly after radiation therapy.

ORAL TONGUE

Most of the T_2 and T_3 oral tongue lesions are treated primarily with radiation therapy, since the radiotherapist is willing to treat more of the tongue than the surgeon is usually willing to excise. T_4 lesions are usually treated by surgery with or without postoperative radiation. Table 9 shows the results (Chu and Fletcher, 1973). Surgery does not salvage more than one third of the failures for any given T stage. The type of surgical procedure necessary can range from intraoral partial glossectomy to a combined tongue, jaw, and neck dissection.

TABLE 9.—ORAL TONGUE, INCIDENCE OF PRIMARY FAILURE
FOLLOWING IRRADIATION (1948 THROUGH 1968)

STAGING	FAILURE BY RADIATION THERAPY		SALVAGE BY SURGERY[*]	ULTIMATE FAILURES
T_1	3/52	6.8%	1/3	5.5%
T_2	17/100	17.0%	5/17	12.0%
T_3	27/66	41.0%	6/27	32.0%
T_4	20/30	67.0%	2/20	60.0%
Total	67/248	27.0%	14/67	20.9%

[*]NED at two years after treatment of failure.

Discussion

Surgical salvage of radiation failures is encouraging, at least in certain sites, particularly the larynx, oral tongue, palate, retromolar trigone, and anterior faucial arch.

Problems in diagnosis occur when there is suspected residual or recurrent disease approximately six weeks after completion of a therapeutic dose of radiation therapy (6,000 rads or more). The surgeon takes a biopsy and the pathologist who examines the tissue sees what he interprets as cancer cells. Can the pathologist distinguish whether the cells are viable or not, and if so, are they able to reproduce? Also, a question may arise when the patient has residual ulceration after radiation therapy. Many times this is delayed healing or radiation necrosis and does not represent a radiation tumor failure. Repeated biopsies often merely add to the extent of nonhealing.

The method of biopsy is of utmost importance in making an early diagnosis of a suspected radiation failure. If there is any residual induration after a period of 12 weeks, a deep incisional-type biopsy should be done.

Most radiation failures occur in the anoxic core of the tumor while the well-oxygenated periphery is sterilized. The biopsy must, therefore, be deep in the central part of the suspected recurrence. Biopsies at the margin of recurrence usually are futile since the surface and surrounding margins will merely show atypia and radiation changes. The surgeon must be aware of this phenomenon if he is to make the early diagnosis of radiation failure. A typical illustration of this common clinical problem would be the patient with a suspected recurrence in the tongue. The tongue is a very muscular, mobile organ, and a deep-seated core of residual tumor can easily be confused with scar tissue and induration, particularly when there is concomitant muscular spasm secondary to pain. Palpating the tongue with the patient under general anesthesia to relax the tongue musculature, will often give a meaningful interpretation of the problem. If there is a questionable or suspicious area, a deep incisional biopsy should be taken.

The length of time after treatment at which recurrence develops affects the ease with which the surgeon can eradicate the disease, since small recurrences are better dealt with than large extensive ones. Late recurrences (after six months) as compared to early recurrences are usually localized and can be excised with better results. In many instances, the type of surgical procedure necessary is rather limited and no real decrease in the cosmetic or functional result is produced. Early recurrences are commonly diffuse and require very radical surgery with complex plastic repair. Healing is impaired, particularly if the recurrence appears before the patient has regained his positive nitrogen balance. However, this can be minimized by modifying our surgical techniques and improving the preoperative nutrition.

Summary

An aggressive team approach to the treatment of patients with head and neck cancer must be utilized if we are to achieve success. Local control is adequate in lesions of oral cavity, faucial arch, and larynx. Local control of a radiation failure is poor in the base of the tongue and the oropharynx. When radiation therapy fails, the surgeon must be prepared and willing to exercise his surgical skill and judgment to achieve the ultimate local control.

REFERENCES

Ballantyne, A. J., and Fletcher, G. H.: Preservation of the larynx in the surgical treatment of cancer, recurrent after radiation therapy. *The American Journal of Roentgenology, Radium Therapy and Nuclear Medicine*, 99:336-339, February 1967.

Chu, A., and Fletcher, G. H.: Incidence and causes of failures to control by irradiation the primary lesions in squamous cell carcinoma of the anterior two thirds of the tongue and floor of mouth. *The American Journal of Roentgenology, Radium Therapy and Nuclear Medicine*, 117:502-508, March 1973.

Horiot, J.-C., Fletcher, G. H., Ballantyne, A. J., and Lindberg, R. D.: Analysis of failures in early vocal-cord cancer. *Radiology*, 103:663-665, June 1972.

Surgical Modifications Necessary after Radiation Therapy in Treatment for Head and Neck Cancer

A. J. BALLANTYNE, M.D.

*Department of Surgery, The University of Texas System
Cancer Center, M. D. Anderson Hospital and
Tumor Institute, Houston, Texas*

As THERE BECOMES more of an interplay between surgery and radiation in the treatment for head and neck cancer, it becomes mandatory that the modifications necessary for the safe accomplishment of surgery in irradiated tissues become understood. Surgery may be employed as part of a planned treatment in which radiation is given to treat the primary and lymph nodes with surgery to follow in the hopes that the control rate and the long-term salvage rate may be increased, or it may be necessary if radiation has been given for cure and has failed. Regardless of the time sequence involved or the original intent of the radiation therapy, certain precautions should be observed if maximum benefit with minimum morbidity is to be obtained. In general, the following criteria must be met:

1. Optimal nutritional and physiological condition must be obtained prior to surgery.

2. Gentle handling and closure of irradiated tissues without tension must be accomplished.

3. Adequate coverage of the carotid and other vital structures such as brain must be secured.

4. The operative procedure must be modified, if necessary, depending upon the amount of radiation, the condition of the tissues, and the nutritional status and age of the patient.

5. Postoperative care must be optimal; antibiotic coverage, blood transfusions, and nutritional support are vitally necessary.

6. There must be some selection of patients, and the safest surgical procedure should be employed.

Optimal Nutritional and Physiological Status Must Be Obtained Prior to Surgery

If irradiation was given preoperatively in high dosage, a four- to six-week rest period for recovery should be allowed. Most patients lose weight during irradiation and they should be allowed to begin to gain weight and feel well before the operative procedure is done. For practical purposes, it can be assumed that the patient is in positive nitrogen balance if he is eating normally, has begun to gain weight and, in general, feels reasonably well. In the patient with recurrent tumor, who has lost a considerable amount of weight, it is vital that he be hospitalized and that either tube feedings with intravenous supplements or intravenous hyperalimentation regimens be employed until such time as it is deemed that the patient is in positive nitrogen balance and is gaining weight.

Gentle Handling and Closure of Irradiated Tissues

Gentle handling and closure of irradiated tissues is necessary for proper wound healing. Irradiated tissues are very susceptible to infection because of their impaired blood supply, and it is essential that they be handled gently and closure be effected without any tension on the wound because they are completely lacking in elasticity. Irradiated tissues closed under tension which do not heal immediately will break down with exposure of whatever structures lie beneath.

Adequate Coverage of the Carotid and Other Vital Structures Such as Brain Must Be Secured

Incisions for neck dissection should not consist of the usual trifurcate incision which places a T over the carotid artery. Suitable incisions for neck dissection may consist of either two parallel transverse incisions, a single curved incision over the carotid artery, or a vertical incision along the trapezius curved inferiorly above the clavicle to allow adequate mobilization of the skin flap (Fig. 1). If the radiation dosage to the skin has been excessively high, the skin is in poor condition, and some skin must be excised, it is sometimes expedient to excise the radiated skin of the neck and replace it with nonradiated skin from the infraclavicular area (Fig. 2).

Following irradiation, the brain must be covered by good nonirradiated

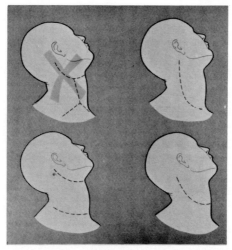

Fig. 1.—Possible incisions for neck dissections following radiation. The one marked with X should never be used.

Fig. 2.—Recurrent reticulum cell sarcoma in neck following radiation. *A*, lines indicate skin to be removed. *B*, appearance after neck dissection and replacement of skin with deltopectoral flap.

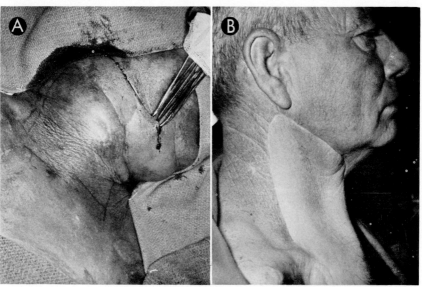

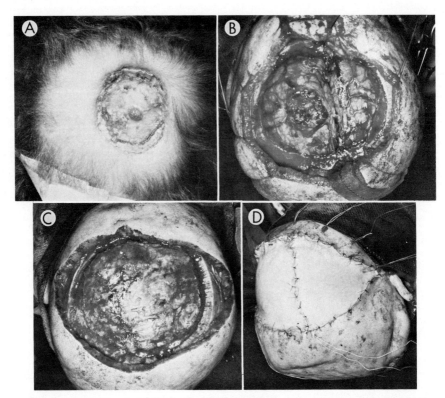

FIG. 3.—Carcinoma involving scalp, skull, and dura. *A*, appearance following radiation. *B*, operative defect. *C*, dural defect with fascia lata graft. *D*, scalp flap mobilized to cover defect in skull.

skin flaps. Although skin grafts will take satisfactorily on nonirradiated brain or dura, it is risky to use the same techniques following radiation therapy. When irradiated skin, bone, and dura have been excised and the brain left exposed, the brain should be covered either with temporal fascia or with a fascia lata graft, and a nonirradiated scalp flap migrated to close the skin defect (Fig. 3).

Modify the Operative Procedures if Necessary, Dependent Upon the Amount of Radiation and Condition of the Tissues, Nutritional Condition, and Age of the Patient

Consider midline incisions for laryngectomy or laryngectomy plus resection of the base of the tongue. Following the operative procedure, the

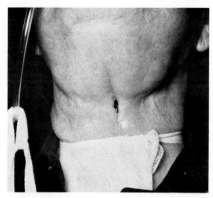

FIG. 4.—Temporary pharyngeal fistula following laryngectomy following radiation.

amount of remaining mucosa and the condition of the tissues should be assessed. It is sometimes feasible to do a primary closure, but if the original tumor dose exceeded 6,000 rads and the tissues are fibrotic, the creation of a temporary midline fistula may add safety to the procedure. A small fistula created well above the stoma is of little inconvenience to the patient and can be closed under local anesthesia in three weeks (Fig. 4).

If inadequate mucosa is left to create a fistula, then the mucosal defect should be replaced with a skin flap. Skin flaps, other than very minor ones which have been irradiated, should not be used. Although it is possible to use small irradiated skin flaps which have been delayed for closure around a pharyngeal stoma, it is unwise to use large radiated flaps for an attempt at closure of large mucosal defects. If the nutrition of the patient is good and there are no complicating factors such as diabetes or old age, nondelayed flaps from the deltopectoral region or from the forehead can be migrated in to close mucosal defects, with great safety. In some instances, if the skin of the neck is so poor that an incision in the lateral neck is inadvisable and a laryngopharyngectomy and resection of the base of the tongue is necessary, the primary incision can be made in the midline of the neck, the operation completed, and a skin flap from the infraclavicular area migrated in through the midline incision (Fig. 5).

If high-dose radiation has been employed preoperatively and the mandible is to be saved, the bone should be covered with either a tongue flap or a skin flap. If the preoperative irradiation has been given only to levels of 4,000 rads and a marginal resection of the mandible is to be done, a split-thickness skin graft might take and the mandible survive. However, if higher dosages have been employed, a forehead flap or other well-nourished skin flap can be expected to give more adequate coverage.

If possible, remove local recurrent cancers of the pharynx and oral cav-

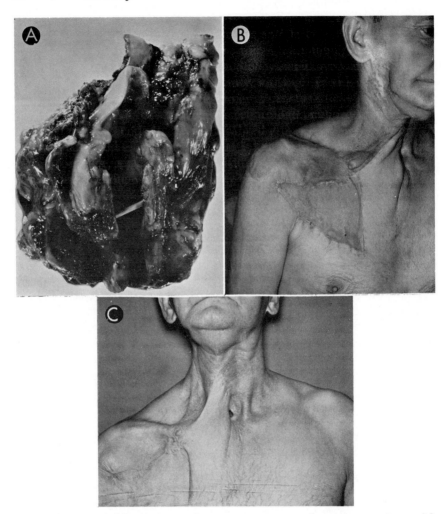

FIG. 5.—Laryngopharyngectomy. *A*, operative specimen of recurrent carcinoma following radiation. *B*, deltopectoral skin flap migrated in to cover pharyngeal wall through midline incision. Note heavily irradiated skin in right upper neck. *C*, after closure of fistula utilizing local skin and deltopectoral flap.

ity through the mouth without entering the neck, if there is no clinically evident tumor in the neck and clinically positive nodes were not present prior to irradiation (Fig. 6). Necrotic mandible should be removed through the mouth without making an incision in the neck. In a recent case, a physician presented with recurrent cancer of the base of the tongue following 7,000 rads tumor dose to the tumor with concomitant use of

5-fluorouracil. The tongue was enormously swollen, the neck extremely fibrotic, and there was necrosis of the right mandible. A laryngectomy and resection of the base of the tongue was done through a midline incision with creation of a midline fistula, and the mandible was removed through the mouth. Healing of wounds was satisfactory, although edema of the tongue and severe fibrosis of the neck persisted.

Consider a modified neck dissection if the entire neck was irradiated and the original palpable nodes were in a localized group. Although such a procedure at first would seem to be heretical, it has found safe, and cosmetically acceptable, and it provides a better functional result. Such procedures are usually done when the primary tumor is small and believed

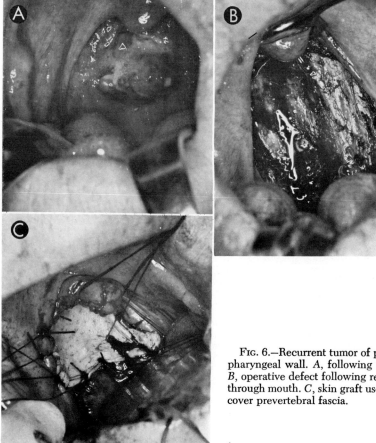

Fig. 6.—Recurrent tumor of posterior pharyngeal wall. *A*, following radiation. *B*, operative defect following removal through mouth. *C*, skin graft used to cover prevertebral fascia.

to be capable of control by irradiation and the nodes present the dominant feature of the disease and are present in a localized group. Following irradiation of the entire neck to at least 5,000 rads with additional localized irradiation to the primary, it is thought that subclinical disease in the neck nodes has been sterilized and it is necessary then only to remove the remaining nodal mass (Fig. 7). It is safe to do a modified bilateral neck dissection following such irradiation at one operative procedure.

Consider staged procedures if the age and nutritional condition of the patient are not suitable for a one-stage procedure. Although the tendency now is to do fewer staged procedures in the treatment for head and neck cancers, they still should play a part in the treatment of the patient with recurrent cancer following irradiation. Many of these people suffer nutritional defects, particularly if they are aged, and the safest procedure and the one which provides the lowest morbidity in the long run may be one which removes the primary tumor with the creation of a simple surgical defect which can be more safely closed at a later date when the nutritional status and general condition of the patient have been improved. Although nondelayed forehead and deltopectoral flaps have a good chance of surviving in the physiologically young individual, such flaps in the poorly nour-

Fig. 7.—*A*, modified neck dissection done following radiation therapy to small primary cancer of pyriform sinus with large cervical metastasis which has been previously biopsied. *B*, incision used for modified neck dissection indicated in *A*.

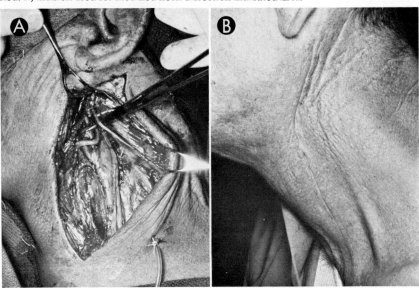

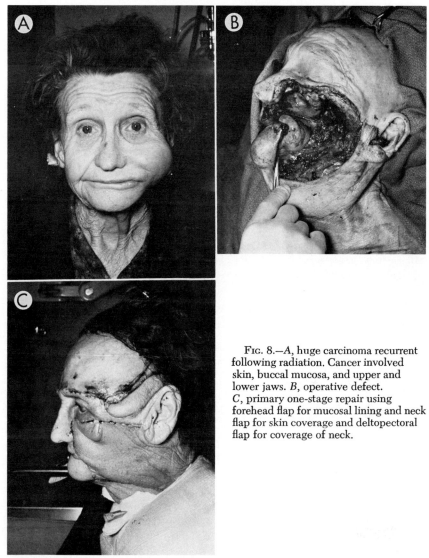

Fig. 8.—*A*, huge carcinoma recurrent following radiation. Cancer involved skin, buccal mucosa, and upper and lower jaws. *B*, operative defect. *C*, primary one-stage repair using forehead flap for mucosal lining and neck flap for skin coverage and deltopectoral flap for coverage of neck.

ished, aged patient may be extremely thin and would prove nonviable if migrated into a previously radiated area. In such situations, either the delayed flap or a tube pedicle should be employed. If the prospects for cure are small, immediate repair should be attempted even in the presence of an unfavorable condition (Fig. 8).

Provide Optimal Postoperative Support

Irradiated tissues are susceptible to infections and in combined procedures, antibiotics should be administered both pre- and postoperatively and continued until the wounds have securely healed. It is also necessary in these patients to check the hemoglobin and, if necessary, the plasma protein levels at frequent intervals because some will have suffered contracted blood volumes. It is not unusual to find that patients having surgery after radiation require considerably more plasma than nonradiated patients. Nutritional supports, either in the form of tube feedings or, if necessary, intravenous hyperalimentation should be resumed as quickly as possible in order to aid the healing process.

Selection of Patients and the Safest Surgical Procedure Should Be Employed

Not every patient with recurrent cancer following irradiation therapy will be benefited by surgical intervention. The patient with fixed nodes following irradiation therapy probably cannot be helped by an attempt to remove these nodes, if they are fixed to the prevertebral muscles, brachial plexus, or vertebrae. Such a situation is illustrated in Figure 9, which shows a patient with metastatic squamous cell carcinoma in the neck fol-

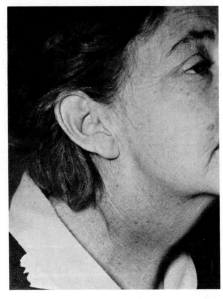

Fig. 9.—Recurrent fixed metastatic squamous cancer of neck following radiation. Surgical intervention failed because of involvement of vertebrae and failure of heavily irradiated skin flaps to adhere.

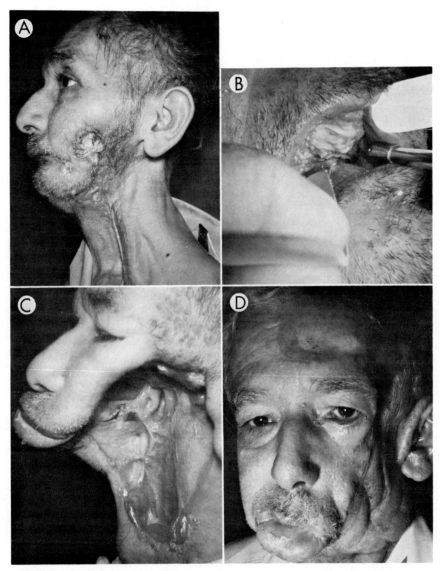

Fɪɢ. 10.—*A*, recurrent cancer of buccal mucosa involving skin of face and neck, upper and lower jaws, and entire tongue. The tumor extended to base of skull. *B*, intra-oral view of same patient showing extensive tumor of upper jaw. *C*, postoperative defect. Base of skull is exposed. Internal carotid artery had to be removed at foramen lacerum. *D*, condition following multistaged repair. Patient remains free of disease.

lowing radiation on two occasions. Because of the patient's severe pain, it was believed that an attempt to remove the tumor might result in relief of pain. However, it was found that the tumor extended into the prevertebral fascia and around the vertebrae and considerable tumor was left. The heavily irradiated skin flaps failed to adhere to the areas of recurrent tumor and a hematoma resulted. Pain was relieved only for a short period of time, but wound problems nullified much of the benefit.

Although caution should be exercised in attempting to remove fixed metastatic tumor after radiation, primary cancers which remain localized can be successfully resected, even though very large and involving multiple areas, providing the surgeon is willing to undertake an operation of sufficient magnitude to remove the tumor and if the patient is fully informed as to the surgery necessary and is willing to undergo the problems of repair. Such a situation is illustrated by Figure 10. This patient had recurrent cancer of the buccal mucosa following irradiation and surgery, but at no time had he had any evidence of regional node metastasis. The tumor invaded the entire tongue, cheek, and hard palate, and surrounded the carotid artery to the base of the skull. There were no neurological complications following resection of the carotid artery, and after multiple surgical procedures for repair of the defect, the patient remains well and free of disease at 10 years.

Summary

Although there are hazards in operating in radiated tissues, if the principles outlined are followed judiciously, it can be expected that surgery can be accomplished in most instances with very low morbidity or mortality. Morbidity may be prolonged if staged procedures are deemed necessary, but these may well be justified if the patient is fully informed beforehand as to what will be necessary and is willing to undergo the procedures required for removing the recurrent tumor, with the anticipated release of pain and other disabling symptoms and the hope of cure. In the author's experience, the employment of these principles has resulted in the absence of carotid perforations in irradiated patients during numerous operations in the past three years.

Papillomas of the Nasal Cavity and Sinuses

BYRON J. BAILEY, M.D., F.A.C.S.

Department of Otolaryngology, The University of Texas Medical Branch, Galveston, Texas

DURING THE PAST DECADE, considerable attention has been focused on the subject of the clinical behavior and management of papillomas of the nasal cavity and paranasal sinuses. Although the medical literature on this subject contains a considerable amount of enlightening information, we can also find an unusual abundance of confusion, contradiction, and varying opinions.

In this paper, we shall discuss our observations in this area and attempt to clarify some of the issues in regard to histopathologic terminology, clinical behavior, and surgical management of nasal papillomas.

We hope that this information, which has been extracted from a careful review of the literature and a series of nine patients treated at The University of Texas Medical Branch during the past four years, will assist the reader in his development of a rational approach to this problem, and perhaps stimulate some to report their experience subsequently.

Historical

Since "those who do not learn history are destined to repeat it," we shall review briefly some of the key reports on this subject.

The earliest reference to nasal papilloma is by Ward in 1854. The next year, Billroth reported two patients, one of whom exhibited repeated recurrences, one of the characteristic problems associated with these lesions. It is probably because of this feature of the disease that Billroth employed the terminology of "villiform cancer" in his writing.

97

In 1883, Hopmann reported his observations and originated the classification system of "hard" and "soft" tumors to which some authors still refer. This observation is related to the amount of fibrous connective tissue in the papilloma and is currently considered irrelevant in terms of prognostic implications.

Hellman in 1897 was the first to write of the apparent potential of these tumors to undergo malignant transformation. This feature of nasal papillomas was of great interest and concern to later authors such as Kramer and Som (1935) and Hall who reported similar observations during the 1930's. It is important for the reader to distinguish carefully between reports of "simultaneous" diagnosis of papilloma and carcinoma, and the documentation of a "malignant transformation" from papilloma to carcinoma. The latter situation appears to have been described in fewer than 20 patients as of the time of this review.

In more recent times, there have been excellent review articles by Lampertico, Russell, and MacComb (1963), Mabery, Devine, and Harrison (1965), Skolnik, Loewy, and Friedman (1966), Osborn (1970), Hyams (1971), and Snyder and Perzin (1972).

Histopathologic Classification of Nasal Papilloma

There is a great deal of significance in regard to subclassification of nasal papillomas into the groups described by Hyams (1971). From his study of 315 cases reviewed at the Armed Forces Institute of Pathology, we observe that these tumors may be grouped into three distinct types: fungiform, inverted papilloma, and cylindrical cell papilloma.

These three types of papilloma differ in terms of their location, gross and microscopic appearance, and clinical behavior. These differences are shown in Table 1. From this tabulation, one can readily appreciate the differences and similarities among these tumors.

The fungiform papillomas are characterized by a septal location, wide-based and cauliflower-like gross appearance, and freedom from association with malignancy.

Inverted papillomas and cylindrical cell papillomas are similar in appearance and clinical behavior. They are found on the lateral nasal wall with frequent involvement of the ethmoid and maxillary sinuses, and appear flat or polypoid. They are associated infrequently with conjoint malignancy and malignant transformation (the incidence of associated malignancy is in the range of 2 to 5 per cent).

Unfortunately, the subclassification can be difficult because of the spec-

TABLE 1.—LOCATION, APPEARANCE, AND CLINICAL BEHAVIOR OF PAPILLOMAS

	MOST FREQUENT LOCATION	GROSS	MICROSCOPIC	CLINICAL
Fungiform	Septum	Exophytic "Cauliflower, verrucous, mulberry" Wide base Grey to pink	Thin central core of stroma Distinct basement membranes Uniformity and polarity of cells Intercellular bridges seen Occasional mitoses; dark nuclei; seldom nucleoli	Males predominantly Younger age group Epistaxis most common Not associated with malignancy
Inverted papilloma	Lateral nasal wall Antrum Ethmoids	Flat or polypoid "Bulky" and firm Vascular Lack of translucence	Stroma from edematous to myxomatous to fibrous Distinct basement membrane Glycogen vacuoles in cytoplasm Occasional goblet cells Numerous micromucous cysts Usually respiratory epithelium	Males predominantly Older age group Obstruction most common symptom Associated with malignancy in 2–5%
Cylindrical cell papilloma	Lateral nasal wall in conjunction with antrum or ethmoids	Flat or polypoid Ragged, beefy papillary surface	Proliferating, multilayered, columnar Well-defined cell borders Many small mucous cysts Eosinophilic cytoplasm Round to oval dark nucleus Infrequent mitoses	Older age group No sex preference Associated with malignancy in 2–5%

trum of changes from one form to another and because of the frequent combination of different subtypes within the same tumor.

Snyder and Perzin (1972) have drawn slightly different conclusions from their study of 39 patients. They believe that the details of epithelial histopathology hold the key to the prognosis in regard to the problems of recurrence and associated malignancy. In their analysis, these authors describe a very high rate of recurrence in patients whose tumors demonstrated cellular atypia or the presence of mucin-producing cells within the epithelial layer.

Clinical Features

There is little in the way of symptomatology to evoke the physician's suspicion in these patients. Nasal obstruction is the most common symptom, with mild epistaxis second in frequency. Nasal pain is a less common symptom.

Anterior and posterior rhinorrhea is noted occasionally. The infrequent findings of orbital swelling, severe headaches, and diplopia suggest the presence of malignant disease.

There does not seem to be a clinical correlation between an allergic history and the development of papilloma. The relationship to chronic infection is disputed by several authors in the light of their contradictory patient groups.

There is also some disagreement concerning the radiographic characteristics of nasal and sinus papillomas. Hyams (1971) and Cody (1967) found occasional thinning or erosion of the bony sinus wall by benign papillomas, but stated that no definite invasion of bone was found unless there was an associated malignancy. Snyder and Perzin (1972) found rarefaction and bone destruction in three patients who had only benign papillomatosis.

The incidence of recurrence is also a subject which is disputed in terms of its incidence. Various authors have observed recurrence rates ranging from 30 per cent to more than 60 per cent. They have differed in their observations concerning the relationship between the histopathologic pattern and the incidence of recurrence. In most series, however, it appears that the fungiform type is less likely to recur than are the inverting and cylindrical cell papillomas.

Snyder and Perzin (1972) stress an important point in their article in this regard. They point out that the incidence of statistical recurrence can vary significantly, depending on how strictly the authors insist upon documentation of previous papilloma excision. If one is willing to accept the patient's history of prior nasal tumor excision, there will be a higher rate of recurrence than if the patient's slides must be obtained and reviewed.

Probably the most important recent statement in regard to recurrence is that made by Hyams in his discussion of the subject. He observed that "in those cases in which attention was directed to assure complete surgical removal of the papilloma, there was an insignificant incidence of recurrence."

Illustrative Case Reports

Perhaps the most useful method for appreciating some of the problems related to the management of nasal papilloma is the elaboration of three descriptive case reports.

CASE 1.—M.T., a 69-year-old man was seen initially in February, 1969, because of progressive rhinophyma of 20 years' duration and partial, left-sided nasal obstruction which had been present for 15 years. He had been bothered by recurrent sinusitis for the preceding 15 years.

The patient had been aware of a seasonal respiratory allergy and was not a smoker. The remainder of his medical history was noncontributory.

On physical examination there were pale, boggy, yellowish-grey polyps in the left nasal cavity. Sinus roentgenograms revealed a left pansinusitis.

Dermabrasion of the rhinophyma was accomplished in conjunction with a left nasal polypectomy. There was more than the customary amount of bleeding with the polypectomy. Microscopic examination of the nasal polyps revealed an associated inverted papilloma.

Two weeks later, the patient was reoperated upon in order to accomplish a complete excision of residual papilloma. The left maxillary antrum was approached via a 3 cm. gingivobuccal incision. The anterior wall of the maxilla was partially eroded and upon removing an adequate portion of this bone, a cystic, polypoid mass was encountered. As this was removed, it became apparent that the tumor in this area extended into the ethmoid sinuses. The medial wall of the maxillary sinus also was dehiscent. An extensive transantral ethmoidectomy was performed, and it seemed that the papilloma was removed along with an adequate margin of normal tissue.

The patient is now three years and seven months postoperative with no evidence of recurrent papilloma. There was no evidence of malignant change in the tissue examined microscopically.

The patient presents a typical picture of inverted papilloma. The histopathologic diagnosis was not suspected prior to the first procedure, and a second operation was necessary in order to accomplish a definitive removal of the papilloma. The approach which was selected afforded adequate visualization, but did not result in postoperative deformity or loss of function.

CASE 2.—K.T., a 77-year-old man presented with a five-mónth history of right infraorbital discomfort and right nasal obstruction. Roentgenograms revealed clouding of the right maxillary antrum and thickening of the mucosa of the left antrum. The patient had smoked one package of cigarettes per day for 20 years.

Right maxillary antral irrigation was performed and returned a scant amount of hemorrhagic fluid. Cytologic examination was reported as Class V with the notation that this cell block suggested "transitional carcinoma, papillary type, with some squamous differentiation." Subsequent cytopathology studies were performed on sputum specimens and were reported as Class I on two occasions and Class II on a third examination.

In April, 1970, a right Caldwell-Luc procedure was performed, and the tissue removed at this time was reported to show "inverted papilloma" without evidence of malignancy in spite of a careful search through numerous tissue sections.

In May, 1970, the antrum was entered by the same approach; the papilloma was arising primarily from the posterior wall, superolaterally, and had eroded the underlying bone in this area. Although the papilloma was said to show some areas of atypia, there was no evidence of malignancy.

The patient was bothered by persistent discomfort in the right infraorbital area and developed signs and symptoms of infection six months postoperatively. Therefore, he underwent a third Caldwell-Luc procedure in December, 1970. This revealed an abscess anterosuperiorly in the right maxillary antrum and fibrosis within the sinus cavity. The pathology report revealed recurrent "maxillary sinus inverted papilloma with foci of transitional cell carcinoma."

Subsequently, the patient received 5,000 rads of ^{60}Co irradiation to the area. The treatment was well tolerated, but the patient began to have recurrent epistaxis 15 months later.

Because of the likelihood of recurrent carcinoma, the antrum was explored again and biopsy disclosed "epidermoid carcinoma." Therefore, in May, 1972, a total maxillectomy was performed, and the patient is now six months postoperative without evidence of recurrence.

This case represents a more complex problem in diagnosis and management. The patient may have had a conjoint malignancy with the inverted papilloma from the first time he was seen, or this may represent malignant transformation of an inverted papilloma. The polypoid lesion in the nose was only an ordinary nasal polyp and did not recur. However, the antral lesion appears to have gone from papilloma, to papilloma with atypia, to papilloma with transitional cell carcinoma, to epidermoid carcinoma over a two-year period.

Case 3.—E.A., a 60-year-old woman was referred for surgical excision of a nasal tumor which had presented as a polypoid mass in the left side of the nose. The patient had smoked one package of cigarettes per day for the past 25 years.

Two prior nasal surgical procedures had been performed by her local otolaryngologist for a posterior nasal tumor involving the septum and the lateral nasal wall as two separate lesions. The first procedure was performed in August, 1971, and was reported as showing an epithelial papilloma without evidence of malignancy.

The patient developed evidence of recurrence and was reoperated upon in February, 1972, at which time the papilloma specimen was noted to contain several areas of squamous carcinoma in situ. This diagnosis was confirmed by pathologists at a leading tumor hospital.

Because of recurrent tumor in the ethmoid sinuses, on the septum, and on the floor of the nose, the patient was readmitted for a definitive excision of the lesion. Biopsy of the lesion on the floor of the nose (and extending anteriorly under the upper lip) revealed transitional cell carcinoma.

Therefore, in July, 1972, the patient underwent a left partial maxillectomy along with an external ethmoidectomy and resection of the septum and the involved palate extending beyond the midline.

The patient has done well postoperatively and has no evidence of persistent or recurrent disease at five months.

This case also appears to represent the progressive change from papilloma, to carcinoma in situ, to invasive transitional cell carcinoma. Complete excision of this malignant disease could be accomplished only by performing a radical resection of the areas of involvement.

Discussion

These case reports have illustrated a few of the problems one encounters in dealing with papillomatous tumors of the nasal cavity and sinuses.

The first problem encountered is that of making the diagnosis with certainty. These tumors are seen infrequently, and therefore are seldom suspected by the surgeon. They frequently resemble ordinary nasal polyps in their gross appearance, and their symptomatology and roentgenographic signs may not give any clear hints concerning their true nature when there is sinus involvement.

Likewise, the pathologist does not encounter these tumors frequently and may not appreciate the significance of certain microscopic features which are of great clinical importance. The specimen should receive a thorough evaluation of many areas, and every effort must be made to subclassify the tumor into its appropriate group.

The next problem is that of selection of the most appropriate management. Failure to appreciate the serious problems which may be associated with inverted papilloma or cylindrical cell papilloma may lead to an incomplete excision of the tumor with subsequent "recurrence." Conversely, some of the information on this subject implies that all inverting papillomas are premalignant or "clinically malignant" and could lead the surgeon into a radical operative procedure which might be deforming and unnecessary.

It appears that conservative management is adequate for fungiform papillomas which characteristically appear on the nasal septum. For inverted or cylindrical cell papillomas, excision with a wider margin of normal tissue is indicated. Careful planning must include the removal of tumor in the ethmoid and maxillary sinuses as well as a careful search for any areas of possible breakthrough of the sinus walls.

This type of surgery is based upon two critical factors. The first is a comprehensive understanding of nasal and sinus surgical anatomy.

The second is adequate visualization (which translates on a practical basis to "exposure" and "hemostasis"). A combination of suction, electrocautery, and packs with vasoconstricting agents is essential. Enhancement of exposure may be accomplished by employing transantral, transethmoid, or transpalatal approaches to the tumor. In special circumstances, a lateral rhinotomy approach may be necessary.

Summary

We have presented a review of the problems associated with the diagnosis and management of papillomatous tumors of the nose and paranasal sinuses.

Our goal has been to clarify some of the confusing terminology related to these neoplasms and their histopathologic subclassification. The long-term prognosis is poorer and the index of suspicion for associated malignancy is greater when the tumor is of the inverted or the cylindrical cell papilloma type.

Radiographic evidence of bone destruction can be associated with benign forms of this disease, but when present should also raise the question of wider excisional margins. A history of numerous prior nasal polypectomies is also associated with a higher incidence of malignant transformation.

Surgical planning must include a thoughtful consideration of the problems associated with obtaining a good exposure, hemostasis, and the ability to excise the tumor along with an adequate margin of normal tissue. Although the surgeon should avoid a deforming surgical procedure in general, he must be aware of the limitations of consistently relying upon intranasal procedures for excision of these papillomas. Sinus exploration and exenteration are often necessary, and lateral rhinotomy must be employed when needed for the above reasons.

Finally, the patient must be instructed carefully regarding the essential nature of close and extended follow-up examinations. Only by attention to all these details of diagnosis and management can we expect to increase the survival of these patients.

REFERENCES

Billroth, T.: As cited by Kramer, R., and Som, M. L.: True papilloma of the nasal cavity. *A.M.A. Archives of Otolaryngology,* 22:22-43, July 1935.

Cody, C. C.: Inverting papillomata of the nose and sinuses. *Laryngoscope,* 77: 584-598, April 1967.

Hall, A.: As cited by Mabery, T. E., Devine, K. D., and Harrison, E. G., Jr.: The problem of malignant transformation in a nasal papilloma: Report of a case. *Archives of Otolaryngology,* 82:296-300, September 1965.

Hellmann, L.: As cited by Kramer, R., and Som, M. L.: True papilloma of the nasal cavity. *A.M.A. Archives of Otolaryngology,* 22:22-43, July 1935.

Hopmann, C. M.: As cited by Kramer R., and Som, M. L.: True papilloma of the nasal cavity. *A.M.A. Archives of Otolaryngology,* 22:22-43, July 1935.

Hyams, V. J.: Papillomas of the nasal cavity and paranasal sinuses. A clinico-pathological study of 315 cases. *Annals of Otology, Rhinology and Laryngology,* 80:192-206, April 1971.

Kramer, R., and Som, M. L.: True papilloma of the nasal cavity. *A.M.A. Archives of Otolaryngology,* 22:22-43, July 1935.

Lampertico, P., Russell, W. O., and MacComb, W. S.: Squamous papilloma of upper respiratory epithelium. *Archives of Pathology,* 75:293-302, March 1963.

Mabery, T. E., Devine, K. D., and Harrison, E. G., Jr.: The problem of malignant transformation in a nasal papilloma. Report of a case. *Archives of Otolaryngology,* 82:296-300, September 1965.

Norris, H. J.: Papillary lesions of the nasal cavity and paranasal sinuses. Part II: Inverting papillomas. A study of 29 cases. *Laryngoscope,* 73:1-17, January 1963.

Osborn, D. A.: Nature and behavior of transitional tumors in the upper respiratory tract. *Cancer,* 25:50-71, January 1970.

Skolnick, E. M., Loewy, A., and Friedman, J. E.: Inverted papilloma of the nasal cavity. *Archives of Otolaryngology,* 84:61-67, July 1966.

Snyder, R. N., and Perzin, K. H.: Papillomatosis of nasal cavity and paranasal sinuses (inverted papilloma, squamous papilloma): A clinicopathologic study. *Cancer,* 30:668-690, September 1972.

Ward, N.: As cited by Hyams, V. J.: Papillomas of the nasal cavity and paranasal sinuses. A clinicopathological study of 315 cases. *Annals of Otology, Rhinology and Laryngology,* 80:192-206, April 1971.

Surgical Technique for Vocal Rehabilitation

ROBERT M. KOMORN, M.D.

*Department of Otolaryngology, Baylor College
of Medicine, Houston, Texas*

NORMAL SPEECH is produced when oropharyngeal structures modify a large, well-controlled, vibrating column of air. After laryngectomy, the primary source for this vibrating column of air is diverted away from the oropharynx to protect the lungs from contamination. Surgical vocal rehabilitation attempts to reconnect the tracheopulmonary system to the oropharynx without producing aspiration.

One of the earliest and most simple methods is found in a report of three patients who spoke with a tracheohypopharyngeal fistula (Guttman, 1935). The first patient created his own fistula with a red-hot icepick and no anesthesia. The other two fistulas were surgically created with a diathermy needle under anesthesia. Because of its lack of acceptance and additional follow-up reports, this technique remains a medical curiosity. We can only speculate as to the causes of its apparent failure.

Beginning in the late fifties, the concept of surgical vocal rehabilitation was reintroduced (Conley, De Amesti, and Pierce, 1958; Asai, 1960; Miller, 1968; Montgomery, 1968; Komorn, Weycer, Sessions, and Malone, 1973). Conley has described several different techniques using either mucosal flaps or autogenous vein that reconnect the trachea to the hypopharynx (Conley, De Amesti, and Pierce, 1958; Conley, 1959, 1969). A specially constructed prosthetic device was frequently needed for phonation. The difficulty of the surgery, stenosis of the tube, awkwardness of the prosthesis, and aspiration have been the major drawbacks to these procedures.

In 1960, Asai described a three-stage laryngoplasty that used regional neck flaps to form a skin-lined tube between a double-barreled tracheostoma and a hypopharyngeal fistula. This technique eliminated the need for a prosthesis. It produced good speech and currently it is the most widely used method for surgical vocal rehabilitation (Asai, 1972; Karlan, 1958; Miller, 1969; Porres and Mersol, 1968). It cannot be performed in patients who have had previous radiation, radical neck dissections, or extensive reconstructive procedures.

Aspiration with this technique frequently occurs, but can be reduced during swallowing by finger pressure over the fistula tract (Miller, 1968; Karlan, 1958). Phonation with the Asai laryngoplasty is sometimes lost because of stenosis or plugging of the tube by granulation tissue and desquamated epithelium.

Attempting to simplify and eliminate the problems of surgical vocal rehabilitation, Calcaterra and Jafek (1971) created a tracheoesophageal (TE) shunt in 10 mongrel dogs by using a full thickness esophageal flap. The technical ease of this procedure, as well as the apparent lack of problems with aspiration and shunt stenosis, prompted us to use this method in human beings.

Clinical Study

Since July 1971, TE shunts have been constructed in 11 patients at the time of laryngectomy and in one patient five months after laryngectomy. Nine patients had en bloc radical neck dissections. One patient was con-

TABLE 1.—CLINICAL MATERIAL

PATIENT	AGE	STAGE OF LESION	XRT TO TE SHUNT AREA Preop.	XRT TO TE SHUNT AREA Postop.	XRT OUTSIDE OF TE SHUNT AREA Preop.	XRT OUTSIDE OF TE SHUNT AREA Postop.
G. C.	42	$T_3N_0M_0$	No	No	No	No
E. P.	47	$T_3N_0M_0$	No	No	No	No
M. H.	55	$T_3N_0M_0$	No	No	Yes*	No
E. C.	50	$T_3N_0M_0$	No	Yes	No	No
H. L.	48	$T_3N_1M_0$	No	Yes	No	No
C. V.	68	$T_3N_0M_0$	No	No	Yes*	No
A. F.	46	$T_3N_0M_0$	No	Yes	No	No
E. C.	49	$T_3N_0M_0$	No	No	No	No
V. P.	65	$T_3N_0M_0$	No	No	No	Yes†
M. R.	51	$T_3N_0M_0$	No	No	No	No
W. C.	68	$T_3N_1M_0$	No	No	No	No
C. G.	48	$T_4N_1M_0$	Yes	No	No	No
Total	12		1	3	2	1

Abbreviations: XRT, radiation therapy; TE shunt, tracheoesophageal shunt.
*Laryngeal field only.
†Lower midline neck shielded during XRT.

sidered for the TE shunt, but extensive scarring from a previous tracheostomy made it technically impossible to create the shunt. All of the patients were men between the ages of 42 and 68 and all had T_3 or larger laryngeal cancers. Radiation therapy that included the area of the TE shunt was given to one patient preoperatively and to three patients after shunt construction. Three additional patients received radiation therapy which did not include the area of the TE shunt (Table 1).

Surgical Technique

The technique of creating the TE shunt has not significantly changed since our last report (Komorn, Weycer, Sessions, and Malone, 1973). Nine shunts were constructed from an inferior medially based flap measuring $2\frac{1}{2} \times 5$ cm. The shunt and esophagus were closed in two layers (Fig. 1A). Three shunts were constructed from an inferior laterally based flap which also measured $2\frac{1}{2} \times 5$ cm. (Fig. 2A). Technically, it is difficult to suture between the shunt and the oblique closure of the esophagus. The medial shunts were connected to the back wall of the trachea (Fig. 1B) and the lateral shunts were connected to the lateral wall of the trachea between

Fig. 1.—Procedure for TE shunt. *A*, inferior, medially based full thickness esophageal flap closed in two layers to form the tracheoesophageal shunt. *B*, medially based tracheo-esophageal shunt sutured to the back wall of the trachea; stent in place. (Courtesy of Komorn, Weycer, Sessions, and Malone, 1973.)

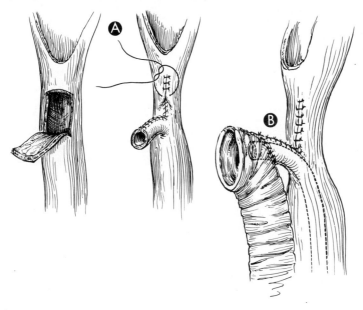

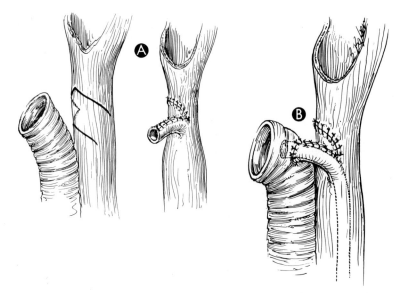

Fig. 2.—*A*, inferior, laterally based full thickness esophageal flap. The esophageal defect is closed obliquely. *B*, laterally based flap sutured to lateral wall of trachea between two tracheal rings; stent in place. (Courtesy of Komorn, Weycer, Sessions, and Malone, 1973.)

two trachea rings (Fig. 2B). A 12 or 14F catheter was used as a stent for approximately two weeks.

Results

Vocal Rehabilitation

Nine patients developed speech 12 to 40 days after surgical treatment; only six patients have retained this speech. TE shunt speech is considerably better than esophageal speech. Using a Multiple Choice Intelligibility Test (Black and Haagen, 1963), TE shunt speakers consistently score above 90 per cent, can sustain an a for a minimum of 15 seconds, and can produce eight to ten words per breath (Komorn, Weycer, Sessions, and Malone, 1973). The average intelligibility score for good esophageal speakers is 60 to 80 per cent (Creech, 1966). Esophageal speakers rarely sustain an a for longer than three to four seconds, and can produce four to nine syllables, not words, per charge of air (Berlin, 1965; Snidecor and Isshiki, 1965) (Table 2).

TABLE 2.—COMPARISON OF AVERAGE TRACHEOESOPHAGEAL SPEECH
WITH AVERAGE ESOPHAGEAL AND NORMAL SPEECH

	TE SHUNT	ESOPHAGEAL[*]	NORMAL[†]
Intelligibility[‡]	>90%	60–80%	100%
Maximum duration of sustained a Count with one breath or charge of air	>15 seconds	3 to 4 seconds	15 to 59 seconds
	20 to 40	8 to 10	40 or >
Words produced with one breath or charge of air	8 to 10	NA	10
Syllables	NA	4 to 9	NA

Abbreviation: NA, information not available.
[*]Adapted from Berlin, 1965.
[†]Adapted from Snidecor and Isshiki, 1965.
[‡]Multiple Choice Intelligibility Test (Black and Haagen, 1963).

WOUND PROBLEMS

Two patients with a laterally based flap and the only patient to receive preoperative radiation therapy to the area of the shunt had wound breakdown and salivary fistulas. All three patients healed spontaneously, but the two patients with the laterally based flap had stenosis of their tracheostoma and TE shunt. One of these two patients also received postoperative radiation therapy and now has an esophageal stricture that requires frequent dilatation. The patient who received preoperative radiation and had a shunt constructed from a medially based flap maintained speech without swallowing difficulties (Table 3).

TABLE 3.—POSTOPERATIVE WOUND PROBLEMS

PATIENT	TYPE OF FLAP	PREOP. XRT TO TE SHUNT AREA	POSTOP. XRT TO TE SHUNT AREA	RESULT
E. C.	Lateral	No	No	Wound breakdown, trachea and TE shunt stenosis, no speech
A. F.	Lateral	No	Yes	Wound breakdown, trachea and TE shunt stenosis, esophageal stricture
C. G.	Medial	Yes	No	Wound breakdown, spontaneous healing, good speech, no swallowing difficulty

Abbreviations: XRT, radiation therapy; TE shunt, tracheoesophageal shunt.

SHUNT STENOSIS

Spontaneous shunt stenosis occurred in two patients who began postoperative radiation therapy after the stent was removed and while granulation tissue was still present around the meatus of the shunt. Stenosis occurred in one patient with generalized arteriosclerosis and a postoperative course characterized by a *Pseudomonas* tracheitis and the need for an aorticofemoral bypass procedure.

Initially, four patients had to use excessive force to talk. Two patients solved this problem by using a 14F catheter to dilate the meatus of the shunt daily for six weeks. The other two patients required a meatoplasty. All four have had excellent speech for 15, 13, 4, and 3 months after shunt construction.

SWALLOWING AND ASPIRATION AFTER SHUNT CONSTRUCTION

Construction of the TE shunt did not interfere with swallowing except in the one patient described above. Immediately after removal of the stent, aspiration of liquids may occur. This usually resolves spontaneously or decreases until there is only an occasional small collection of moisture around the meatus of the shunt. Neither aspiration pneumonia nor tracheobronchial infection has occurred.

Two patients with symptomatic hiatal hernia, however, aspirated with liquids. Surgical revision of the angle of the shunt eliminated the problem in one and reduced it in the other. Despite one year of excellent speech, no weight loss, and no pulmonary infection, this latter patient requested closure of his shunt. This was done as an office procedure.

The isoperistaltic inferiorly based design of the shunt probably accounts for the low incidence of aspiration. Cinefluoroscopic studies show that a bolus of material will initially flow past the opening of the shunt without entering it. As the normal esophageal peristaltic wave passes the area of the shunt, the bolus of material is compressed and some of it may enter the shunt. This reflux frequently occurs after removal of the stent, but seems to persist only if a hiatal hernia is present.

Discussion

A TE shunt provided rapid and apparently permanent vocal rehabilitation in 6 of 12 laryngectomized patients (Table 4). The limitations and causes of failure appear to be related to either technique or patient selection. Wound breakdown with fistula formation occurred with two of three

TABLE 4.—SUMMARY OF RESULTS

PATIENT	MONTHS POSTSHUNT	INITIAL TE SHUNT SPEECH	RETAIN TE SHUNT SPEECH	COMMENTS
G. C.	15	Yes	Yes	No postop. problems
E. P.	14	Yes	Yes	Hiatus hernia. Needed revision of shunt
M. H.	13	Yes	No	Hiatus hernia. Shunt surgically closed
E. C.	11	Yes	No	Stenosis of shunt during postop. XRT
H. L.	11	No	No	Stenosis of shunt during postop. XRT
A. F.	10	Yes	No	Lateral based flap. Wound breakdown and fistula
C. V.	9	Yes	Yes	Lateral based flap. No postop. problems
E. C.	8	No	No	Lateral based flap. Wound breakdown and fistula
V. P.	6	Yes	Yes	Shunt constructed five months post-laryngectomy
M. R.	5	No	No	Tracheitis and arteriosclerosis
W. C.	4	Yes	Yes	No postop. problems
C. G.	3	Yes	Yes	Preop. radiation
Total		9	6	

Abbreviations: TE shunt, tracheoesophageal shunt; Postop. XRT, postoperative radiation therapy.

laterally based flaps. This flap is technically more difficult to construct and, until further evaluation is completed in the dog laboratory, its use has been discontinued. The only wound breakdown that occurred with the medially based flaps was when preoperative radiation therapy was used for a $T_4N_1M_0$ transglottic cancer. Stenosis occurred only in the two patients who had received postoperative radiation therapy and the one patient who had a postoperative tracheitis. In retrospect, leaving the stent in place or delaying the start of radiation may have prevented the stenosis in the two irradiated patients.

The advantages of this technique are that it can either be performed at the time of laryngectomy or as a one-stage secondary procedure. The medially based flap is easy to construct and can be used except when the lower cervical esophagus is excessively scarred. Radical neck dissections have not interfered with creation of the shunt.

The speech produced with a TE shunt is similar to esophageal speech. Both methods depend on air passing through the cricopharyngeus into the oropharynx. TE shunt speech has several advantages. Duration of speech is increased because the source of air is the tidal volume and not a small bolus of trapped air. Volume and pitch ranges are increased. In esophageal speech, the air is passively released when the cricopharyngeal muscle relaxes. In TE shunt speech, the air is forced through the cricopharyngeal muscle, by thoracic and abdominal muscles, as it would be forced through the vocal cords. Even though patients with TE shunts learn to speak after simple instruction on how to close the tracheostoma with a finger, work with a speech pathologist improves the quality until it closely resembles laryngeal speech (Malone and Komorn, in preparation).

Summary

The tracheoesophageal shunt is indicated for vocal rehabilitation whenever a total laryngectomy with or without a radical neck dissection offers the patient the best chance for long-term survival. It is also indicated in previously laryngectomized patients who have failed to achieve vocal rehabilitation by nonsurgical means. Based on our experience with 12 patients, specific contraindications are:

1. Planned pre- or postoperative radiotherapy which includes the lower neck or upper mediastinum.

2. Extensive resections requiring flap reconstruction of the hypopharynx.

3. Pre-existing esophageal disease.

4. Hiatus hernia with reflux.

5. Extensive scarring of the upper cervical esophagus from previous surgical procedures.

6. Anticipated poor wound healing from diabetes mellitus, arteriosclerosis, or active bronchopulmonary infection.

Patients must understand that this is a new procedure and that other means of vocal rehabilitation are available. They must also understand and be willing to accept the risk of failure and be intelligent enough to recognize and care for any special problems that may arise. This procedure should not be done without careful and close clinical follow-up.

REFERENCES

Asai, R.: Laryngoplasty. *Journal of the Japan Bronchoesophageal Society*, 12: 1-3, 1960.

——: Laryngoplasty after total laryngectomy. *Archives of Otolaryngology*, 95:114-119, February 1972.

Berlin, C. I.: Clinical measurement of esophageal speech: 3. Performance of non-biased groups. *Journal of Speech and Hearing Disorders*, 30:174-183, May 1965.

Black, J. W., and Haagen, C. H.: Multiple-choice intelligibility test, forms A and B. *Journal of Speech and Hearing Disorders*, 28:77-86, February 1963.

Calcaterra, T. C., and Jafek, B. W.: Tracheo-esophageal shunt for speech rehabilitation after total laryngectomy. *Archives of Otolaryngology,* 94:124-128, August 1971.

Conley, J. J.: Vocal rehabilitation by autogenous vein graft. *Annals of Otology, Rhinology and Laryngology,* 68:990-995, December 1959.

————: Surgical techniques for the vocal rehabilitation of the post-laryngectomized patient. *Transactions of the American Academy of Ophthalmology and Otolaryngology,* 73:288-299, March-April 1969.

Conley, J. J., De Amesti, F., and Pierce, M. K.: A new surgical technique for the vocal rehabilitation of the laryngectomized patient. *Annals of Otology, Rhinology and Laryngology,* 67:655-664, September 1958.

Creech, H. B.: Evaluating esophageal speech. *Journal of Speech and Hearing Association of Virginia,* 7:13-19, 1966.

Guttman, M. R.: Tracheohypopharyngeal fistulization; new procedure for speech production in laryngectomized patient. *Transactions of the American Laryngological, Rhinological and Otological Society,* 41:219-226, 1935.

Karlan, M. S.: Two stage Asai laryngectomy utilizing a modified Tucker valve. *American Journal of Surgery,* 116:597-599, October 1958.

Komorn, R. M., Weycer, J. S., Sessions, R. B., and Malone, P. E.: Vocal rehabilitation with a tracheo-esophageal shunt. *Archives of Otolaryngology,* 97:303-305, April 1973.

Malone, P., and Komorn, R. M.: Vocal rehabilitation techniques used following construction of a tracheo-esophageal shunt. (In preparation.)

Miller, A. H.: Further experiences with the Asai technique for vocal rehabilitation after laryngectomy. *Transactions of the American Academy of Ophthalmology and Otolaryngology,* 72:779-781, September-October 1968.

————:Surgery for vocal rehabilitation after laryngectomy. In *Proceedings of the Centennial Symposium,* Manhattan Eye, Ear and Throat Hospital. St. Louis, Missouri, C. V. Mosby, 1969, Vol. II, pp. 311-317.

Montgomery, W. W., and Toohill, R. J.: Voice rehabilitation after laryngectomy. *Archives of Otolaryngology,* 88:499-506, November 1968.

Porres, R., and Mersol, V. F.: Tracheohypopharyngeal shunt after total laryngectomy. *Archives of Otolaryngology,* 88:413-418, October 1968.

Snidecor, J. C., and Isshiki, N.: Vocal and air use characteristics of a superior male esophageal speaker. *Folia Phoniatrica,* 17:217-232, 1965.

Advances in Anesthesiology for Surgery of the Head and Neck

WILLIAM S. DERRICK, M.D.

Department of Anesthesiology, The University of Texas System Cancer Center, M. D. Anderson Hospital and Tumor Institute, Houston, Texas

CERTAIN ASPECTS OF ANESTHESIA for surgery of the head and neck provide the anesthesiologist with problems not encountered in the therapy for neoplasia located elsewhere in the body. In surgery of the head and neck, it is often necessary that the surgical team virtually surround the head and neck area, and it is therefore difficult for the anesthesiologist to maintain contact with and control of the patient's airway. Airway problems arise especially in peroral endoscopic procedures where it is virtually impossible to insure a patent airway and normal pulmonary ventilation with conventional anesthetic drugs and procedures. Another problem area relates to the treatment by radiation therapy of pediatric patients, where it is exceedingly difficult to maintain proper positioning throughout the course of radiation therapy. It is my purpose in this brief communication to discuss two relatively new drugs which have been extremely helpful to us in these problem areas. These two drugs are Innovar and ketamine.

Innovar is a combination of a tranquilizer, droperidol, and a narcotic analgesic, fentanyl, in a 50:1 ratio so that each milliliter of Innovar solution contains 2.5 mg. of droperidol and 0.05 mg. of fentanyl. Droperidol produces general quiescence, a reduced responsiveness to environmental stimuli, has a strong antiemetic effect, and may cause some lowering of the blood pressure. It tends to potentiate the action of barbiturates and narcotics. Fentanyl is a potent, rapid-acting, morphine-like narcotic analgesic. It produces respiratory depression and reduces respiratory minute volume, primarily because of a decrease in the respiratory rate. With rapid intravenous administration, bradycardia may occur which is of vagal origin and may be quickly reversed with intravenous atropine administration. Occasionally, rapid intravenous administration of Innovar may cause severe rigidity of the abdominal and thoracic musculature. This rigidity may be overcome by the intravenous administration of a muscle relaxant such as tubocurarine.

The depth of Innovar anesthesia is usually indicated, in a spontaneously breathing patient, by an increase in the respiratory rate and depth. In an apneic patient, lightening of anesthesia is usually indicated by the elevation of the pulse rate and blood pressure. Lacrimation may also occur.

Innovar produces a notable decrease in the reflex irritability of the respiratory and upper alimentary tracts. This property, when used with topical anesthesia, makes Innovar an ideal anesthetic for endoscopic examination of the larynx, pharynx, tracheal-bronchial tree, or esophagus. At the same time, the patient will ordinarily maintain spontaneous respirations. In certain procedures where the patient's cooperation is necessary, Innovar will provide a state of somnolence with profound analgesia. The patient is able to respond to commands and to cooperate, yet is usually amnesic for the procedure. Innovar is nonexplosive, reduces postoperative nausea and vomiting, is not hepatotoxic, and provides a smooth recovery from anesthesia, with the patient remaining tranquil and cooperative.

The induction dose of Innovar is 1 ml. per 20 to 25 pounds of body weight given slowly intravenously. For maintenance, 0.5 to 1 ml. of Innovar, or fentanyl alone, may be given when the patient shows signs of lightening of the depth of anesthesia.

Innovar is therefore a useful drug to provide sedation and analgesia or to supplement local anesthesia for a wide range of procedures in which patient cooperation is necessary. It may also be used to supplement nitrous oxide-oxygen anesthesia with muscle relaxants if required.

The second drug, ketamine, is a nonbarbiturate, nonnarcotic anesthetic. It produces a state of general anesthesia which differs from that produced by conventional anesthetic agents. The term "dissociative" has been given to this state, because ketamine appears to interrupt association pathways of the brain selectively.

Induction of ketamine anesthesia is characterized by horizontal or vertical nystagmus and the abrupt opening of the eyes. This state is further characterized by profound analgesia with normal or slightly increased muscle tone, including the intraoral muscles and the tongue, so that the airway usually remains unobstructed in spite of changes in position. Pharyngeal reflexes are usually maintained, and therefore mechanical stimulation of the pharynx should be avoided unless adequate muscle relaxants are used. Except with overdosage, respiration is very little affected. When respiratory depression occurs, it is usually of short duration and is easily treated by supportive pulmonary ventilation.

Ketamine stimulates the cardiovascular system and results in an acceleration of the cardiac rate and an increase in the systolic and diastolic blood pressure. Excessive salivation may occur when atropine or another drying agent has not been administered preanesthetically.

During emergence from ketamine anesthesia, the patient may experience vivid dreams, with or without psychomotor activity. These phenomena are observed much more frequently in adults than in children, and often follow premature stimulation in the recovery period while the state of dissociation still exists. When this side effect appears troublesome, a small intravenous dose of a rapid-acting barbiturate is helpful in abolishing it.

Ketamine is rapid-acting. An intravenous dose of 1 mg. per pound of body weight usually produces anesthesia within 30 seconds and lasts 5 to 10 minutes. If longer effects are required, additional doses of one-half the induction dose may be given. It may also be given intramuscularly in a dose of 5 mg. per pound and will produce surgical anesthesia within 3 to 4 minutes following injection. By this route, anesthesia lasts from 12 to 25 minutes.

Ketamine is extremely valuable in pediatric anesthetic problems and is recommended for short, painful diagnostic or surgical procedures. It may also be used for induction of anesthesia prior to the administration of other general anesthetic agents. Ketamine has been found to be an extremely useful anesthetic drug, especially to maintain quiescence in small children who are receiving radiotherapy. With proper dosage and management, it is possible to maintain an immobile state during treatment while still providing safety for the patient.

Both Innovar and ketamine are easy to administer and have proved to be excellent drugs for special anesthetic problems and indications. It should be borne in mind, however, that they are both potent agents and require the same degree of attention and support as do other anesthetic drugs.

REFERENCES

Corssen, G., Groves, E. H., Gomez, S., and Allen, R. J.: Ketamine: Its place in anesthesia for neurosurgical diagnostic procedures. *Anesthesia and Analgesia,* 48:181-188, March-April 1969.

Corssen, G., Miyasaka, M., and Domino, E. F.: Changing concepts in pain control during surgery: Dissociative anesthesia with CI-581: A progress report. *Anesthesia and Analgesia,* 47:746-759, November-December 1968.

Fox, J. W., and Fox, E.: Neuroleptanalgesia: A review. *North Carolina Medical Journal,* 27:471-475, October 1966.

Martin, S. J., Murphy, J. D., Colliton, R. J., and Zeffiro, R. G.: Clinical studies with Innovar. *Anesthesiology,* 28:458-463, March-April 1967.

Wilson, G. H., Fortias, N. A., and Dillon, J. B.: Ketamine: A new anesthetic for use in pediatric neuroroentgenologic procedures. *The American Journal of Roentgenology, Radium Therapy and Nuclear Medicine,* 106:434-439, June 1969.

Wilson, R. D., Traber, D. L., and McCoy, N. R.: Ketamine—(2-(0-chlorophenyl)-2-methyl aminocyclohexanone hydrochloride)—a new anesthetic for use in children. (Abstract) *Clinical Research,* 16:92, January 1968.

Recent Developments in Chemotherapy for Head and Neck Cancer

JEFFREY A. GOTTLIEB, M.D.,
M. ANDREW BURGESS, M.D.,
GERALD P. BODEY, M.D., AND
ROBERT B. LIVINGSTON, M.D.

*Department of Developmental Therapeutics, The University of
Texas System Cancer Center, M. D. Anderson Hospital
and Tumor Institute, Houston, Texas*

CHEMOTHERAPY for head and neck neoplasia has generally been relegated to palliative efforts for the patient with advanced disease. Numerous clinical trials, most of them empirical, have shown several agents, notably methotrexate and 5-fluorouracil, capable of producing significant, although short-lasting, tumor regressions in this advanced setting. Other agents, such as hydroxyurea, have often been given in conjunction with radiotherapy. Some others have been given as intra-arterial infusions, and while response rates have improved in some series with this technique (Sullivan *et al.*, 1960), the over-all duration of response has remained brief. Some physicians may question whether the palliation achieved with these trials is worthwhile when balanced against expense, patient inconvenience, and complications. However, it must be remembered that the natural duration of life for patients failing primary surgical or radiotherapeutic procedures may not be short. During this period, the pain from bone involvement and local extension of rapid, invasive growth may be considerable, and in this setting even moderate palliation may be extremely gratifying.

Over the last several years, new agents have been developed based on the results of screening against animal tumor models which mimic the slower growth patterns of the advanced carcinomas. New approaches to chemotherapy have also developed which utilize kinetic and biochemical principles rather than relying on empiricism alone. This paper will concentrate on some of these new efforts, emphasizing the collated data from recent clinical trials, many of which are still in progress.

Bleomycin

Bleomycin, an antitumor antibiotic produced by a strain of *Streptomyces verticillus* isolated from the soil of Japanese coal mines, was first discovered in 1962 by Umezawa and his colleagues in Japan (Umezawa, Ishizuka, Maeda, and Takeuchi, 1967). The drug consists of a group of water-soluble basic peptides composed mainly of one component, bleomycin A_2. Extensive pharmacological studies in Japan in the 1960's showed that bleomycin was concentrated in skin and other squamous cell tissue (Umezawa, Ishizuka, Maeda, and Takeuchi, 1967). In 1969, Ichikawa first reported an impressive response rate with squamous cell carcinoma involving the penis (Ichikawa, Nakano, and Hirokawa, 1969). Other studies soon followed and showed that squamous cell carcinoma of the head and neck (Takeda, Sagawa, and Arakawa, 1970), uterine cervix (Suzuki, Murai, Watanabe, and Nunokawa, 1970), and esophagus (Wada, 1970) also had a high response rate to this agent. The drug was introduced into the United States in March of 1970 by Bristol Laboratories. Approximately 1,500 patients have since received this agent in various clinical trials in different chemotherapeutic centers. Table 1, which is compiled

TABLE 1.—BLEOMYCIN IN SQUAMOUS CELL CARCINOMA OF THE HEAD AND NECK: SUMMARY OF AMERICAN EXPERIENCE

SITE	NUMBER OF EVALUABLE PATIENTS	NUMBER OF RESPONSES
Larynx and paralarynx	62	20 (32%)
Tongue	52	15 (29%)
Floor of mouth	32	19 (59%)
Nasopharynx	27	9 (33%)
Tonsil	24	7 (29%)
Oropharynx	18	7 (39%)
Sinuses	15	6 (40%)
Palate	13	6 (46%)
Buccal mucosa	12	6 (50%)
Epiglottis	9	5 (56%)
Lip	8	2 (25%)
Gingiva	7	3 (43%)
Other	3	1 (33%)
Total	282	106 (37.6%)

from the records of Bristol Laboratories (Magers and Agre, 1972), is a compendium of the results of bleomycin treatment for squamous cell carcinoma of the head and neck in the United States. In all, 282 patients have received an evaluable course of therapy (generally defined as three or more weeks of treatment) and 106 (37.6 per cent) of them have achieved a 25 per cent or greater decrease in the size of their tumors. As shown in Table 1, the response rate of the various sites of involvement is relatively similar, with perhaps carcinoma of the mouth somewhat more responsive than the other sites. The median durations of response have been short— on the order of six to eight weeks in the experience of most clinicians. It should be emphasized, however, that all patients receiving bleomycin had advanced disease, no longer amenable to surgical or radiotherapeutic approaches. Many had also failed on initial chemotherapeutic efforts, predominantly with methotrexate or 5-fluorouracil. Although brief, many of the responses were quite dramatic, thus producing significant symptomatic and objective palliation.

The usual treatment program consists of twice-weekly intravenous injections utilizing a dose of 15 mg.* per square meter of body surface area or approximately 30 mg. Therapy has generally continued for six to eight weeks and has then been discontinued because of the increased risk of pulmonary toxicity seen with high accumulative dosage (see below). The drug, which has become commercially availtble (Blenoxane, Bristol Laboratories), is supplied as a white crystalline powder in a 15-mg. ampule which is readily dissolved with sterile distilled water or saline. Bleomycin has also been given intramuscularly, but in a randomized study performed by the Southwest Cancer Chemotherapy Study Group, the response rate in squamous cell carcinoma of the head and neck was considerably less when given intramuscularly (5 per cent) than when given intravenously (22 per cent) (Luce, 1972). Prolonged intra-arterial infusions with bleomycin have also been successful in a number of patients with head and neck carcinoma, as have several adjuvant studies combined with radiotherapy, but the over-all efficacy of these methods has not yet been fully evaluated. Yagoda and his co-workers have attempted to increase the duration of response by giving very small doses (0.5-2.0 mg.) subcutaneously daily for periods up to nine months (Yagoda, Krakoff, LaMonte, and Tan, 1971). In this study, patients were instructed to give their own injections, much like diabetics, and no major complications were observed with this self-administration program. While encouraging results were seen in lymphomas, tumors extremely sensitive to this agent, responses with head and

*Bleomycin has been released commercially in units rather than milligrams. One unit of bleomycin is the equivalent of 1.012 mg. of bleomycin A_2 hydrochloride.

neck carcinoma patients have been relatively few, and further evaluation of this technique is required before it can be recommended.

Several studies employing new kinetic data concerning bleomycin have recently been performed at M. D. Anderson Hospital and Tumor Institute. Barranco and Humphrey (1971), studying Chinese hamster cells in vitro, demonstrated that bleomycin was most capable of causing cell death when the tumor cell was in the process of mitosis (Fig. 1). This study suggested that if the number of cancer cells in mitosis could be increased, the efficacy of bleomycin would be increased. Previous observations by Frei and his co-workers had shown that the antitumor vinca alkaloid, vincristine (Oncovin), was capable of increasing the number of mitoses in human bone marrow by its stathmokinetic effect (Frei *et al.*, 1964). Figure 2 demonstrates that approximately six to 12 hours after an intravenous injection of vincristine, the number of human bone marrow cells in mitosis had

Fig. 1.—The effects of increasing doses of bleomycin on the survival of Chinese hamster cells *in vitro*. The lowest cell survival rate (*i.e.*, the greatest cell kill) is seen when cells are in mitosis. (From Barranco and Humphrey, 1971; reproduced by courtesy of *Cancer Research*.)

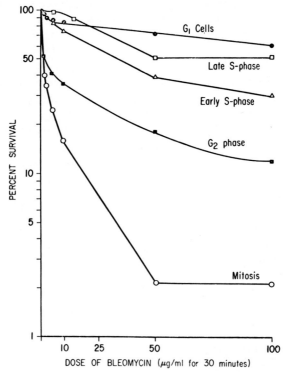

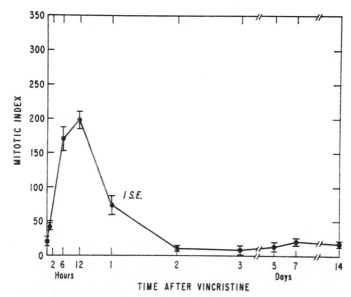

Fɪɢ. 2.—The effects of single doses of vincristine (0.01–0.1 mg./kg.) on the mitotic index in the human bone marrow after increasing amounts of time. Each mitotic index represents the average number of mitoses seen in 1,000 nucleated cell counts. The peak index occurs 6 to 12 hours after injection. (Adapted from Frei *et al.*, 1964.)

increased approximately 10-fold. Similar results have been seen in squamous tumors of the oral cavity in man (Meyer and Donaldson, 1969). As a result of these observations, two studies, one preclinical and one clinical, were started. The preclinical study showed that bleomycin administered six hours after a vincristine injection in the rodent bearing Lewis lung carcinoma was more potent than either drug administered alone (Schabel, personal communication). A similar study in man utilizing 1 mg. of vincristine six hours before 30 mg. of bleomycin, both administered intravenously twice weekly, was associated with a considerable improvement in the response rate. Thus, while the response rate for carcinoma of the lung was 3 of 60 (5 per cent) with bleomycin used alone, the response rate with bleomycin used at the same dose but potentiated by vincristine as described above was 4 of 15 (27 per cent), with a doubling of the median duration of response as well (Livingston, Bodey, Gottlieb, and Frei, 1973). Further studies utilizing this kinetic principle are in progress.

Toxic side effects from bleomycin have been relatively minor. One notable asset of this agent is its lack of significant hematopoietic toxicity. Thus, patients with extensive previous therapy with inadequate bone mar-

TABLE 2.—INFLUENCE OF AGE ON BLEOMYCIN
PULMONARY TOXICITY

AGE OF PATIENTS	NUMBER OF PATIENTS	PATIENTS WITH PULMONARY TOXICITY
Under 50 years	16	3 (19%)
50 years or older	40	16 (40%)

row reserve may receive bleomycin without risk of overwhelming myelo-suppression. This attribute of the drug has prompted its use in a number of combinations with potent myelosuppressive chemotherapeutic agents, notably in patients with lymphoma. Combination trials in head and neck cancer have thus far been relatively limited, but studies utilizing metho-trexate and bleomycin are currently being evaluated by a number of treatment centers (Mosher, DeConti, and Bertino, 1972).

Side effects seen with more regularity include a fever following administration and a desquamative dermatitis involving predominantly the extensor surfaces. The mechanism by which bleomycin induces fever is poorly understood, but simultaneous administration of antipyretics or corticosteroids along with bleomycin can generally ablate any febrile episode. The skin changes, while annoying, are rarely severe and are completely reversible. Hyperpigmentation, loss of hair, mucosal ulceration, and gastrointestinal disturbances have also been observed in varying percentages in different trials (Bonadonna *et al.*, 1972). None of these changes is usually serious enough to warrant discontinuation of therapy.

The major dose-limiting toxicity with bleomycin has been an insidious onset of pulmonary fibrosis associated with respiratory insufficiency and even occasional deaths. As data collected in our department indicate (Table 2), the incidence of any pulmonary toxicity is increased in patients 50 years or older, suggesting the need for careful follow-up of elderly patients. In Table 3, it is shown that the incidence of toxicity is also related to dose, with patients receiving a total dose of less than 200 mg./M^2

TABLE 3.—RELATIONSHIP OF DOSE TO
BLEOMYCIN PULMONARY TOXICITY

DOSE OF BLEOMYCIN RECEIVED	NUMBER OF PATIENTS	PATIENTS WITH PULMONARY TOXICITY
Under 200 mg./M^2	22	5 (23%)
200 mg./M^2 or more	34	14 (41%)

(or approximately 300 to 400 mg.) having less pulmonary toxicity than that seen in patients receiving higher doses (Salem, 1971). These observations have prompted most investigators to limit the total dose of bleomycin administered to approximately 350 mg. However, it is necessary to follow patients carefully with pulmonary function tests and blood gases as well as physical examination, since occasional patients may show evidence of pulmonary toxicity at a lower dose, particularly if they are elderly. De Lena and his co-workers have recently reported that the first evidence of pulmonary toxicity may be fine crackling rales in the bases of the lungs. If bleomycin is discontinued when this sign first appears and systemic corticosteroid therapy instituted, the pulmonary toxicity may be completely reversible (De Lena, Guzzon, Monfardini, and Bonadonna, 1972). Studies in dogs have shown that the process of pulmonary fibrosis is similar to an interstitial pneumonitis and relatively responsive to high doses of corticosteroids (Fleischman *et al.,* 1971). Nevertheless, irreversible changes in the lung produced by bleomycin have been observed, and careful monitoring of pulmonary function as described above remains obligatory for all patients receiving this new antitumor agent. Bristol Laboratories has also noted that 12 of 1,568 evaluable patients (0.77 per cent) have developed a sudden anaphylactoid-like reaction, which was fatal in eight (Magers and Agre, 1972). However, all of these reactions occurred in patients with malignant lymphoma, and the risk of this serious side effect in patients with head and neck neoplasia appears minimal.

Adriamycin

Another agent which has recently undergone extensive clinical trials is the new anthracycline antibiotic, adriamycin. This drug, which differs from its parent compound daunorubicin by the substitution of a hydroxyl group on the number 14 carbon (Fig. 3), has shown activity in a number of experimental and human neoplasms. Unlike daunorubicin, which has its major activity limited to the chemotherapy of leukemias, adriamycin has shown activity in a wide variety of solid tumors including soft tissue sarcoma, breast carcinoma, bladder cancer, and squamous cell carcinoma (Gottlieb *et al.,* 1972; Middleman, Luce, and Frei, 1971).

Table 4 summarizes the results recorded in the treatment of patients with squamous cell carcinomas of the head and neck. Although the experience with this new agent is relatively limited, the response rate is encouraging, especially since most of the patients receiving this drug have had disease even further advanced than those receiving bleomycin. Another promising aspect of the responses to adriamycin is their duration. Unlike

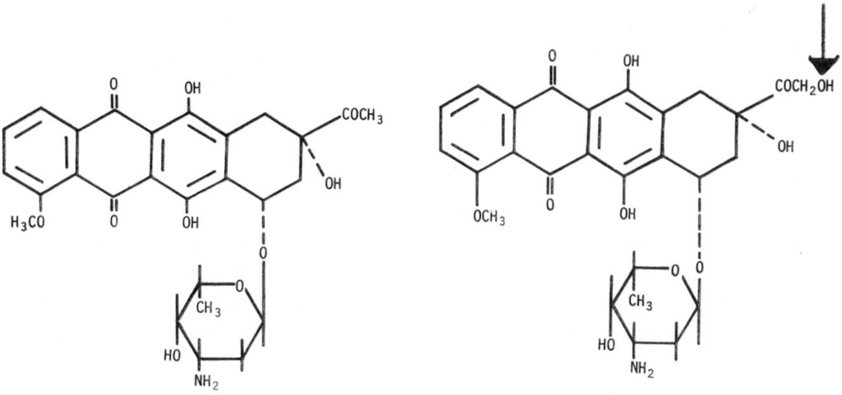

Daunorubicin
NSC-82151

Adriamycin
NSC-123127

Fig. 3.—Chemical structures of daunorubicin and adriamycin. Arrow indicates the hydroxyl substitution which is the only structural difference in the two compounds.

bleomycin, where durations longer than two months are unusual, the duration of many responses to adriamycin may be in excess of six months, and if the response is complete, considerably longer.

Adriamycin is supplied in a 10-mg. ampule containing an orange-red powder. The drug is currently available only on a research basis, but is expected to be commercially available soon. It is reconstituted with normal saline or distilled water and given as a rapid intravenous injection or infusion, taking care to avoid extravasation which will cause necrosis. The usual dose is 60 to 75 mg./M^2 of body surface area given every three weeks or as blood count recovery permits. Toxicity from adriamycin is limited predominantly to a predictable leukopenia and a near-complete alopecia. The fall in white count reaches its maximum approximately two

TABLE 4.—EFFICACY OF ADRIAMYCIN IN SQUAMOUS CELL
CARCINOMA OF THE HEAD AND NECK

NUMBER OF PATIENTS EVALUATED	NUMBER OF RESPONSES (>50% REGRESSION)	REFERENCE
13	6	O'Bryan et al. (1973)
9	4	DiPietro, DePalo, Molinari, and Gennari (1970)
4	1	Middleman, Luce, and Frei (1970)
4	2	Bonadonna et al. (1970)
30	13 (43%)	

weeks after drug administration, with rapid recovery thereafter. Alopecia begins approximately three weeks after the first dose and is often complete including axillary, facial, and pubic hair. With cessation of adriamycin therapy, hair regrowth has been noted in all cases. Other less common side effects include nausea, stomatitis, and a fever limited to the day of administration (Middleman, Luce, and Frei, 1971).

Although transient EKG changes are observed in approximately 10 per cent of patients receiving adriamycin, these changes appear to be readily reversible and are usually insignificant. A rare, more serious form of cardiotoxicity, congestive heart failure, appears to be directly dose-related. Thus congestive failure occurred only once in 366 patients who were treated with less than 550 mg./M^2 of adriamycin (0.27 per cent), but we observed 10 cases in the 33 patients who received more than 550 mg./M^2 of this drug (30 per cent). As a result of these observations, we currently limit our patients to no more than a total cumulative dosage of 550 mg./M^2 of adriamycin (Lefrak, Pitha, Rosenheim, and Gottlieb, 1973).

Combination chemotherapy with adriamycin has been most encouraging. The reproducibility of the myelosuppressive pattern of adriamycin has made it relatively simple to add adriamycin to other drugs, including cyclophosphamide, vincristine, and methotrexate. Trials of adriamycin in combination with these and other agents are currently in progress in several of the cooperative study groups, and further data concerning their efficacy in squamous cell carcinoma of the head and neck can be expected shortly.

One of the major reasons for including adriamycin in this article is that it may have great potential as a possible radiotherapeutic potentiator. Like actinomycin D, the mechanism of action of the anthracyclines (including adriamycin) appears to involve intercalation with nucleic acids (Calendi *et al.*, 1965). Observations of patients undergoing simultaneous radiotherapy and adriamycin chemotherapy have shown a greater skin reaction than that anticipated with radiotherapy alone (Gottlieb, unpublished data). Trials in several institutions are in progress, evaluating simultaneous administration of adriamycin and radiotherapy. The preliminary reports are encouraging, and these studies, when completed, may have great applicability to therapy for patients with carcinoma of the head and neck.

Other Drugs

While adriamycin and bleomycin are the most encouraging of the recently developed antitumor drugs currently in clinical trial, a number of other agents have also shown evidence for possible usefulness in therapy for metastatic squamous cell carcinoma. Among these are the nitrosoureas, particularly bis-choroethyl-nitrosourea (BCNU), which has been noted to produce two complete and two partial remissions in 25 patients with head and neck cancer. Several new oral nitrosoureas, including cyclohexyl-chloroethyl-nitrosourea (CCNU) and methyl CCNU, have recently begun clinical trials, and studies in laboratory animals suggest that these agents may be even more potent than BCNU (Carter, Schabel, Broder, and Johnston, 1972). Cytosine arabinoside, an antileukemic drug noted for its ability to inhibit DNA polymerase, has also shown promise in a limited study of patients with head and neck carcinoma. In one series of 20 patients, there were four responders. This agent may be particularly effective in rapidly growing tumors where the majority of cells are synthesizing DNA (Papac and Fischer, 1971).

Two other agents which have just entered clinical studies are the antibiotic, azacytidine, and the bacteriostatic agent, cis-dichlorodiammineplatinum. Among the first patients treated with these agents were several with squamous cell carcinoma, and a few responses have been recorded. It is too early to determine whether these agents will have therapeutic usefulness in carcinoma of the head and neck, but their lack of cross-resistance with conventional agents will make further studies with these two drugs of interest (Soper, 1972).

In addition to studies with new agents, a number of investigators have returned to some of the older agents in hope of exploiting new methods of utilizing these drugs. A notable example is methotrexate, where pioneer work by Djerassi (1967) and by Bertino (Bertino, Levitt, McCullough, and Chabner, 1971) has shown that extremely high doses of methotrexate can be tolerated by the patient if the normal tissue cells are rescued from methotrexate toxicity by citrovorum factor. This process, called "citrovorum rescue," has been intensively investigated by Bertino with encouraging results in head and neck carcinoma. In his studies, doses of methotrexate as high as several grams/M² have been well tolerated with less toxicity and better efficacy than that seen with conventional methotrexate therapy (Bertino, Levitt, McCullough and Chabner, 1971). A number of investigators have also explored methotrexate and 5-fluorouracil in adjuvant studies prior to or after radiotherapy and/or surgery (Friedman, DeNarvaes, and Daly, 1970; Vermund, Gollin, and Ansfield, 1969). Adjuvant studies offer the advantage of initiating therapy when there is relatively little residual tumor tissue remaining, thus increasing the likelihood of complete cell eradication with antitumor agents. This method of therapy may be one of the most promising, but further evaluation, especially with the newer agents, is still required.

Conclusions

Although many of the studies reported above must be considered preliminary, they indicate the steady improvement in chemotherapeutic techniques, as well as the increasing number of agents effective in treatment for advanced carcinoma of the head and neck. If the results of these early investigations are confirmed by the more extensive studies now in progress, then hopefully, goals beyond just palliation can be anticipated.

Acknowledgments

This investigation was supported by CA-05831, CA-10379, and CA-03754 from the National Cancer Institute.

Dr. Bodey is a Scholar of The Leukemia Society of America, Inc.

REFERENCES

Barranco, S. C., and Humphrey, R. M.: The effects of bleomycin on survival and cell progression in Chinese hamster cells *in vitro. Cancer Research*, 31:1218-1223, September 1971.

Bertino, J. R., Levitt, M., McCullough, J. L., and Chabner, B.: New approaches to chemotherapy with folate antagonists: Use of leucovorin "rescue" and enzymic folate depletion. *Annals of the New York Academy of Sciences*, 186:486-495, November 30, 1971.

Bonadonna, G., De Lena, M., Monfardini, S., Bartoli, C., Bajetta, E., Beretta, G., and Fossati-Bellani, F.: Clinical trials with bleomycin in lymphomas and in solid tumors. *European Journal of Cancer*, 8:205-215, August 1972.

Bonadonna, G., Monfardini, S., De Lena, M., Fossati-Bellani, F., and Beretta, G.: Phase I and preliminary phase II evaluation of adriamycin (NSC 123127). *Cancer Research*, 30:2572-2582, October 1970.

Calendi, E., Di Marco, A., Reggiani, B., Scarpinato, B., and Valentini, L.: On physico-chemical interactions between daunomycin and nucleic acids. *Biochimica et biophysica acta*, 103:25-49, May 11, 1965.

Carter, S. K., Schabel, F. M., Jr., Broder, L. E., and Johnston, T. P.: 1,3-Bis(2-chloroethyl)-1-nitrosourea (BCNU) and other nitrosoureas in cancer treatment: A review. *Advances in Cancer Research*, 16:273-332, 1972.

De Lena, M., Guzzon, A., Monfardini, S., and Bonadonna, G.: Clinical, radiologic and histopathologic studies on pulmonary toxicity induced by treatment with bleomycin (NSC-125066). *Cancer Chemotherapy Reports*, 56:343-356, June 1972.

Di Pietro, S., de Palo, G. M., Molinari, R., and Gennari, L.: Clinical trials with adriamycin by prolonged arterial infusion. *Tumori*, 56:233-244, 1970.

Djerassi, I.: Methotrexate infusions and intensive supportive care in the management of children with acute lymphocytic leukemia: Follow-up report. *Cancer Research*, 27:2561-2564, December 1967.

Fleischman, R. W., Baker, J. R., Thompson, G. R., Schaeppi, U. H., Illievski, V.

R., Cooney, D. A., and Davis, R. D.: Bleomycin-induced interstitial pneumonia in dogs. *Thorax,* 26:675-682, November 1971.

Frei, E., III, Whang, J., Scoggins, R. B., Van Scott, E. J., Rawl, D. P., and Ben,
M.: The stathmokinetic effect of vincristine. *Cancer Research,* 24:1918-1925,
December 1964.

Friedman, M., DeNarvaes, F. N., and Daly, J. F.: Treatment of squamous cell
carcinoma of the head and neck with combined methotrexate and irradiation.
Cancer, 26:711-721, September 1970.

Gottlieb, J. A.: Unpublished data.

Gottlieb, J. A., Baker, L. H., Quagliana, J. M., Luce, J. K., Whitecar, J. P., Jr.,
Sinkovics, J. G., Rivkin, S. E., Brownlee, R., and Frei, E., III: Chemotherapy
of sarcomas with a combination of adriamycin and dimethyl triazeno imidazole
carboxamide. *Cancer,* 30:1632-1638, December 1972.

Ichikawa, T., Nakano, I., and Hirokawa, I.: Bleomycin treatment of the tumors
of penis and scrotum. *The Journal of Urology,* 102:699-707, December 1969.

Lefrank, E. A., Pitha, J., Rosenheim, S., and Gottlieb, J. A.: A clinicopathologic
analysis of adriamycin cardiotoxicity. *Cancer,* 32:302-314, 1973.

Livingston, R. B., Bodey, G. P., Gottlieb, J. A., and Frei, E., III: Kinetic schedul-
ing of vincristine (NSC-67574) and bleomycin (NSC-125066) in patients
with lung cancer and other malignant tumors. *Cancer Chemotherapy Reports,*
57:219-224, April 1973.

Luce, J. K.: Clinical trials of bleomycin in solid tumors and lymphomas. (Abstract) *Proceedings of the American Association for Cancer Research,* 13:38,
1972.

Magers, C. F., and Agre, K.: Clinical summary on bleomycin. New drug application report of Bristol Laboratories to the Food and Drug Administration, September 1972.

Meyer, J. S., and Donaldson, R. C.: Growth-kinetics of squamous cell carcinoma
in man. A study of 4 squamous cell carcinomas using stathmokinetic effect of
vinblastine *in vivo. Archives of Pathology,* 87:479-490, May 1969.

Middleman, E., Luce, J., and Frei, E., III: Clinical trials with adriamycin. *Cancer,* 28:844-850, October 1971.

Mosher, M. B., DeConti, R. C., and Bertino, J. R.: Bleomycin therapy in advanced Hodgkin's disease and epidermoid cancers. *Cancer,* 30:56-60, July
1972.

O'Bryan, R. M., Luce, J. K., Talley, R. W., Gottlieb, J. A., Baker, L. H., and
Bonadonna, G.: Phase II evaluation of adriamycin in human neoplasia. *Cancer,*
32:1-8, July 1973.

Papac, R. J., and Fischer, J. J.: Cytosine arabinoside (NSC-63878) in the treatment of epidermoid carcinomas of the head and neck. *Cancer Chemotherapy
Reports,* 55:193-197, April 1971.

Salem, P. A.: Pulmonary changes and bleomycin. *The Cancer Bulletin,* 23:68-69,
November-December 1971.

Schabel, F. M., Jr.: Personal communication.

Soper, W. T., Editor: Proceedings of the phase I-phase II liaison meeting. Bethesda, Maryland, Cancer Therapy Evaluation Branch, National Cancer Institute,
March 9, 1972.

Sullivan, R. D., Miller, E., Wood, A. M., Clifford, P., Duff, J. K., Trussell, R., and
Burchenal, J.: Continuous infusion cancer chemotherapy in humans—effects of

therapy with intra-arterial methotrexate plus intermittent intramuscular citrovorum factor. *Cancer Chemotherapy Reports*, 10:39-44, December 1960.

Suzuki, M., Murai, A., Watanabe, T., and Nunokawa, O.: Treatment of cancer of the female genital organs with a new anti-cancer agent, bleomycin (BLM). *Acta medica et biologica*, 17:259-275, April 1970.

Takeda, K., Sagawa, Y., and Arakawa, T.: Therapeutic effect of bleomycin for skin tumors. *Gann*, 61:207-218, June 1970.

Vermund, H., Gollin, F. F., and Ansfield, F. J.: Clinical studies of 5-fluorouracil as adjuvant to radiotherapy. *Frontiers of Radiation Therapy and Oncology*, 4:132-158, 1969.

Umezawa, H., Ishizuka, M., Maeda, K., and Takeuchi, T.: Studies on bleomycin. *Cancer*, 20:891-895, 1967.

Wada, T.: Chemotherapy for esophageal cancer by bleomycin. (Abstract) *Tenth International Cancer Congress Abstracts*. Houston, Texas, The Medical Arts Publishing Co., 1970, pp. 492-493.

Yagoda, A., Krakoff, I., LaMonte, C., and Tan, C.: Clinical trial of bleomycin. (Abstract) *Proceedings of the American Association for Cancer Research*, 12: 37, 1971.

Panel Discussion: Cancer of the Larynx

MODERATOR: RICHARD H. JESSE, M.D.

Chief, Section of Head and Neck Surgery, Department of Surgery, The University of Texas System Cancer Center, M. D. Anderson Hospital and Tumor Institute, Houston, Texas

Dr. Jesse: We have selected cases of carcinoma of the larynx which, in some areas, are slightly controversial in the attempt to bring out various points. Four of the six cases were constructed to stress certain points.

CASE 1.—This 49-year-old man is in good general condition. He smokes 15 cigars a day. He does not drink alcohol. A verrucal lesion of the right vocal cord crosses the commissure and slightly infiltrates the anterior third of the left cord. There is little, if any, mobility change. There are no positive nodes. The laryngogram shows only slightly impaired motion of the left cord and some disease on the surfaces of both the right and left cords. A bulky lesion of the right cord bulges into the ventricle, but the cord is not fixed (Fig. 1A). The biopsy was invasive grade II, squamous cell carcinoma.

Dr. Roy B. Sessions, Associate Professor of Otolaryngology, Baylor College of Medicine, Houston, Texas: To manage this patient, other than the routine preoperative type of chest film, etc., I would have both a laryngogram and tomogram made before doing a biopsy. The radiotherapist and I see the patient together after the laryngograms and tomograms and before the biopsy. With the patient in the operating room and under general anesthesia, I would do a direct laryngoscopy and biopsy. The biopsy of this mucoid-looking tumor is very important. There is little doubt that it is neoplastic in origin, but the definition between a true histological verrucous carcinoma and squamous cell carcinoma is important. The laryn-

135

goscopy adds to the knowledge about the tumor and aids in studying the subglottic area anteriorly.

Dr. Jesse: Dr. Guillamondegui, would you have any other work-up procedures?

Dr. Oscar M. Guillamondegui, Assistant Professor of Surgery, Section of Head and Neck Surgery, The University of Texas System Cancer Center, M. D. Anderson Hospital and Tumor Institute, Houston, Texas: Assuming that the tomographic studies were done, the laryngogram would be important. It will show how much the vocal cords move. We should know if mobility is impaired and, if so, if it is caused by tumor bulk or cord fixation.

Dr. Byron J. Bailey, Department of Otolaryngology, The University of Texas Medical School, Galveston, Texas: The reason that it is important to make the differentiation between verrucous carcinoma and a verrucoid-appearing epidermoid carcinoma, is that radiation therapy is notoriously ineffective and is perhaps contraindicated in verrucous carcinoma. We have a situation where the anterior commissure of the larynx is involved and the vocal ligaments are attached anteriorly to the thyroid cartilage. If a conservative surgical procedure is done, it must be one of the anterior commissure procedures. The procedure should be one that allows us to remove most of one cord if necessary, and at least two thirds of the opposite cord all the way back to the opposite arytenoid. We must spare the arytenoid on one side and the posterior commissure and must remove a central segment of thyroid cartilage. The first goal obviously is to remove all malignant disease. The role of conservation surgery is to preserve as much laryngeal function as possible, including speech, swallowing, and the larynx's sphincteric function. If major parts of the larynx are resected, we must have a reliable reconstructive method and always remember that preserving the patient is the first goal and preserving the voice and the larynx and its other functions is the second goal. For this patient, at The University of Texas Medical School at Galveston, we would make a high thyroid incision which would allow us to be able to visualize and palpate the jugular lymph chains in order to be sure that there was no unsuspected metastatic disease. We then would come down on the midline on the thyroid cartilage and elevate the external perichondrium. We would elevate this very carefully since it will be used to line laryngeal lumen after reconstruction.

We then would make parallel cartilage cuts about 3-5 mm. from the midline of the thyroid ala, so we have a strip of cartilage 6-10 mm. wide. This is left with the specimen so the anterior commissure ligaments are not violated. The internal perichondrium inside of the thyroid ala is elevated back to the posterior margin of the thyroid ala on the side of lesser involvement, and at that point, the larynx is entered.

We would then make superior and anterior cuts and fold the larynx open, so we can visualize the tumor. Exposure and hemostasis, careful visualization, and careful outlining of the tumor are the keys to successful resection. After we have elevated the internal perichondrium on the opposite side, we can resect a great deal of the interior of the larynx with adequate margins. We then can reconstruct the interior of the larynx with sternohyoid muscle flaps, each of which has a covering of external thyroid perichondrium to provide a lining for the laryngeal lumen. This will prevent the formation of much granulation tissue and subsequent postoperative stenosis. The perichondrium muscle flap provides a cushion for the opposite cord to meet when only one arytenoid is left. It helps preserve an effective glottic sphincter mechanism to prevent aspiration, retards the medial collapse of the thyroid cartilage, and provides a good lining.

Dr. Joseph H. Ogura, Professor and Head of Otolaryngology, Washington University School of Medicine, St. Louis, Missouri: I would handle this somewhat differently. I would use the same approach that Dr. Bailey would except for one thing. On the major side of the lesion, I would resect the thyroid cartilage and swing this cartilage cut over 4 mm. Because we know the arytenoid was not invaded, I would leave the vocal process alone. For repair, I would use a McNaught Keel (a tantalum metal with three prongs) on the outside of the muscles and allow the vocal cord to reconstitute itself. It does and has very good mobility. Both cords can be resected just above the vocal process on either side and still maintain good glottic function.

Dr. Gilbert H. Fletcher, Professor of Radiotherapy, The University of Texas System Cancer Center, M. D. Anderson Hospital and Tumor Institute, Houston, Texas: You see in Figure 1A an anterior lesion with slight subglottic extension for which we would give 7,000 rads as indicated in Figure 1B. Through the years we have irradiated a number of lesions in which we cannot prove invasive squamous cell carcinoma. We keep on with irradiation because when we analyzed our results in 42 patients with similar lesions we found only two failures. In other words, we pay no attention to the verrucous disease with the exception of that on the buccal mucosa or the gum. One would not irradiate in situ carcinomas of the gum or of the buccal mucosa, but those on the vocal cord are different. When you remove that much larynx, as Dr. Ogura suggested, I really don't see how one could really and truly have a normal voice; maybe they do, I don't know. Anyway, at M. D. Anderson Hospital, we think they have a better voice if

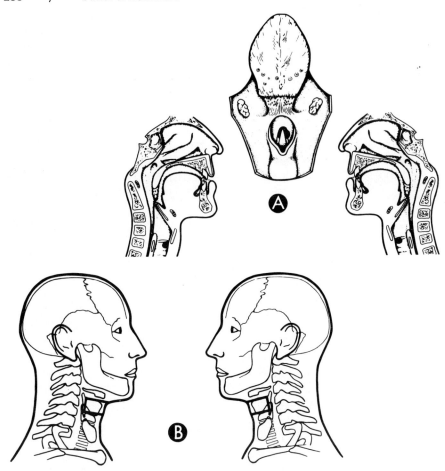

Fig. 1.—*A*, verrucal lesion in 49-year-old man, CASE 1; right vocal cord crossing the anterior commissure with no mobility change. *B*, area of application of 7,000 rads ⁶⁰Co in 6½ to 7 weeks using 5 × 4 inch lateral portals.

they are treated by radiation and if there is a failure, the surgical procedure is still available to salvage the patient.

Dr. Jesse: How many failures do you have—25%?

Dr. Fletcher: This is a T_2 lesion, and it is a large lesion. If it was a T_1, failure rate is exactly 10%, and it makes no difference whether the commissure is involved as long as the lesion is T_1, that is on the cord. Now, this is a T_2 lesion and it is off the cord; it is bulky and there is also partial loss of mobility. The failure rate is 25% in such lesions, but the 75% of patients in whom we succeed will have a normal voice in contrast to the less than optimal voice after partial laryngectomy.

Dr. Jesse: All right, now, let's say this happens to be one of those 25% which were radiation therapy failures. Dr. Ogura, what can you do now? Do you conserve the larynx or do you do a total laryngectomy?

Dr. Ogura: When you try to do postradiation surgery on cordal lesions, there are several things that you must bear in mind. (1) Is this a lesion that is on the cord? (2) Is this a T_2 lesion which is subglottic? Now, I have operated on many postradiation recurrences and I find the greatest difficulty is determining the exact site of the original tumor. When it recurs, the recurrence usually extends submucosally, making it difficult to clear the disease. We have some 30 postradiation cord recurrences that we have treated by hemilaryngectomy; I have failed in about 30% of these when the lesion was primarily extending 5 or 6 mm. subglottically and recurred. They recur just in the subglottic area and it's very deceptive when you do a hemilaryngectomy. I request frozen sections of the adjacent tissue before I decide to close the wound. In about half of the instances, they say it's negative; later they come back with a positive diagnosis and I must do a total. I always have to assume when you are close to a radiation recurrence, that it recurs in the original area; usually it does in the patients treated by radiation therapy. For a lesion of this magnitude which originally goes from vocal process to vocal process, I would not attempt conservative resection after radiation recurrence unless the recurrent cancer is limited to the cord. If it recurs only on one membranous cord, that's a different story. But since both cords are positive postradiation, I would do a total laryngectomy.

Dr. Jesse: I will now present the follow-up on this patient.

Twenty-seven months after radiation therapy, there was a recurrence on the anterior left cord and impaired motion. We performed an anterior lateral laryngofissure and attempted an extended frontolateral partial laryngectomy. Because the recurrence extended through the commissure and into cricoid thyroid membrane, total wide field laryngectomy was done with a left thyroid lobectomy and subtotal right thyroid lobectomy. The pathology report showed extension of cancer into the subglottic area on the left, to the right thyroid cartilage under an intact cord, and extension into the left thyroid lobe and isthmus. There were no positive nodes.

Dr. Fletcher: We have had 68 failures in 470 patients with T_1 and early T_2 vocal cord cancer. Of those, we have lost 6 patients to the disease, 6 only.

Dr. Jesse: Six is all we've lost, including both radiation therapy and surgery.

Dr. Fletcher: Right.

Dr. Sessions: One should recognize the tumor may quickly get out the weakest area.

Dr. Joe Selmer, Tyler, Texas: Is there any value in observing the mobility of cords with an image-intensifying fluoroscope?

Dr. Fletcher: I don't think so. The laryngogram, with the various maneuvers, is really the best study. You may not see much motion by indirect laryngoscopy. Referring to the lesion in Figure 1A, we now would treat it somewhat differently than shown in Figure 1B, because, with or without invasion of the commissure, when the disease extends subglottically, it does make a difference. Failure jumps from 10 to 25%. In the more recent years, we have extended our treatment fields downward and never give less than 7,000 rads.

Dr. Sam Jampolis, M. D. Anderson Hospital: With the type of surgery that was originally proposed, what would be the functional result as far as speech is concerned?

Dr. Bailey: Dr. Ogura mentioned that he allows the area to granulate. He and others have reported that functional result is good. With the more classical type of hemilaryngectomy with a mucosal closure, the voice was very weak and the patients have a tendency to aspirate. The use of the bipedicle muscle flap seemed to result in a considerably stronger voice, particularly when the patient was willing to go through a fairly rigorous course of speech therapy.

Dr. Michael Flynn, Louisville, Kentucky: If you use a keel and leave both arytenoids, the voice is excellent. It is not normal, but it is a little husky.

Dr. Sessions: When you take out both vocal cords and put a keel in, a new vocal cord is formed. It is a brand new sort of cord that moves in and out and they have a nice voice. Now, if you do a hemilaryngectomy, their voice is hoarse. If you put a muscle pedicle flap in, then you get a good voice, because a new pseudocord is formed. If the arytenoid is removed, the bulk must be filled in. If not, the patient has no voice. Hence, I fill it up as if I'm creating a new false cord, or pseudocord.

Dr. Flynn: Dr. Ogura, what percentage of patients with T_1 and T_2 lesions treated by partial laryngectomy come to total laryngectomy either because of recurrences or functional problems?

Dr. Ogura: The difference is 92 or 93% for T_1 lesions and 80% for T_2 lesions.

Dr. Flynn: What percentage eventually ends with total laryngectomy?

Dr. Ogura: About 10% of that group come back with recurrence and a total laryngectomy is done. The rest die of other diseases; this is an absolute mortality because I calculate all death rates.

Dr. Fletcher: But you can't have 90% at five years, Joe. Some must die of coronary disease.

Dr. Jesse: I think the answer there is that you, Dr. Ogura, get a little different group of patients in that the population that comes to your private office is medically a better group than those Dr. Fletcher sees. Is your patient population from your VA Hospital in your series?

Dr. Ogura: Oh, no, not the VA. Mine are younger patients.

Dr. Jesse: I think that's the answer. Let's go to the second case.

CASE 2.—This patient has a T_2N_0 lesion of the right vocal cord with moderate but not complete fixation. The arytenoid is not involved (Fig. 2). The laryngogram shows the lesion going to the commissure and coming back on the cord, and going subglottically down to just above the cricoid cartilage.

Dr. Jesse: Dr. Bailey, what work-up would you want here other than the mirror examination and laryngogram, and how would you do it?

Dr. Bailey: Certainly the next step would be a very careful direct laryngoscopy to determine the exact extent of subglottic extension. This is not easy because you are looking down a 17- or 18-cm. long tube. We believe that we can do a better examination under general anesthesia using a very small cut in the tracheal tube. With the patient asleep, he is free from any coughing reflex and does very little swallowing. We are then able to use an anterior commissure laryngoscope to determine quite accurately

FIG. 2.—T_2N_0 squamous cell carcinoma right vocal cord with subglottic extension (CASE 2). Partial fixation of right cord is shown.

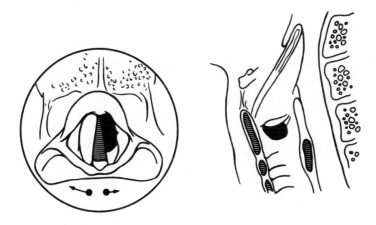

whether it is a 7-, 10-, or 13-mm. subglottic extension. We immediately
have two or three separate examiners diagram their impression of the extent of the lesion on forms that are present in the operating room. These
are the most important documents to which we can refer during the course
of treating a patient. Other things that we will look for are other areas of
tumor extension, second primaries, and the degree of cord mobility. In
other words, we don't go directly to the obvious lesion and then stop; but
we go through a thoroughly planned, orderly sequence of examination.

Dr. Jesse: Dr. Sessions, how would you handle this problem?

Dr. Sessions: I think that it is important to recognize what type of patient that you are dealing with who has this particular lesion. Let us
assume, first, that we have a reliable patient whose personal life regarding
use of cigarettes and alcohol is reasonable. With this type of patient we
can use the indirect mirror to examine him quite well. With this patient,
at Baylor, we would want to begin radiotherapy, using the philosophy of
going up to a moderate dose; if there is obvious tumor regression and if,
hopefully, mobility returns, we carry him to a therapeutic dose of between
6,000 and 7,000 rads. The radiotherapist would be able to decide. If there
is not obvious tumor regression, or if cord mobility does not improve, the
difficulty then begins. The problem becomes one of evaluation. The fact
that the cord does not move after say about 4,000 rads of cobalt doesn't
mean that the tumor is necessarily out of control. It may be fibrosis and
scarring that causes this lack of mobility. What it does, I think, is impair
your judgment ability and lessens your ability to follow this tumor during
the course of radiotherapy. I think that in the patient in whom significant
progress is not made after a moderate dose of radiotherapy has been given
and, if the subglottic extension is of a posterior type, a total laryngectomy
should be done. If the patient has anterior type subglottic extension, where
it is easier to encompass surgically, I would do a conservative hemi-type
laryngectomy.

Dr. Jesse: At what dose would you make the decision?

Dr. Sessions: In talking with the radiotherapist, we think that at about
4,000 rads we have a dose level at which we can make some judgment as
to the regression of tumor growth. If this is an unreliable patient or a
patient who is difficult to examine, my feeling would be to begin with a
hemilaryngectomy. The point is that cord immobility, or at least decreasing cord mobility, certainly doesn't necessarily contraindicate either surgery or radiotherapy, but is a real danger sign. Impaired mobility indicates, obviously, some sort of muscle involvement. This may be tumor just
adjacent to muscle causing myositis from the tumor edge. It may be super-

ficial invasion of the thyroid cartilage or fixation as the tumor gradually moves medially and subglottically.

Dr. Fletcher: I think we would treat that case by irradiation and I agree with Dr. Sessions that we, with the head and neck surgeon, would take another look at it at the 4,000 rad level. I think that that way the mobility can be better evaluated with the laryngogram. At 4,000 rads, if the lesion has completely disappeared, you know it was exophytic and then complete the radiation therapy. We would, of course, extend the radiation field down to include the entire cricoid and perhaps even include part of the trachea. You might as well be generous with it. And we would go to 7,000 rads; but after the dose reaches 5,500 rads the arytenoid would be left out of the field. In this way no edema develops. In the last 250 patients so treated for vocal cord lesions, only two patients developed edema and in both there were some extenuating circumstances.

Dr. Jesse: Dr. Guillamondegui, would you do a partial hemilaryngectomy or something like that on the 25% of patients in whom radiotherapy failed?

Dr. Guillamondegui: No, I don't think so, for this type of lesion. If treatment of the lesion failed when adequate radiation therapy was given, I would be very suspicious of the type of lesion it is and I would rather do a total laryngectomy.

Dr. Fletcher: When there are other extensive lesions, limited to the cord or the anterior commissure, of 68 recurrences in some 400 plus patients, 55 were right in the middle of the cord. This is why some had cordectomies and some had partial laryngectomies. We were dealing with lesions which were not early vocal cord cancers.

Dr. Sessions: I wouldn't do a partial laryngectomy with irradiation recurrence after the initial lesion looked like this.

Dr. Andrew Jensen, San Antonio, Texas: I would like to refer the question to Dr. Bailey. He referred to an adequate examination of the subglottic area and referred to millimeters. Do you use a microscope, some type of measuring apparatus, or how do you measure in millimeters?

Dr. Bailey: We have the ability to work from a fixed point in most cases, usually from the upper central incisors and by positioning the anterior commissure laryngoscope exactly at the level of the uninvolved cord. We then advance this laryngoscope, keeping the lesion in view until we reach its inferior margin. We then can measure on the scope pretty accurately how far we've gone. This is not possible using the Jako Laryngoscope usually employed with microscopic laryngoscopy, but it is possible with the small anterior commissure scope.

Dr. Fletcher: The best way is to measure it on the lateral laryngogram. By knowing the magnification factor you can very simply measure the exact lower limit.

Dr. Sessions: We use the opposite cord. We take into account the method of taking pictures and assume that it is a 12 to 10 times magnification. This would take into account that the image is larger. This may vary depending on tube distance. I think Dr. Fletcher is quite right that we can measure accurately the exact lower limit. The only other thing you have to be sure of is that on direct laryngoscopy the tumor is not posterior and subglottic. This is a very important matter of differentiation.

Dr. A. Fletcher Clark, San Antonio, Texas: Does any panel member use suspension laryngoscopy in the right-angled bronchoscope for evaluation of subglottic lesions?

Dr. Sessions: I don't. But I'll tell you another way you can evaluate the lesion but it is a little risky. In Europe, they use what is called transconioscopy. They stick a perforator below the cricoid and then they inspect it from below. I don't think we're doing this in America but they use this particularly in Sweden.

Dr. Goldstein, Lycea, California: I want to know if I did right or wrong. Apparently I did wrong. Just last week, I saw a 25-year-old Spanish male who had had hoarseness for seven months. He was on heroin for several years but is on methadone now. His whole larynx was filled. I could not identify anything. Just a few days before, a general surgeon did a surgical exploration because he thought the patient had thyroiditis or something in the thyroid. The surgeon found a fistulous tract going up into the larynx through the cartilage. When we did the thyroidotomy, we found an extensive lesion destroying one true cord, half of the other cord, and extending down really past the cricoid. We, of course, did a complete laryngectomy. There were no positive nodes; we took out the two upper tracheal rings leaving about a 5 mm. or so margin and we only took out half of the thyroid lobe on the side where we thought the lesion had originated. This was an exophytic type of squamous cell carcinoma. Should I have done more or less? No radiotherapy was given.

Dr. Jesse: I think the answer is that until you were in, you didn't know with what you were dealing. Apparently, the lesion was so big that there was no way to really find out what it was. Isn't that what you are saying? I think most of us would probably have done what you did.

CASE 3.—This is a T_3N_{2B} transglottic lesion involving the true and false cords, the laryngeal face of the epiglottis, and the interarytenoid area (Fig. 3). It crosses the midline at that point. The aryepiglottic fold was involved to the rim and the right side of the larynx was fixed. There are

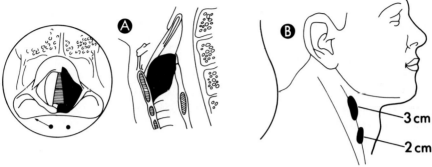

Fig. 3.—case 3. *A*, T_3N_{2B} transglottic lesion involving true and false cords crosses the posterior midline with the right side of larynx fixed. *B*, two ipsilateral nodes were clinically positive.

two ipsilateral movable nodes. The lesion comes down to the bottom of the thyroid cartilage, goes up on to the epiglottis and goes back on the ary-epiglottic fold. The patient with this bulky lesion is breathing somewhat poorly.

Dr. Jesse: Dr. Guillamondegui, what would you do with this man?

Dr. Guillamondegui: Well, this patient probably needs a laryngectomy and seems to have respiratory problems. Initially the laryngectomy should be done. I would not consider doing a tracheostomy and waiting for a period of time. I prefer to do the tracheostomy and then immediately do the laryngectomy and the radical neck dissection, unless, of course, his general physical condition was so poor that we would prefer not to operate on him at all.

Dr. Jesse: So, Dr. Guillamondegui, you would do the laryngectomy as an emergency, if he was breathing poorly, rather than doing a tracheostomy?

Dr. Guillamondegui: Yes, since the lesion was described as being a carcinoma.

Dr. Jesse: You made the assumption that it was carcinoma. What if you saw him in the middle of the night? Would you still do the laryngectomy?

Dr. Guillamondegui: I think it would be a pleasure to get the pathologist into the operating room in the middle of the night.

Dr. Jesse: That's exactly what I'd hoped you'd say. Dr. Sessions, what would you do? Anything new or different?

Dr. Sessions: First of all, the treatment that I would ultimately do would be a little different. I would certainly do a total laryngectomy and right neck dissection but I think on N_2 necks it has been shown that postoperative radiotherapy in the range of 5,500 rads in five or six weeks is very beneficial. So, I would follow the total laryngectomy and neck dissection with postoperative radiation. I would include the stoma in the field of therapy.

Dr. Jesse: You would include the stoma?

Dr. Sessions: I would. Regarding the preoperative tracheostomy, I really don't know about this. My feeling is that I think the incidence of stoma recurrence is related more to the subglottic location, and their size is of more importance, rather than the time sequence of tracheostomy and laryngectomy. That may not be so true without postoperative radiotherapy. I don't know.

Dr. Jesse: Do I understand that you are more worried about the cells in the lymphatics of the mucosa than you are about contamination of an emergency tracheostomy?

Dr. Sessions: All I am saying is that I'm not convinced that theoretical seeding from a tracheostomy exists. It does exist when you have an exophytic tumor. It exists all the time. So, if a man is breathing poorly, I am certainly not against doing the laryngectomy if it is convenient. If for some reason, nutritionally or something else, we have to put off the laryngectomy but have to tracheostomize this patient, I don't see any great harm.

Dr. Jesse: Dr. Ogura, either you or one of your men wrote something about stoma recurrence, didn't you, in relation to tracheostomies at one time?

Dr. Ogura: Yes, stomal recurrence was predominately associated with lesions in the subglottis, transglottic lesions or glottic lesions that extend subglottically. We never did see any with pure supraglottic lesions or those of the pyriform fossa. The incidence of seeding is not that high. Recurrence has been variously reported anywhere from 7 to 40% in the stoma. We didn't have anything like that.

Dr. Fletcher: You did not even have 7%?

Dr. Ogura: We did have 7%, but did not have 40%. Stomal recurrence has been reported 40% in other series and has been related to the tracheostomy. Our pathologists, Ackerman and Bauer, have never been able to determine whether they are lymphatics or nodes or what they are. You have a problem with a patient who has a poor airway. I don't like to do laryngectomies and neck dissections without a biopsy.

Dr. Jesse: Do you get Dr. Ackerman up in the middle of the night?

Dr. Ogura: No, I don't think so. If this patient came in at midnight, obviously you'd have to do a tracheotomy on this patient and not get a pathologist up in the middle of the night. If the patient needs a tracheotomy, you have to do it, that's all. Then, in our institution, we would start with irradiation first in a large lesion that extends subglottically even though our data show that preoperative radiation does not help transglottic lesions. We are not sure that it doesn't help the nodes. I think it does in higher doses. After surgery we complete our radiation, split the dose.

Dr. Jesse: So, you would give what, 3,000 rads, then operate and then give another 2,000 rads?

Dr. Ogura: Right.

Dr. Jesse: Dr. Bailey, what would you do?

Dr. Bailey: Well, I would not do an emergency laryngectomy and neck dissection. I think that Dr. Ogura's study and those of others have indicated that the stoma recurrence is associated with the size and the subglottic extension of the tumor and not to the fact that you have done a tracheotomy. At least that is the impression that I have. I would like to have even more than a biopsy. I would like to have a day or two to study this patient and get some blood studies and find out whether his heart, lungs, liver, and kidneys are functioning as well as I would like them to be. I would then proceed with total laryngectomy and radical neck dissection on the involved side. I have not had any experience with postoperative radiation.

Dr. Jesse: Let me ask you a question. Suppose you did come in the middle of the night and did a tracheostomy because your pathologist wouldn't get out of bed. How long would you wait until you did the definitive procedure? Would it make any difference to you?

Dr. Bailey: If you ask me, I would like to do it as soon as the patient's general medical condition was known and was stable. I'd like to do it within two or three days.

Dr. Jesse: Some of the older literature says that you should wait a minimum of two weeks probably because of infection at that time. Do you think that is still valid?

Dr. Bailey: I certainly don't understand the rationale for waiting.

Dr. Jesse: Dr. Fletcher, would you accept this patient? Two or three want to give him to you for postoperative radiation. Would you treat him postoperatively or would you want him to have radiation primarily?

Dr. Fletcher: Not primarily, but I'd accept him for postoperative treatment under certain circumstances. Were the nodes positive?

Dr. Jesse: Yes.

Dr. Fletcher: We do not routinely do postoperative radiotherapy in such cancer patients. We would if the nodes are positive in the surgical specimen. We would not if the nodes are negative or if the subglottic extension doesn't extend below the level of the thyroid cartilage. Certainly, the stoma recurrences are direct function of the extent of the subglottic disease. So if there is extensive subglottic disease you have to include the stoma in the radiation field, otherwise in such patients, in our experience, recurrence has been 25%. It creates some problem, but it is a must. When there is a stoma recurrence, the patient has had it; the disease goes down along the trachea and mediastinum. Now, the fact that he had nodes presenting in the neck would be a reason in itself to use postoperative radiation because two nodes were positive and you'd expect 50% recurrence in the radically dissected neck. Now, another indication for postoperative radiation is in the even more extensive cases where the disease has gone through the cartilage into the tissues of the neck. That is connective tissue infiltration, so of course, you would use radiation. Only one patient in three gets postoperative radiation for extensive vocal cord cancer for these reasons. In patients who receive radiation, we would give 6,000 rads to the upper neck and 5,000 rads to the lower neck (Fig. 4). Perhaps, at times, if there were very bad subglottic extension we may use the electron beam and give another 1,000 rads over the stoma. Why the electron beam? Because if you use cobalt or 6 MeV initially without the larynx being present, the spinal cord is only something like 3.5 to 4 cm. deep and if you give 5,000 rads to the spinal cord one risks chronic myelitis. One must be careful of the spinal cord dose.

Question from Audience: Considering that this lesion extended across the midline and the nodes on the dominant side were positive nodes, would you consider doing an elective surgical procedure on the contralateral neck?

Dr. Fletcher: There is no need for that if you use postoperative radiation.

Dr. Jesse: We would probably do a jugular node dissection on the other

FIG. 4.—CASE 3, areas of postoperative radiation. *A*, upper neck field, 6,000 rads ⁶⁰Co. *B*, anterior lower field, 5,000 rads ⁶⁰Co or a combination of ⁶⁰Co and electron beam.

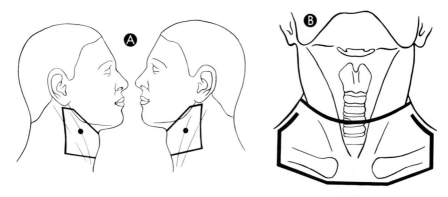

side. We would take out the midjugular and low jugular nodes. That gets the first echelon. But Dr. Fletcher is right; the postoperative radiation treatment obviates the necessity for doing the second neck.

Dr. A. J. Ballantyne, M. D. Anderson Hospital: I haven't heard anyone say anything about the paratracheal nodes or the metastasis into the thyroid in a situation like this.

Dr. Guillamondegui: We routinely try to include those nodes in the wide field laryngectomy so if there is a question of metastasis in the chain of nodes, they can be removed at the time of the surgical resection.

Dr. Ballantyne: I think that many of the stoma recurrences are actually due to paratracheal nodes which are missed at the time of surgery. Also, in a lesion of this character, the tumor tends to stream out between the cricoid and along the recurrent laryngeal nerve, so I think it's very important to resect the thyroid on that side plus the recurrent laryngeal nerve and the paratracheal nodes way down into the mediastinum.

Dr. James Harrington, Arlington, Texas: Back to the midnight laryngectomy. I don't think this is good. In the middle of the night I am not at peak efficiency; the operating room staff is not at peak efficiency. You get less than the best results under these circumstances. When you do a tracheotomy, a high tracheotomy should be done, and this lends itself to further therapeutic procedures. You can resect the temporary stoma later if necessary.

Dr. Pete Naman, Lamesa, Texas: Would the panel approach the neck any differently if you had the same primary lesion but no clinically palpable nodes?

Dr. Sessions: I would not do a radical neck dissection on an N_0 neck.

Dr. Jesse: Would you do a wide field laryngectomy?

Dr. Sessions: I would do a wide field laryngectomy and I would most assuredly give postoperative radiation therapy up to about 5,500 rads or so. In N_0 necks, 5,500 rads cuts down the incidence of nodes appearing later in the neck by 90% or so.

Dr. Bailey: I don't agree, but I also would like to ask another question of the panel. There has been a good discussion about positive nodes in the neck and good discussion about subglottic extension, but I have read and heard that the most serious prognostic sign in any carcinoma of the larynx, and I think it is reflected in the new TNM system, is the fixed cord. With the fixed cord I would expect occult metastasis and I would expect that my fingers are not talented enough to feel some of the nodes, particularly paratracheal nodes, so I would do a neck dissection. I wonder if Dr. Ogura has any comments about what degree of seriousness cord fixation has when compared to positive nodes or subglottic extension.

Dr. Ogura: Initially we reported on a series on transglottic lesions which we did not radiate; the incidence of occult nodes was high, about 50%. With the advent of 3,000 rads of preoperative radiation, I continued to do elective neck dissections. The incidence of occult nodes dropped to about half. I suppose this means that this dose of irradiation at least causes difficulty for a pathologist in finding whether those nodes are positive. Our present concepts regarding these transglottic lesions are that only for these massive lesions would we do an elective neck dissection. When you have a big lesion, you should do an elective neck dissection. I don't consider that a contralateral neck dissection is indicated for a transglottic lesion, because our series shows that contralateral metastases are practically zero.

Dr. Jesse: Even when the lesion crosses the posterior midline?

Dr. Ogura: We would consider giving postoperative radiation at the time of elective surgery if the lowest nodes are positive. I would warn against doing a high tracheotomy through tumor tissue. I don't think it is a good policy to do a high tracheotomy. If you do one through the first tracheal ring, the lesion might extend below that. If you do it unknowingly, that's another matter, but I still prefer a low tracheotomy.

Dr. Robert Komorn, Baylor College of Medicine, Houston, Texas: Dr. Guillamondegui, you didn't discuss the possibility of distant metastasis. If a distant metastasis were found in the posttracheostomy workup, would you manage the laryngeal lesion any differently than you described? When you plan to do an emergency laryngectomy, do you have time to find a lung or liver metastasis? Are you concerned about this when you do your emergency laryngectomy?

Dr. Guillamondegui: I am not talking about an emergency laryngectomy in the emergency room. The patient is in the hospital and has been here for a couple of hours. In this time he has had time to have a chest x-ray film taken, etc. This is essentially the same type of workup that he would have routinely or electively. If we find he has a couple of lung shadows, then we must decide whether it is worth trying to prove these shadows to be metastases and whether they will change our approach to the larynx. He is obstructed and has a large lesion. I would probably go ahead with the laryngectomy. This does not mean that the presence of distant metastases should not be investigated. In some types of patients with a smaller lesion, probably a tracheostomy would suffice. I believe this man will have problems swallowing and talking and he will eventually have a necrotic mass in the neck. He will therefore have benefit from a laryngectomy even if he eventually dies of his distant metastases.

Dr. Jesse: Let's go on to the next case.

CASE 4.—This patient is 66; he drinks a wee bit and he smokes a fair number of cigars. He has a lesion of the false cord with extension to the arytenoid. The lesion is not on the true cord nor at the commissure. The motion of the larynx is good; squamous cell carcinoma Grade II has been found and there are no positive nodes in the neck (Fig. 5).

Dr. Ogura: There's no question in my mind. I would do a conservative operation on this patient. I would do an elective neck dissection because in such cases, the incidence of occult metastases is high in our series. I would not treat this man with full irradiation.

Dr. Jesse: You wouldn't use radiation at all?

Dr. Ogura: We reviewed the preoperative irradiation group and found that radiation didn't influence the course of the disease. Biologically these tumors behave pretty well. They're not very aggressive at this point unless the nodes have appeared. The occult nodes surprise me. The cure rate for such patients is very high when treated surgically. I do an elective neck dissection simply because of the continuing incidence of occult nodes. If the lesion were higher than this and less than 2 cm. we don't do a neck dissection, for example, on the petiolus epiglottis. You should expect an 80% survival rate with such patients.

Dr. Bailey: Occasionally the lesions involving the lower third of the false cord and extending over to the arytenoid may be amenable to treatment by a vertical rather than the supraglottic procedure. The postoperative recovery period, at least in my patients, is much easier for patients who have undergone a vertical procedure with a reconstructive component. I do keep my eyes peeled for the occasional false cord lesion that can be so treated.

Dr. Ogura: Would you, though, in this case?

Dr. Bailey: No, I wouldn't. The lesion is too high and too far posteriorly.

Fig. 5.—CASE 4, illustration showing area of involvement of squamous cell carcinoma of the right false cord. Carcinoma bulges into the ventricle and comes up to the arytenoid, but does not extend over to the pyriform fossa. The commissure is clear and motion is normal.

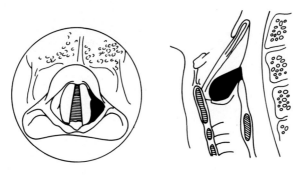

Dr. Guillamondegui: The good mobility of the cord seems to indicate that this is a rather superficial lesion. I would have this patient treated by radiation and I think that the success in this type of treatment for a T_2 lesion is pretty good. At least it is over 80%.

Dr. Jesse: Dr. Fletcher, would you accept this patient for primary treatment?

Dr. Fletcher: We would be delighted. We would expect an 80% survival just like Dr. Ogura indicated for his partial laryngectomy. We do have one benefit, however; if we irradiate the neck, we would expect the sterilization of the occult metastases that Ogura says are present.

Dr. Jesse: How would you treat the patient, Dr. Fletcher?

Dr. Fletcher: The field that we would treat the patient with is shown in Figure 6. Perhaps the field would include a little more of the upper and midjugular nodes than is shown in the diagram. We would treat the subdigastric and midjugular nodes to 5,000 rads and then reduce the field over the primary area and go to 6,500 rads in 6½ weeks as you see here.

Dr. Jesse: You wouldn't treat the lower neck?

Dr. Fletcher: There is no point to that. The nodes in the lower neck are rarely positive and irradiating the lower neck will increase our complications. If we use the fields shown in Figure 6, patients have perfect function.

Dr. Jesse: Dr. Ogura would do it with radical neck dissection and a partial laryngectomy. Dr. Fletcher would do it with radiation alone and include a portion of the neck where the occult nodes grow, and Dr. Sessions would do the supraglottic laryngectomy and leave the neck for his radiotherapist to treat.

Fig. 6.—CASE 4, treatment area for a T_2N_0 squamous cancer of the false vocal cord.

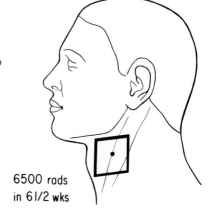

6500 rads
in 6 1/2 wks

Dr. Eleanor Montague, The Methodist Hospital, Houston, Texas: I wouldn't irradiate the neck. We have heard a great deal about surgical salvage of radiation therapy failures. Dr. Fletcher, could you tell us about radiation therapy salvages of surgical failures? Another question relates to the conservative procedure. Everyone now wants the better part of two worlds. They want to do the conservative procedure and they want the irradiation because they are convinced that it is good and reduces the local recurrence problem, both in the neck and at the primary site. But, how feasible is it to treat with high doses a larynx which has had conservative procedure?

Dr. Fletcher: If you wait for a gross recurrence, radiation salvage is next to zero. One must not wait for surgical recurrence. The patient must be treated postoperatively very quickly. Of all the lesions of the supraglottic larynx, the false cords are the better ones from the standpoint of fewer ipsilateral and contralateral metastases. This is not true of the epiglottis. Such lesions do have a fair number of contralateral metastases. The lesions of the false cords produce fewer metastases of any site within the supraglottic larynx. I don't mean they don't metastasize; it's just that the metastasis is less than in the aryepiglottic fold and the epiglottis.

Dr. Ogura: One big problem is comparing staging systems. The radiotherapist compares it with his tomogram and his indirect film. The surgeon or the plastic surgeon or otolaryngologist stages it as he sees the lesion and as the specimen comes out. There are two different things.

Dr. Fletcher: I might hasten to add that we don't change the staging, not even to coincide with the pathological staging later on.

Dr. Robert Steckler, M. D. Anderson Hospital, Houston, Texas: I would like to ask Dr. Ogura about the supraglottic laryngectomy in a 66-year-old man whom Dr. Jesse described as "drinks a bit." I think a pint a day is a good bit, even in Texas. What percentage of your patients wind up with radiologic evidence of aspiration following the supraglottic, especially in the older age group like this patient?

Dr. Ogura: Well, I make sure that the patient is not a pulmonary cripple. If he is, he doesn't get the conservative operation. I'd use the stair test, walking up two flights. If he can do this without getting short of breath, he is a good candidate. Of course, like anybody else, I have to be sure that the patient doesn't have liver disease. If the patient has, we get our best internist, who is a surgical internist. In this case, as you have depicted it, I would take the arytenoid out and I would fix the vocal process in the midline. I lighten the anesthesia and put a catheter down the tracheal bronchial tree and make absolutely certain that I had the cord in the midline without a triangular chink. In my earlier cases, I would get a little chink and then I would have to do some modification by injecting Teflon to get glottic closure. The function for these patients is excellent.

CASE 5.—This patient has a T_2N_{3B} lesion of the suprahyoid epiglottis with extension to the right arytenoid, but not into the valleculum (Fig. 7A). There are two movable nodes on the right and one on the left (Fig. 7B).

Dr. Jesse: Dr. Bailey, what would you do with this one?

Dr. Bailey: We would approach this with a supraglottic laryngectomy and a neck dissection on the side of greater involvement and come back later, if those were, indeed, histologically positive nodes, with a second neck dissection on the contralateral side in a period of six weeks.

Dr. Jesse: You'd do a staged neck procedure, then.

Dr. Bailey: Yes.

FIG. 7.—CASE 5. *A*, squamous cell carcinoma of suprahyoid epiglottis with extension to the right arytenoid. *B*, bilateral clinically positive movable nodes.

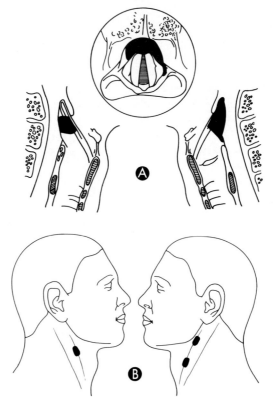

Dr. Ogura: Well, I know how this case was treated but I don't agree with it. I would give this patient 4,000 rads to the nodes. I wouldn't worry about the primary and I would go in on the lesser side and do a neck dissection, leaving one internal jugular vein. The node is not big, so I'd strip the vein. Then I'd do a complete neck dissection on the opposite side, do a supraglottic procedure and then close up.

Dr. Jesse: When you say strip, what do you mean?

Dr. Ogura: You just strip the nodes and do a radical neck dissection, leaving the internal jugular veins. The morbidity rate of taking both internal jugular veins is quite significant.

Dr. Jesse: Would you take the 11th nerve and the muscle out on both sides?

Dr. Ogura: Well, in a classical neck dissection that is done. According to the nodes shown in Figure 7B the spinal accessory would be posterior. One could take it out and put a nerve graft in on both sides if he wanted. I would, in essence, do a bilateral neck dissection and a partial supraglottic.

Dr. Sessions: There is no question about the bilaterality of the metastasis and the nodes are hard. I think the significant point about this case is the fact that this tumor is biologically a bad tumor. You have a patient who has a lesion in an area that is a unilateral type structure and yet the main element of metastasis is contralateral. The tone of the therapy here should be the most aggressive therapy that you can possibly deliver. This is a combination of surgical resection plus high-dose postoperative radiation therapy. In order to deliver all the radiotherapy that I think is indicated, I would do a total laryngectomy with bilateral neck dissection and postoperative radiotherapy. I think I would do a modified neck dissection on the left, perhaps. The lesion is resectable by a partial laryngectomy but in order to deliver the amount of radiotherapy that I would want, I would do a total because postoperatively the supraglottis wouldn't tolerate the amount of radiotherapy.

Dr. Guillamondegui: I agree that some of these lesions are biologically very active. It would seem to me that this lesion could conceivably be radiated and followed by a modified neck dissection if the nodes are persistent or large enough to justify doing that. If the lesion is not controlled by radiation, although I think it has a fair chance of being controlled, then of course, a total laryngectomy would be the procedure.

Dr. Jesse: We would treat the primary area and both sides of the neck as indicated in Figure 8. In order to sterilize those nodes, the radiation dose would have to be very high, in which case the fibrosis and trouble rates would be much higher. So we would go in and do a modified neck dissection bilaterally after we are sure the radiation therapy has secured the primary. If the primary is positive, a total laryngectomy is also done with the modified neck dissection.

Dr. Luis Krause, Mexico City: I heard Dr. Bailey say that he would do a staged neck dissection. I want to ask him if he wouldn't worry about waiting six weeks when he knows there is tumor in the nodes in the neck?

Dr. Bailey: No, I would not worry about the six-week wait because if you have a large series of patients, the morbidity and mortality will be lower by waiting that period of time than they would be if you did both sides of the neck at the same time, even though you save the jugular vein on the second side with two operations.

Dr. Michael Flynn, Louisville, Kentucky: What percentage of patients receiving a conservative supraglottic operation on the larynx have functional problems and what percentage of these eventually go on to total laryngectomy?

Dr. Ogura: I have done 500 of these, excluding hemilaryngectomies. In only two cases have I had to remove the larynx because of functional problems.

Dr. Fletcher: In all of these patients, the neck has been much neglected. Nobody mentions recurrences in the neck. I mean if one side was positive for two nodes and assuming they would be positive surgically, that means that according to data of Memorial Hospital, there is at least a 50% risk of recurrence in that neck, plus the other neck is also positive, another 36%.

Dr. Bailey: I am sorry that I can't give you the exact percentage, but I would estimate that taking all cases it wouldn't be more than 20%.

Dr. Jesse: Dr. Fletcher, what kind of results can you expect with irradiation?

Fig. 8.—case 5. A, fields shown receive 5,000 rads of ^{60}Co in five weeks—come down so that epiglottis receives 7,000 rads in seven weeks. B, anterior lower field is given 5,000 rads in five weeks.

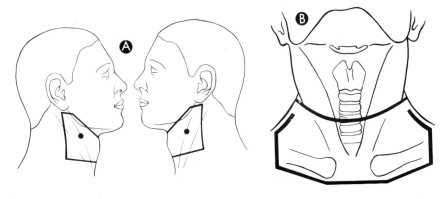

Dr. Fletcher: Well, the suprahyoid epiglottic lesions actually do quite well with the radiation, even more extensive ones. We would give 5,000 rads to the upper neck and then reduce the field to give 7,000 rads on the epiglottis itself (Figs. 8A and 8B). The lower portion of the neck is given 5,000 rads in five weeks through an anterior portal. We would expect 75% control of the local lesion and practically no failures in the neck if followed by modified neck dissection.

Dr. Jesse: Local control by irradiation or local control by surgery after irradiation?

Dr. Fletcher: No, no, sir. Seventy-five per cent local control by radiation to the primary and 8% failure in the neck if you follow it by a modified neck dissection. I don't treat the neck entirely by irradiation; we would do a modified neck dissection.

The Value of Angiography in Head and Neck Tumors

SIDNEY WALLACE, M.D., AND
HECTOR MEDELLIN, M.D.

*Department of Diagnostic Radiology, The University of Texas
System Cancer Center, M. D. Anderson Hospital and
Tumor Institute, Houston, Texas*

IN THE MORE COMMON malignant diseases of the head and neck, angiography usually adds little to the diagnosis or the management of patients with such diseases. These neoplasms are, for the most part, squamous cell carcinomas and are usually relatively hypovascular. However, they do invade or distort the normal vasculature, information necessary prior to biopsy or definitive surgery (Berrett, 1965) (Fig. 1).

With the increasing utilization of transphenoidal biopsy of lesions of the sphenoid sinus and pituitary fossa, it is of considerable value to determine the position of the cavernous portion of the carotid artery. Displacement, distortion, and invasion of the carotid artery by a squamous cell carcinoma of the sphenoid sinus are illustrated in Figure 2. Obstruction of the cavernous sinus and orbital vein by a sphenoid and ethmoid sinus carcinoma is demonstrated by orbital venography (Fig. 3).

Occlusion or rupture of the common or internal carotid artery following radical cervical lymph node dissection and radiotherapy has occurred in 73 patients during a 15-year period at M. D. Anderson Hospital. The demonstration of this impending catastrophe by carotid arteriography provides an adequate opportunity for a more vigorous approach.

Thyroid and Parathyroid Tumors

The superior thyroid branch of the external carotid artery and the inferior thyroid branch of the thyrocervical trunk make up the vascular supply

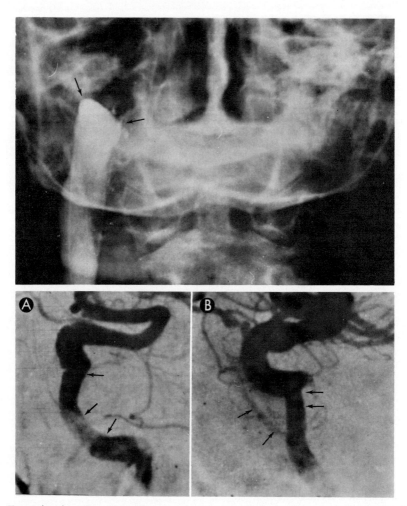

FIG. 1 (*top*).—Metastatic carcinoma (*arrows*) to the base of the skull obstructing the jugular vein.

FIG. 2 (*bottom*).—Squamous cell carcinoma of the sphenoid sinus. A, distortion of the cavernous portion of the internal carotid artery produced by a carcinoma of the sphenoid sinus. B, irregularity of the proximal portion of the cavernous segment of the carotid artery and enlargement of the inferior hypophyseal artery as the result of a carcinoma of the sphenoid sinus.

to the thyroid and parathyroid glands. Selective injection of these vessels leads to exquisite demonstration of lesions of these glands.

The normal thyroid, as well as thyroid and parathyroid adenomas, may opacify making differentiation difficult at times (Capps and Hipona, 1963). Comparison must be made with a radioactive thyroid scan to determine the contour of the thyroid gland. Large malignant lesions of the thyroid may distort, invade, and obstruct the normal brachiocephalic vessels (Fig. 4).

The parathyroid glands, usually four, are located in the posterior aspect of each pole of the thyroid. The two superior parathyroids are at the level

FIG. 3.—Carcinoma of the sphenoid and ethmoid sinuses. *A*, tomogram revealing destruction (*arrows*) of the right ethmoid and sphenoid sinuses, anteroposterior view. *B*, tomogram in the base view. *C*, orbital venogram demonstrating obstruction of the ophthalmic vein (*arrow*).

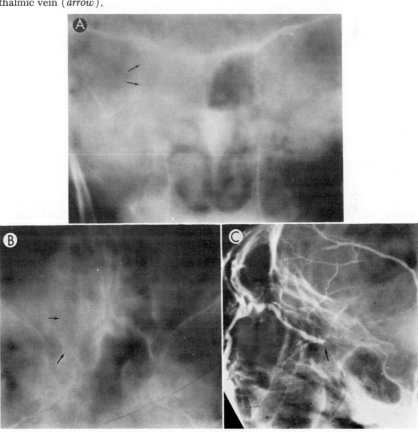

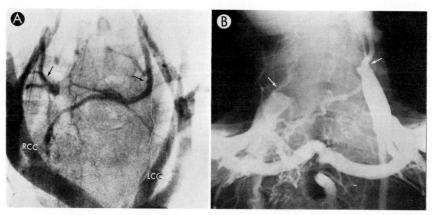

Fig. 4.—Carcinoma of the thyroid. *A,* displacement of the common carotid arteries (RCC and LCC) as well as the thyroidal arteries. *B,* obstruction of the jugular veins (*arrows*) with opacification of collateral vessels.

of the inferior border of the cricoid cartilage; the lower two lie in the vicinity of the lower pole of the thyroid. Five parathyroid glands have been found in 25 per cent of individuals.

The blood supply of the parathyroid glands originates in the inferior thyroid branch of the thyrocervical trunk; one small tributary supplies each gland. Anomalous parathyroid tissue in the mediastinum is supplied by branches from the inferior thyroid artery, the innominate artery, the internal mammary artery, or the aortic arch.

In evaluating the patient with hypercalcemia in search for a parathyroid lesion, thermography, venous sampling and venography, and arteriography are utilized for localization. Thermography may be of value (Fig. 5). The demonstration of a local area of increased heat emission is enhanced by cooling with a preliminary alcohol wash of the neck.

Parathormone assay of venous blood has been the most reliable method of localization (Powell *et al.,* 1972). Catheterization performed via the basilic veins or, preferably, the femoral vein enables the collection of multiple venous samples from the inferior vena cava, superior vena cava, and both innominate and jugular veins. Selective catheterization of the thyroidal vein is most revealing. The inferior thyroid veins may drain into the left innominate vein and lead to some confusion in localization. Mediastinal parathyroid lesions also require arteriography for more specific delineation of the involved gland. Of 20 patients with parathyroid lesions, 19 have been accurately diagnosed by selective venous sampling.

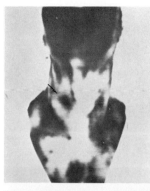

Fig. 5 (*left*).—Thermogram of the neck. An area of increased heat emission, localizing the site of the parathyroid adenoma (*arrow*).

Fig. 6 (*below*).—Parathyroid adenoma: *A*, selective catheterization of the left inferior thyroidal artery demonstrated accentuation of the caudal curve of the vessel (*arrows*). *B*, the parathyroid adenoma (*arrows*) was opacified in the capillary phase. (Courtesy of K. Kuroda, Philadelphia, Pennsylvania.)

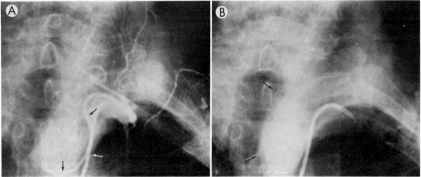

Selective opacification of the thyrocervical trunk is an important complementary procedure in detecting enlargement of the parathyroid glands (Doppman *et al.*, 1969; Hardy, Snavely, and Langford, 1964; Seldinger, 1954; State, 1964). The inferior thyroidal artery is frequently dilated in the presence of adenomas or hyperplasia, and a tumor blush may delineate the enlarged gland (Fig. 6). Normally, the inferior thyroidal artery takes a cephalad and then a caudad direction. In the absence of tumor stain, the mass may be detected by distortion of the cephalic and caudal curves. Opacification of the esophageal and tracheal branches should not be mistaken for abnormal vessels. Arteriography has not been as consistent as venous sampling but these procedures should be used in combination.

Far more rewarding is angiography in benign tumors of the head and neck, angiofibromas, chemodectomas, and hemangiomas. In these lesions, angiography can (1) establish a definitive diagnosis, (2) delineate the blood supply, (3) demonstrate the extent of neoplasm, and (4) determine the presence of residual or recurrent disease.

Angiofibroma of the Nasopharynx

Juvenile angiofibroma (nasopharyngeal angiofibroma, fibroid of the nasopharynx, juvenile basal fibroma, and myxofibroma) is a highly vascular, essentially benign neoplasm arising from the basilar fibrocartilage and occurring in the nasopharynx or posterior nasal cavity of pubescent boys (Bhatia, Mishra, and Prakas, 1967; Conley, Healey, Blaugrund, and Perzin, 1968; Holman and Miller, 1965). Although a relatively uncommon tumor, it is still the most common benign tumor of the nasopharynx in adolescent males. Angiofibromas are rarely seen in females. Approximately 15 per cent occur in patients over 20 years of age; there is a 35 per cent incidence of local recurrence and an over-all mortality rate of 30 per cent (MacComb, 1963).

Histologically, the tumor is composed of large vascular spaces with varying amounts of fibrous stroma. A malignant counterpart, either sarcomatous or carcinomatous, has been reported but is rare (Hormina and Koskinen, 1969; Sharma, Gupta, Sanyal, and Kasliwal, 1968).

Angiofibromas are locally invasive, erode adjacent sinuses, and penetrate into normal fissures and foramina. Because of these properties, the radiologic picture is relatively characteristic (Fitzpatrick, 1967). The mass is fairly well circumscribed, originating in the posterior superior nasopharynx and extending into the neighboring structures. The posterior wall of the maxillary sinus may be bowed anteriorly; a sphenoid hole may result from superior extension; erosion may occur into the hard palate, pterygoid plates, and clivus; and enlargement of the basilar foramina, sphenoidal fissure, and nasal cavity may be sequelae of the slow progressive growth of these neoplasms (Fig. 7).

A specific radiologic diagnosis can be made by carotid angiography because of the vascular nature of these neoplasms (Thibaut, 1963; Wilson and Hanafee, 1969). Rosen, Hanafee, and Nahum (1966) have described the angiographic appearance as being characterized by considerable enlargement and displacement of the internal maxillary arteries with opacification of numerous dilated vessels, a homogenous blush, and an absence of venous filling. In small lesions, the blood supply is almost exclusively from the ipsilateral internal maxillary artery and the ascending pharyngeal branches of the external carotid artery (Fig. 8A). As extension occurs into the orbit, the cranial vault, or the sphenoid sinus, additional blood supply may be derived from the ophthalmic and cavernous branches of the internal carotid artery (Fig. 8B). Therefore, bilateral carotid angiography with selective opacification of the external and internal carotid arteries is essential.

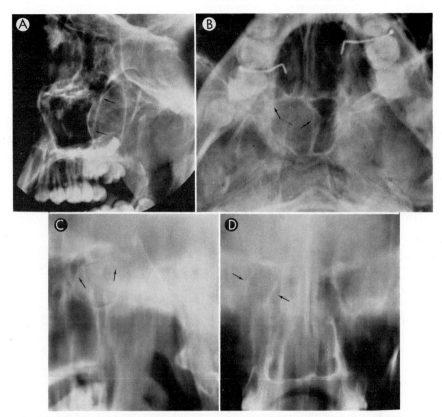

Fig. 7.—Angiofibroma of the nasopharynx. *A*, anterior bowing (*arrows*) of the posterior wall of the maxillary sinus, lateral view. *B*, erosion (*arrows*) of the right sphenoid sinus, base view. *C*, tomogram, lateral view. Erosion and upward bowing (*arrows*) of the inferior wall of the sphenoid sinus by the nasopharyngeal angiofibroma. *D*, tomogram, anteroposterior view. Erosion and enlargement (*arrows*) of the right superior and inferior orbital fissures. The nasal cavity is also expanded on the right.

With recurrences, especially after ligation of major vessels, the muscular branches of the vertebral artery and the cervical branch of the thyrocervical trunk contribute to the supply of the angiofibroma, necessitating visualization of these vessels. The total vascular supply must be appreciated prior to attempts at surgical ablation, if this is to be the therapeutic management. After therapy, residual disease can best be demonstrated by angiography.

A mass in the posterior nasopharynx in an adolescent female is usually something other than a juvenile angiofibroma. The angiogram reveals

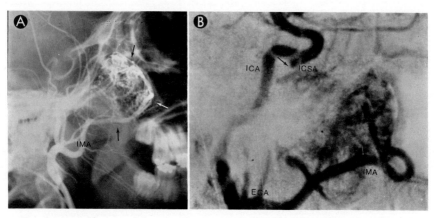

Fɪɢ. 8.—Angiofibroma of the nasopharynx. *A*, the highly vascular lesion is supplied by the internal maxillary artery (IMA). *B*, additional blood supply may be derived from the inferior cavernous sinus branch (ICSA) of the internal carotid artery (ICA). IMA = internal maxillary artery, ECA = external carotid artery.

sparse vascularity of an embryonal rhabdomyosarcoma in contrast to the angiofibroma (Fig. 9).

Chemodectomas

Tumors arising from chemoreceptor tissue are known as chemodectomas (nonchromaffin paragangliomas) and are believed to be of neural crest origin and related to neoplasms of the adrenal medulla. This tissue is found in many sites throughout the body, but is most prevalent in the head and neck (Bateson and Bull, 1967).

The common locations in the head and neck include:
(1) In the temporal bone:
   Superior ganglion
   Jugular ganglion
   Auricular branch of the vagus nerve (nerve of Arnold)
   Tympanic branch of the glossopharyngeal nerve of Jacobson—
      glomus jugulare and glomus tympanicum
(2) In the neck:
   Inferior ganglion of the vagus nerve (vagal body)
   Cervical portion of the vagus nerve (glomus intravagale)
   Bifurcation of the common carotid artery (carotid body tumor)
   Adjacent to the larynx—glomus laryngicum

(3) In the orbit:

Ciliary ganglion (ciliary body)

(4) In the mandible:

The alveolar body

These tumors are histologically identical and are believed to represent hyperplasia rather than neoplasia (LeCompte, 1951). Chemodectomas may be familial and multiple. Bilateral chemodectomas are found in 10 per cent of patients. Malignant change occurs in 5 per cent and local recurrence is seen in 10 per cent (Bradshaw, 1961).

Once again angiographic findings are diagnostic. A well-circumscribed network of tortuous arteries is opacified which originates primarily from the external carotid artery. The tumor capillary blush is intense with eventual drainage into the dilated veins. Arteriovenous shunting was seen recently in only one case and because of this, the possibility of malignant disease was considered.

The angiographic picture in the usual location of a chemoreceptor organ permits a specific diagnosis, thereby negating a biopsy which, because of the vascular nature of these lesions, is fraught with the danger of exsanguination.

The more common chemodectomas of the head and neck are carotid body tumors, glomus jugulare tumors, and glomus intravagale tumors.

Carotid Body Tumors

The carotid bodies are located on each side of the neck at the bifurcation of the common carotid. Physiologic activity is mediated through the ninth and tenth cranial nerves.

Carotid body tumors are by far the most common chemodectomas; approximately 500 cases have been reported (Cordell, Myers, and Hightower, 1967; LeCompte, 1951; Rao and Narayanan, 1969; Rosenfield, 1967). Eighteen carotid body tumors have been seen at M. D. Anderson Hospital (Westbrook *et al.*, 1972). The family history was positive in two while five patients had multiple lesions. They are more frequently seen in females, with an average age on admission of 50 years. One of these patients demonstrated definite malignant disease with recurrence and bony metastases (Reese, Lucas, and Bergman, 1963).

A carotid body tumor frequently presents as a palpable neck or pharyngeal mass. Some patients complained of discomfort, pain, dysphagia, hoarseness, or syncope.

Radiography of the neck reveals a soft tissue mass which may impinge

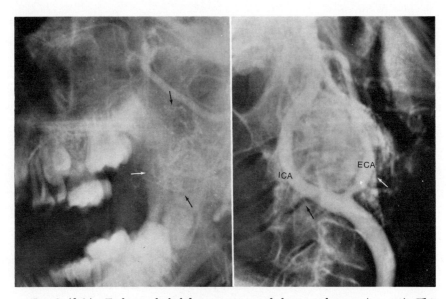

Fig. 9 (*left*).—Embryonal rhabdomyosarcoma of the nasopharynx (*arrows*). This lesion in an adolescent female was far less vascular and less well defined.

Fig. 10 (*right*).—Carotid body tumor. The internal (ICA) and external (ECA) carotid arteries are displaced around a richly vascular carotid body tumor (*arrows*).

upon the pharynx and, on rare occasions, contains calcification. Carotid arteriography opacifies a vascular mass at the bifurcation of the common carotid artery which splays the external and internal carotid arteries (Bosniak, Seidenberg, Rubin, and Arbeit, 1964) (Fig. 10). The internal carotid artery is displaced laterally and posteriorly. The external carotid is anterior and either medial or lateral in location. Aside from establishing a specific diagnosis, the demonstration of invasion of the major vessels is necessary prior to determining the therapeutic approach. The morbidity of surgical therapy has frequently been related to the presence and extent of vascular involvement.

Tumors of the Glomus Jugulare and Glomus Tympanicum

These two varieties of chemodectomas differ only in location: one involves the tympanic cavity (glomus tympanicum) and the other develops from the jugular bulb (glomus jugulare) (Rucker, 1963; Schermer *et al.*, 1966). Other lesions of the chemoreceptor cells in the temporal bone may originate in the auricular branch of the vagus nerve (nerve of Arnold) or

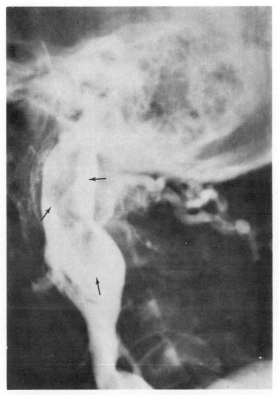

Fig. 11.—Glomus jugulare tumor. The intraluminal mass in the jugular vein (*arrows*) was a downward extension of the tumor at the base of the skull.

the superior ganglion of the vagus nerve, and these are not readily distinguishable from the glomus jugulare (Simonton, 1968). These chemodectomas may extend into the middle ear, erode the petrous and mastoid portions of the temporal bone, compress and obstruct the sphenoid sinus, and invade the jugular vein; the seventh, eighth, ninth, tenth, and eleventh cranial nerves may be involved.

Asymmetry of the jugular foramina is not unusual under normal circumstances. However, a loss of the distinct margins and irregular enlargement of the jugular foramina, especially in the pars nervosa, is significant. This may be accompanied by erosion of the petrous pyramid and the mastoid process. Tomography of the petrous pyramid is essential for the more complete demonstration of the presence and extent of destruction.

Selective external carotid angiography enhanced by subtraction tech-

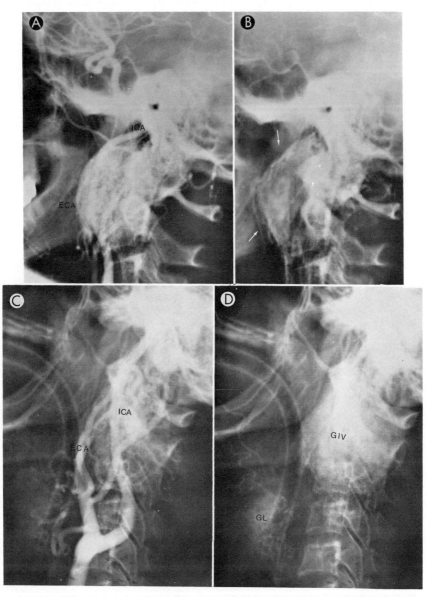

Fig. 12.—Glomus intravagale tumor. *A*, the highly vascular lesion displaced the internal (ICA) and external (ECA) carotid arteries anteriorly. *B*, the glomus tumor (*arrows*) was located above the carotid bifurcation and below the base of the skull. *C* and *D*, glomus intravagale (GIV) and glomus laryngicum (GL). Multiple tumors are not uncommon. The vascularity of these lesions is similar; the location determines the type. ECA = external carotid artery, ICA = internal carotid artery.

nique will best visualize these glomus tumors. In one patient, an arteriovenous shunt was seen. Prior to the angiogram, a biopsy was performed which might explain the shunting. The possibility of malignant disease was considered because of this unusual phenomenon in a glomus lesion.

Glomus jugulare tumors may narrow, compress, obstruct, or invade the jugular vein, presenting as an intraluminal mass (Fig. 11). Jugular venography may be accomplished by selective catheterization on puncture and injection of the jugular vein. If there is no defect in the jugular bulb, the glomus tumor is more likely to have arisen from the glomus tympanicum.

On occasion, the glomus jugulare tumor projects downward and presents as a neck mass. Differentiation from a glomus intravagale is made by the finding of a normal jugular foramen as well as the lack of an intracranial component of the lesion. Glomus intravagale seldom, if ever, extends above the base of the skull.

Glomus Intravagale Tumors

The inferior ganglion of the vagus nerve (vagal body) or the cervical portion of the vagus nerve may be the site of origin of the glomus intravagale tumors (Westbury, 1967). These lesions involve the ninth and tenth cranial nerves but seldom the seventh and eighth. The mass displaces the pharynx medially. A palpable thrill and a bruit may be present.

Once again, biopsy is fraught with danger. Angiograms will demonstrate the highly vascular lesion above the carotid bifurcation. The internal and external carotid arteries are displaced anteriorly and medially. The tumor stain may extend up to the base of the skull but seldom beyond it (Fig. 12). The jugular venogram may show displacement.

The specific diagnosis of the different glomus tumors is based on their location and extent, and on their effect on the carotid arteries. The differential diagnosis includes parotid tumors, neurogenic tumors, lymph node enlargement of any etiology, branchial cleft cysts, chordomas, aneurysms, etc. Angiography may be extremely helpful in establishing the diagnosis.

Hemangiomas

Other vascular lesions such as hemangiomas, hemangioendotheliomas, and angiosarcomas may be seen in the head and neck. Extensive erosion of the bones of the face and skull may accompany the lesions. Phleboliths may be seen which suggest their angiomatous nature. When such lesions present as a mass, biopsy may be complicated by excessive bleeding.

Complete opacification of the vascular supply of these lesions frequently includes bilateral carotid, vertebral, and thyrocervical angiography (Fig.

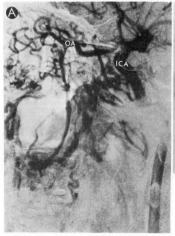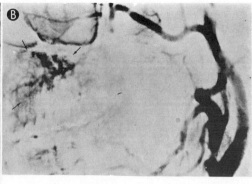

FIG. 13.—Hemangioma. A, hemangioma of the face, fed by the ophthalmic artery (OA), a branch of the internal carotid artery (ICA). B, hemangioma of the maxilla (arrows) supplied by the internal maxillary artery, a branch of the external carotid artery.

13). This is especially essential if surgical treatment is contemplated. Recurrences are usually the rule because of the difficulty of complete excision.

REFERENCES

Bateson, E. M., and Bull, T.: Two unusual tumours of the chemoreceptor system with angiographic demonstration. *British Journal of Radiology,* 40:120-124, February 1967.

Berrett, A.: Value of angiography in the management of tumors of the head and neck. *Radiology,* 84:1052-1058, June 1965.

Bhatia, M. L., Mishra, S. C., and Prakash, J.: Lateral extensions of nasopharyngeal fibroma. *The Journal of Laryngology and Otology,* 81:99-106, January 1967.

Bosniak, M. A., Seidenberg, B., Rubin, I. C., and Arbeit, S.: Angiographic demonstration of bilateral carotid body tumors. *The American Journal of Roentgenology, Radium Therapy and Nuclear Medicine,* 92:850-854, October 1964.

Bradshaw, J. D.: Radiotherapy in glomus jugulare tumours. A review of cases seen at the Christie Hospital, Manchester, from 1943 to 1959. *Clinical Radiology,* 12:227-228, July 1961.

Capps, J. H., and Hipona, F. A.: Visualization of thyroid tissue by contrast angiography. *Radiology,* 81:619-623, October 1963.

Conley, J., Healey, W. V., Blaugrund, S. M., and Perzin, K. H.: Nasopharyngeal angiofibroma in the juvenile. *Surgery, Gynecology and Obstetrics,* 126:825-837, April 1968.

Cordell, A. R., Myers, R. T., and Hightower, F.: Carotid body tumors. *Annals of Surgery,* 165:880-885, June 1967.

Doppman, J. L., Hammond, W. G., Melson, G. L., Evens, R. G., and Ketcham, A. S.: Staining of parathyroid adenomas by selective arteriography. *Radiology,* 92:527-530, March 1969.

Fitzpatrick, P. J.: The nasopharyngeal angiofibroma. *Clinical Radiology,* 18:62-68, January 1967.

Hardy, J. D., Snavely, J. R., and Langford, H. G.: Low intrathoracic parathyroid adenoma. *Annals of Surgery,* 159:310-315, February 1964.

Holman, C. B., and Miller, W. E.: Juvenile nasopharyngeal fibroma; roentgenologic characteristics. *The American Journal of Roentgenology, Radium Therapy and Nuclear Medicine,* 94:292-298, June 1965.

Hormina, M., and Koskinen, O.: Metastasizing nasopharyngeal angiofibroma. A case report. *Archives of Otolaryngology,* 89:523-526, March 1969.

Kim, S. K., and Capp, M. P.: Jugular foramen and early roentgen diagnosis of glomus jugulare tumor. *The American Journal of Roentgenology, Radium Therapy and Nuclear Medicine,* 97:597-600, July 1966.

Kircher, K.: Chemodectoma of the vagus nerve. *Radiology,* 88:94-95, January 1967.

LeCompte, P. M.: Tumors of the carotid body and related structures. In *Atlas of Tumor Pathology,* Section 4, Fascicle 16, Washington, D. C., Armed Forces Institute of Pathology, 1951.

MacComb, W. S.: Juvenile nasopharyngeal fibroma. *American Journal of Surgery,* 106:754-763, November 1963.

Powell, D., Shimkin, P. M., Doppman, J. L., Wells, S., Aurbach, G. D., Marx, S. J., Ketcham, A. S., and Potts, J. T., Jr.: Primary hyperparathyroidism. Preoperative tumor localization and differentiation between adenoma and hyperplasia. *The New England Journal of Medicine,* 286:1169-1175, June 1, 1972.

Rao, P. B., and Narayanan, P. S.: Carotid body tumour. *The Journal of Laryngology and Otology,* 83:837-842, August 1969.

Rees, H. E., Lucas, R. N., and Bergman, P. A.: Malignant carotid body tumors. Report of a case. *Annals of Surgery,* 157:232-243, February 1963.

Rosen, L., Hanafee, W., and Nahum, A.: Nasopharyngeal angiofibroma, an angiographic evaluation. *Radiology,* 86:103-107, January 1966.

Rosenfield, L.: Discussion of carotid body tumors (article by Cordell, A. R., Myers, R. T., and Hightower, F.) *Annals of Surgery,* 165:886-887, June 1967.

Rucker, T. N.: Radiology of glomus jugulare tumors in the temporal bone. *Radiology,* 81:807-816, November 1963.

Schermer, K. L., Pontius, E. E., Dziabis, M. D., and McQuiston, R. J.: Tumors of the glomus jugulare and glomus tympanicum. *Cancer,* 19:1273-1280, September 1966.

Seldinger, S. I.: Localization of parathyroid adenomata by arteriography. *Acta radiologica,* 42:353-366, November 1954.

Simonton, K. M.: Paraganglioma (chemodectoma) of the middle ear and mastoid. *Journal of the American Medical Association,* 206:1531-1534, November 11, 1968.

Sharma, U., Gupta, P. K., Sanyal, B., and Kasliwal, K. C.: Case reports. Carcinoma in recurrent nasopharyngeal fibroma. *The British Journal of Radiology,* 41:625-628, August 1968.

State, D.: The enlarged inferior thyroid artery, a valuable guide in surgery of parathyroid adenomas. *Surgery,* 56:461-462, September 1964.

Thibaut, A.: Angiographie carotidienne éléctive dans le diagnostic et le traitement des angiofibromes nasopharyngiens. *Acta radiologica,* 1:468-480, January 1963.

Westbrook, K. C., Guillamondegui, O. M., Medellin, H., and Jesse, R. H.: Chemodectomas of the neck: selective management. *American Journal of Surgery,* 124:760-766, December 1972.

Westbury, H.: Case reports. Glomus intravagale tumour. *British Journal of Radiology,* 40:148-150, February 1967.

Wilson, G. H., and Hanafee, W.: Angiographic findings in 16 patients with juvenile nasopharyngeal angiofibroma. *Radiology,* 92:279-284, February 1969.

The Place of Diagnostic Radiology in Diagnosis and Treatment for Head and Neck Cancer

GERALD D. DODD, M.D., AND
BAO-SHAN JING, M.D.

*Department of Diagnostic Radiology, The University of Texas
System Cancer Center, M. D. Anderson Hospital and
Tumor Institute, Houston, Texas*

THE MANAGEMENT PROBLEMS presented by malignant tumors of the head and neck are complex and may require a multidisciplinary approach to achieve the best results. This statement implies more than a close working relationship between the surgeon and radiotherapist. Depending upon the individual patient, such disciplines as otolaryngology, vascular surgery, neurosurgery, plastic surgery, maxillofacial surgery, radiotherapy, diagnostic radiology, psychiatry, speech therapy, and physiatry may be involved.

It is not uncommon for the potential of diagnostic radiology to be minimized. The correct diagnosis is often evident on clinical examination and, with the exception of the exclusion of pulmonary metastases or the confirmation of clinically suspected bone destruction, radiologic procedures are often neglected. The referring physician may be unfamiliar with the natural history of the tumors and may not appreciate that selection of the proper therapeutic regimen is often based upon a precise knowledge of the origin of the tumor as well as its extent. For example, small exophytic carcinomas of the vocal cord tend to grow slowly and invade the regional lymphatics at a relatively late date. These may be managed by the radiotherapist with preservation of the patient's voice. Conversely, the seemingly small cancer of the vocal cord which extends inferiorly to involve the subglottic space does not respond well to irradiation and should be managed by laryngectomy. Subglottic extensions are difficult, if not impossible, to detect without adequate tomographic or laryngographic studies.

Although the importance of the pretreatment localization and staging of tumors cannot be overemphasized, the relationship of diagnostic radiology to the quality of survival should not be neglected. Adequate documentation of the extent of the disease may prevent overly enthusiastic treatment for the potentially curable patient as well as for the patient with hopelessly advanced disease.

In 1948, Dr. Gilbert H. Fletcher introduced to M. D. Anderson Hospital and Tumor Institute the techniques of Coutard, Baclesse, and LeBorgne as a routine part of the clinical evaluation of patients with tumors of the head and neck. This policy has remained in force for the past 24 years, with the techniques being augmented and diversified as our experience has increased or new approaches have become available. To obtain the most detailed information, a variety of radiographic and contrast media

FIG. 1.—Lateral soft tissue film of the nasopharynx. *A*, normal lateral soft tissue study showing the characteristically smooth concavity of the roof and posterior wall. The pharyngeal orifice of the eustachian tube, bounded posteriorly by the torus tubarius, is readily identified (*arrow*). *B*, a huge carcinoma of the nasopharynx which bulges anteriorly into the nasal cavity and oropharynx. The normal concavity of the posterior nasopharyngeal wall is reversed, and lateral wall detail is obliterated.

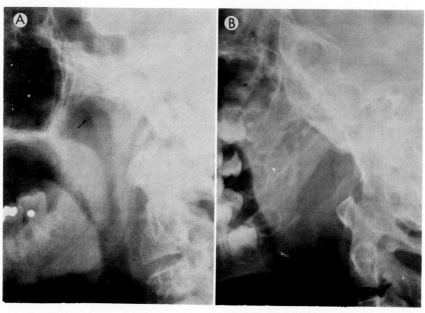

must be employed. These range from simple lateral soft tissue films of the neck to selective and subselective contrast studies of the regional circulation. Although there are well-defined indications for each procedure, tomography is probably the most useful and may be employed in a variety of situations. The introduction of multidirectional tomographs has greatly increased the amount of information that may be obtained, and the complex and closely related structures of the head and neck are ideally suited for the application of precise body section techniques.

Although radiologic examinations may be employed with profit in many types of head and neck tumors, their most frequent use occurs in the diagnosis and mapping of tumors of the nasopharynx, paranasal sinuses, and laryngopharynx. While time and space do not permit a complete discussion of the findings in each area, it is hoped that the following brief discussions will illustrate the need for routine use of these procedures.

Tumors of the Nasopharynx

The nasopharynx is an anatomic blind spot which is not readily examined clinically. A roentgen examination consisting of a single lateral soft

Fig. 2.—Midline sagittal tomogram of the nasopharynx. *A*, normal study illustrating the clear delineation of the posterior nasopharyngeal wall and adjacent structures obtainable with tomographic techniques. Although visualization is improved over the lateral soft tissue study, it must be remembered that multiple sections are required to detail all anatomic structures. *B*, carcinoma of the nasopharynx. The tomogram clearly demonstrates an irregular mass which projects into the airway. The normal concavity of the posterior wall is obliterated.

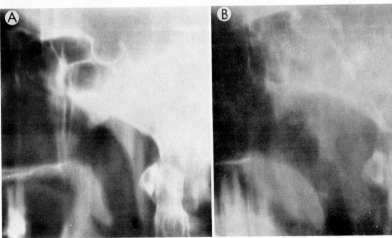

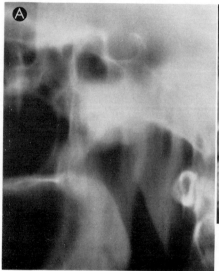 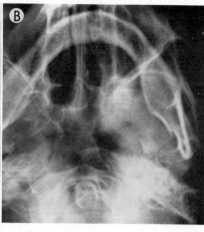

FIG. 3.—Carcinoma of the lateral wall of the nasopharynx. *A*, a midline sagittal tomogram showing only slight straightening of the normal posterior concavity and minimal irregularity of the air-soft tissue interface. The extent of the tumor is not appreciable. *B*, base view of the same patient showing a large mass arising from the left lateral wall of the nasopharynx. The en face mass is hidden in the lateral projection. Note the sclerotic reaction in the left pterygoid plates, a fairly common finding in tumors of the nasopharynx and paranasal sinuses. The sclerosis may be secondary to long-standing infection or may represent osteoblastic response to invading tumor cells.

tissue film of the nasal and oral pharynx will frequently confirm or exclude the presence of a nasopharyngeal mass, particularly of the exophytic or ulcerative type (Fig. 1). However, there are multiple bony and soft tissue structures superimposed upon the nasopharyngeal fossa in the conventional radiogram, and sagittal tomograms are of great assistance in evaluating the presence and extent of a mass lesion (Fig. 2). When the tumor arises from the lateral wall or is infiltrative in nature, stereoscopic base views of the skull are mandatory (Fig. 3), and a contrast nasopharyngogram may prove most useful in the delineation of minimal infiltration. This is particularly true of those tumors which tend to produce only minor alterations in the air-soft tissue interface of the nasopharynx (Fig. 4). If the tumor is extensive and involves the floor of the middle fossa, plain films and/or tomograms in the coronal projection as well as of the base of the skull are required for both diagnostic and staging purposes. Both blastic and lytic changes may be seen in the neighboring structures (Figs. 3B and 5).

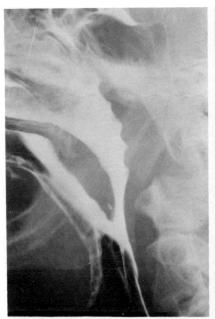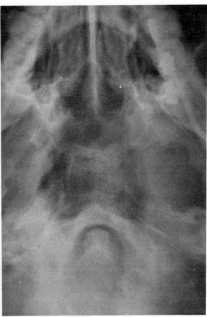

Fig. 4 (*left*).—Contrast nasopharyngogram. An infiltrating tumor is clearly demonstrated by the mucosal irregularity of the posterior wall. The normal concavity is only minimally altered.

Fig. 5 (*right*).—Invasion of the base of the skull. Extensive carcinoma of the nasopharynx with destruction of the floor of the left middle fossa, the left petrous tip, and the left lateral aspect of the basisphenoid. Relatively early destructive changes may also be seen in the region of the right foramen ovale.

Tumors of the Paranasal Sinuses

The majority of malignant tumors of the paranasal sinuses are indolent by nature. Unfortunately, the initial symptoms are vague and the more disturbing complaints may not develop until extensive invasion of bone, lymphatics, or regional nerves has occurred. The delay is often compounded by physicians or dentists, particularly when superimposed inflammatory disease responds transiently to symptomatic therapy. It does not seem unreasonable to recommend that any patient with symptoms which do not respond rapidly and adequately to the usual medications be subjected to roentgen examination. If the findings are normal but the symptoms persist, the patient should be reexamined at frequent intervals or submit to operative visualization and biopsy. This routine is especially

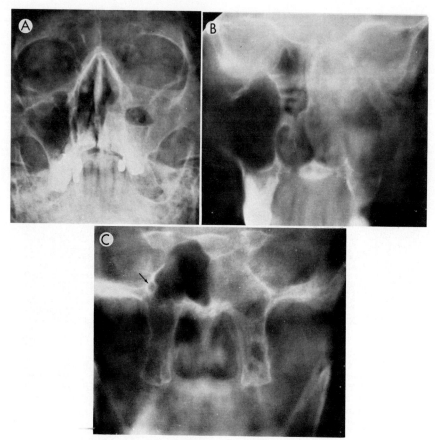

Fig. 6.—Carcinoma of the left maxillary antrum. *A*, a conventional Waters view of the facial bones showing opacification of the left maxillary antrum with a small air-fluid level centrally. The right maxillary sinus is clear and the lateral and superior walls of the opacified chamber are seemingly intact. *B*, coronal tomogram at the midsinus level. Note that the fluid level is no longer apparent, but thickened and irregular internal wall margins are demonstrated. The lateral wall of the sinus is destroyed anteriorly and there is extension of the tumor into the right nasal fossa and superiorly to involve the right ethmoid cells and orbit. *C*, coronal tomogram at the level of the pterygoid fossae. Note the intact foramen rotundum on the right (*arrow*) and the absence of the foramen on the left, plus invasion of the adjacent pterygoid plates. The obliteration of the foramen implies neural invasion. In this case, the tumor is not only more extensive than anticipated from conventional films, but involvement of the superior recess and the regional nerves substantially affects the treatment plan and prognosis.

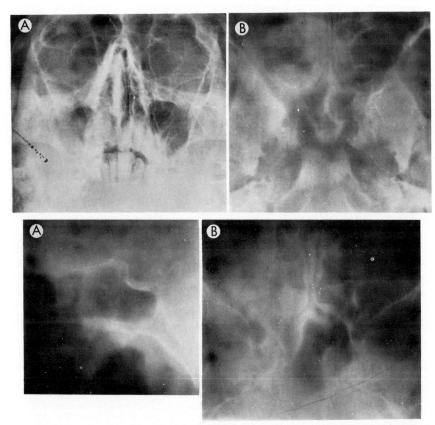

FIG. 7 (*top*).—Adenoid cystic carcinoma of the right maxillary antrum. *A*, conventional Waters' view showing minimal bone destruction in the inferior recess of the right maxillary antrum. This is seemingly early disease which should respond well to surgical extirpation. *B*, tomogram of the base of the skull in the same patient. There is enlargement of the right foramen ovale, indicating erosion by adjacent mass. This finding implies metastases to the gasserian ganglion and indicates that a specific treatment pattern should be followed and that the prognosis for this patient is relatively hopeless.

FIG. 8 (*bottom*).—Assessment of tumor origin on the basis of the distribution of the disease. *A*, sagittal tomogram of the nasopharynx demonstrating destruction of the anterior wall of the sphenoid sinus. The adjacent soft tissues of the posterosuperior wall of the nasopharynx are slightly irregular. The appearance suggests a primary nasopharyngeal tumor. *B*, basilar tomogram showing the bulk of the mass originating from the posterior ethmoid cells and extending caudally toward the sphenoid. This finding indicates a probable ethmoid origin of the disease.

applicable to the person over 40 years of age with no antecedent history of sinus disease.

Roentgen diagnosis of malignant tumors depends upon the demonstration of bone destruction. While conventional films may suffice for diagnostic purposes in the typical advanced case, they often do not reveal minimal to moderate destruction which may be completely or partially masked by superimposed intact bone. Although tomography is recommended for early diagnosis, it is regrettable that few patients are referred for roentgen examination at a sufficiently early date to make it particularly useful in this respect. At present, the most important use of tomography is the mapping and classification of these tumors. The extent of the disease as shown tomographically commonly exceeds that appreciable clinically (Fig. 6), and conclusions as to the advisability of radical surgery, irradiation, or both can often be reached without preliminary exploratory procedures. However, it must be emphasized that the typography of disease is of secondary importance if clinically detectable node metastases are present.

In general, it can be stated that identification of tumor in the posterior wall of the maxillary antrum, the pterygopalatine fossae, or the floor of the middle fossa offers a very poor prognosis (Figs. 6C and 7). Surgery and radiation are at best palliative in this group.

The poor results of treatment for malignant tumors of the paranasal sinuses are then mainly attributable to: (1) late diagnosis and (2) improper assessment of the origin and extent of the disease with subsequent inadequate or poorly planned therapy. Although routine radiographic mapping of the disease has its limitations, it is our belief that it is indicated in every instance (Fig. 8). Better palliation may be expected in the advanced case, and cures may be anticipated in a higher percentage of patients.

Tumors of the Larynx and Hypopharynx

Most tumors of the larynx and hypopharynx can be detected by mirror and/or endoscopic examination. The value of the roentgen examination lies in the determination of the precise anatomical location of the lesion as well as its extent and size. The degree of functional impairment of the involved structures may also be demonstrated.

The most commonly employed technique is the lateral soft tissue film of the neck. Its value is limited to the detection of involvement of the postpharyngeal soft tissues, the thyroid cartilage, the laryngeal surface of the epiglottis, and the pre-epiglottic space (Fig. 9).

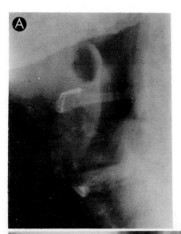

FIG. 9.—Lateral soft tissue films of the neck. *A*, in the normal study, the pre-epiglottic space, post-pharyngeal soft tissues, and thyroid cartilage are clearly delineated. Air may also be seen within the laryngeal ventricles, and the anteroposterior contours of the subglottic space are well defined. Of primary importance is the integrity of the pre-epiglottic space, thyroid cartilage, and subglottic space. *B*, carcinoma of the laryngeal surface of the epiglottis. The mass is obvious, but the area of ulceration and necrosis inferiorly could not be appreciated clinically (*arrow*). *C*, lateral soft tissue xerogram of the neck. Recently we have been utilizing this technique in preference to the conventional soft tissue film. Detail of the thyroid cartilage is very well seen and the soft tissue planes are clearly delineated. Relatively minor calcification in the cricoid cartilage is well shown and the hyoid bone is sharply defined. A carcinoma of the pharyngeal wall is seen posteriorly.

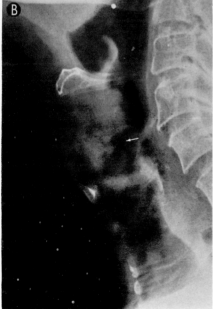

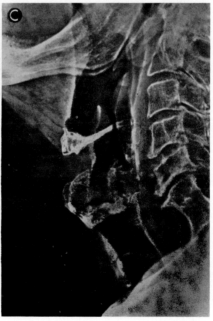

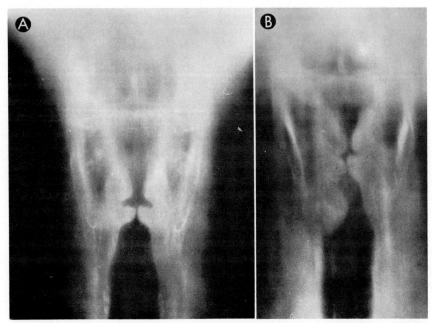

FIG. 10.—Tomographic examination of the larynx. *A*, normal study. In the anteropos-terior plane, the pyriform sinuses, true cords, laryngeal ventricles, false cords, subglottic space, and aryepiglottic folds are clearly demonstrated. In a complete study, sections are made at 0.5-cm. intervals throughout the entire larynx. *B*, carcinoma of the true cord with supra- and subglottic extension. The tomogram clearly illustrates a massive sub-glottic spread on the right as well as extension superiorly to involve the ventricle, false cord, and medial aspect of the right pyriform sinus. The approximate equality of the dis-ease on either side of the true cord indicates an origin in the true cord. Clinically, sub-glottic disease is difficult to demonstrate, and these tumors are frequently considered of supraglottic origin.

Frontal tomograms of the hypopharynx and larynx allow the laryngeal and hypopharyngeal structures to be visualized free of the shadows of the cervical spine. Good visualization of the pyriform sinuses, false cords, ven-tricles, and true cords can often be obtained. The subglottic space and aryepiglottic folds are also shown to good advantage (Fig. 10). Occasion-ally, destruction of the lateral lamina of the thyroid cartilage may be shown. In general, the frontal tomogram is very useful in the diagnosis of tumors of the larynx and hypopharynx, but is of limited value in those areas in which the tumor cannot be seen in profile, *i.e.*, lesions located on the anterior and posterior walls. It is also often impossible to visualize a small lesion of the cord, to differentiate a cancer from inflammatory edema of the cord, or to determine the degree of functional impairment of the

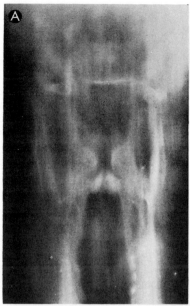
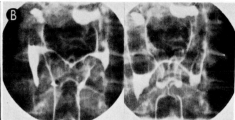

Fig. 11.—Early carcinoma of the left true cord. *A*, the tumor is difficult to visualize tomographically. *B*, contrast laryngogram. With performance of the inspiration maneuver (*left*), a slight loss of mobility of the left cord is demonstrated. On phonation maneuver (*right*), encroachment of tumor upon the left ventricle is evident as well as a roughening of the superior surface of the true cord. Contrast studies are generally preferable to tomograms and lateral soft tissue films for the demonstration of early lesions, both morphologically and functionally.

larynx and hypopharynx (Fig. 11). Under these circumstances, a contrast laryngogram is of great value. It is capable of demonstrating not only minor anatomical abnormalities, but also a clear assessment of function (Fig. 12).

Summary

Radiographic procedures play an integral part in the diagnosis and staging of tumors of the upper respiratory and alimentary tracts. In the head and neck, the diagnosis of cancer is obvious from the clinical examination in the majority of cases. However, detailed knowledge of the extent of the disease, often based upon radiographic findings alone may be the deciding factor in the development of a proper treatment plan. For the diagnostic radiologist to properly evaluate the roentgen findings, he must have a working concept of the implications of his observations. Without this understanding, he cannot function effectively as a member of the team and therefore will have little chance to influence the basic therapeutic approach. Regrettably, although the methodology and diagnostic information necessary to make these techniques effective have been placed on a firm scientific basis during the past 50 years, they are still not regularly

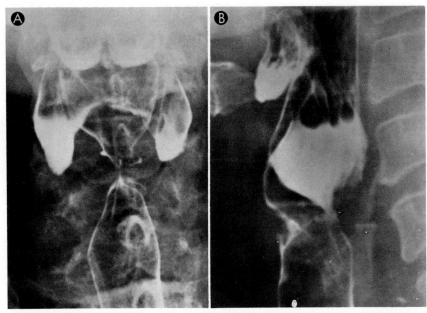

Fig. 12.—Carcinoma of the right true cord with subglottic extension. *A*, contrast laryngography in the anteroposterior phonation projection, demonstrating an infiltrative tumor mass arising from the right true cord with obliteration of the ventricle and extension to the right lateral subglottic region. There is a considerable loss of mobility of the right cord. *B*, lateral contrast laryngogram shows that the tumor involves the anterior commissure and extends into the anterior subglottic space. This finding significantly alters the treatment of this patient.

employed in many institutions which treat head and neck cancer patients. This deficit is primarily traceable to the radiologist who does not have an adequate clinical knowledge of cancer. It is hoped that this and similar seminars will eventually result in their more widespread application.

Surgical Treatment of Patients with Advanced Cancer of the Paranasal Sinuses

ALFRED S. KETCHAM, M.D.,
PAUL B. CHRETIEN, M.D.,
LIONEL SCHOUR, M.D.,
JEAN R. HERDT, M.D.,
AYUB K. OMMAYA, M.D., AND
JOHN M. VAN BUREN, M.D.

*National Cancer Institute and National Institute of Neurological
Diseases and Stroke, National Institutes of Health,
Bethesda, Maryland*

THE INFREQUENT OCCURRENCE of certain cancers in no way lessens the critical need for the same satisfactory treatment modalities as are available or needed for the commonly encountered cancers. In addition, the therapy regimes that are utilized must be under continual critical evaluation if inadequacies are to be identified and survival results are to be improved (Martin, 1948). The treatment of neoplasms arising in or extending into the paranasal sinuses has wanted for techniques which would favorably alter the alarmingly high local recurrence rate that follows the usual attempts at operative resection (Watson, 1942; Wilkins, 1952). This is particularly so when tumor involves the ethmoid or frontal sinuses, a commonly suspected occurrence at that time when the diagnosis of sinusitis is altered by the delayed identification of tumor (Schall, 1948; Tabah, 1962; Salem, Zaharia, and Travezan, 1963).

Eighty per cent of tumors of the paranasal sinus arise in the maxillary sinus (Ashley and Schwartz, 1964), an area which is surgically accessible. However, unless recognized while small in size, it is common to find direct extension through the thin bony partitions into the ethmoid sinus (Mac-Comb and Martin, 1942). Once cancer has arisen in or extended to the ethmoid sinus, there is little resistance to direct and rapid extension to the roof of this structure which serves as the thin olfactory nerve, perforated partition into the anterior cranial fossa. Rarely can this portion of the floor of the anterior fossa, called the cribriform plate, be resected or tumor excised or curetted out of the ethmoid by the usual transfacial approach without creating cerebral complications (Frazell and Lewis, 1963). In addition, the true extent of intracranial tumor invasion cannot be accurately determined unless the frontal lobe of the brain itself, with its adherent dura at the cribriform area, is adequately mobilized and exposed. The transfacial approach to this ethmoid cribriform area usually results in undue cosmetic alterations which should be avoided if tumor cure can be equalled or bettered by another approach or another therapeutic modality.

Primary radiation therapy to this area is also fraught with difficulties (Devine, Scanlon, and Figi, 1957), because of the proximity of the orbital contents, brain, and pituitary. Complications related to bone necrosis are to be expected and often require surgical drainage (Gibb, 1957). This mode of therapy is preferred by some (Dalley, 1957), and up to 40 per cent survival rates have been reported (Gibb, 1957; Snelling, 1957). Yet it appears that these figures may well include patients who actually have no tumor invasion into the ethmoids but who are suspected of having such because of the X-ray studies. One of the most distressing of diagnostic problems in cancer of this area concerns the accuracy of determining, preoperatively, whether the usually seen X-ray appearance of ethmoid, sphenoid, or frontal sinus opacity is the result of direct tumor invasion, infection, or blockage related to the tumor mass in the nasopharynx or maxillary sinus. Such questions may be answered with difficulty by transnasal biopsy, but are truly settled by adequate surgical exposure.

The neurosurgical exposure to the contents of the orbital ethmoid anatomy roofed by the anterior cranial fossa was shown to be feasible as early as 1941 (Dandy, 1941), and later by others who found this a realistically safe approach to the frontal and paranasal sinus (Malecki, 1959; Pool, Potanos, and Krueger, 1962; Tym, 1961). In his traditionally innovative manner, Klopp joined with Smith in 1954 (Smith, Klopp, and Williams, 1954) and reported an instance of complete ethmoid cancer resection by combined transfacial, intracranial, separate incision approach (Smith, 1957). The first series of 19 patients who underwent this procedure was reported in 1963 (Ketcham, Wilkins, Van Buren, and Smith, 1963), but with limited follow-up on a portion of the case material. A subsequent paper dealt with the complications of such surgical treatment (Ketcham, Hoye, Van Buren, Johnson, and Smith, 1966), followed by a report dealing primarily with the neurosurgical aspects of this operation (Van Buren, Ommaya, and Ketcham, 1968).

This report will detail an encompassing 14-year experience with the combined transfacial, intracranial surgical approach to cancer of the ethmoid frontal and sphenoid sinuses in 48 patients in whom there is a minimum three-year follow-up.

Patient Material

More than 110 patients have been evaluated for intracranial, transfacial resection based upon referring physicians' suspicions that advanced tumor growth involved more than one anatomical location in the nasal, paranasal, orbital areas. This does not include many patients seen and not admitted after an outpatient screening workup, in that such outpatient records are not retrievable by diagnosis. The 48 patients in this series include six who underwent surgical procedures performed by surgeons who recently left the National Cancer Institute but whose criteria for evaluation, surgery, and follow-up were identical to those for patients operated on at the Clinical Center.

Of the 29 males and 19 females, only 12 had received no previous treatment. Eight were surgical failures, 12 had full-course radiation, and 16 had been resistant to both surgery and radiation previous to being admitted to the study (Table 1). Thirty-one patients (age range of 16 to 75 years) were diagnosed as having various types of carcinoma, 14 patients (age range of 6 to 73 years) had sarcomas (Ketcham, Chretien, and Pilch, 1969), and three patients had esthesioneuroblastoma (Table 2). The majority of patients studied were over 45 years of age, with the median age being 57 years. All patients were followed from three to 14 years; none were lost to follow-up.

The most critical evaluation made in determining the extent of tumor

TABLE 1.—TREATMENT PREVIOUS TO ADMISSION FOR 48 PATIENTS WITH CANCER OF PARANASAL SINUSES INVOLVING THE ETHMOID AREA

PATHOLOGY	NONE	SURGERY	RADIATION	BOTH
Epidermoid carcinoma (17)	3	1	6	7
Other carcinomas (14)	5	2	3	4
Sarcoma (14)	4	5	2	3
Esthesioneuroblastoma (3)	0	0	1	2

TABLE 2.—Survival Free of Disease, by Pathological Classification, of 48 Patients*, Followed 3 to 14 Years, with Cancer which Involved the Ethmoid Sinuses and Treated by Cranial Facial Exenteration of Sinuses

	No. of Pts. Treated	No. of Pts. Free of Disease
Carcinoma	31	15
Epidermoid	13	7
Undifferentiated	5	3
Adenocarcinoma	6	2
Transitional cell	3	1
Adenoid cystic	2	1
Basal cell	2	1
Sarcoma	14	6
Undifferentiated	5	1
Fibrosarcoma	3	2
Rhabdomyosarcoma	3	1
Chondrosarcoma	2	2
Leiomyosarcoma	1	0
Esthesioneuroblastoma	3	0
Total	48	21

*Includes two hospital deaths as a result of surgical complications; four deaths of other causes, patients free of disease; and two deaths of unrelated second primary cancer.

invasion was by roentgenographic exam (Dodd, Collins, Egan, and Herrera, 1959). Routine tomograms in the sagittal and transverse plane accompanied stereoscopic Waters views, both anterior, posterior, and lateral, as well as the routine X-ray studies of the skull. Patients were deemed incurable by surgery if they exhibited good evidence of tumor invasion into the sphenopalatine fossa with distinct loss of the pterygoid plates (Coleman and Ruffin, 1962). Sphenoid sinus clouding and bilateral ethmoid opacity were common but usually could not be confirmed as being tumor without actual surgical exploration. Bony erosion of the medial walls of the orbit was taken as confirmation of ethmoid involvement with tumor, as was also the loss of bony definition in the cribriform plate area. Pneumoencephalography, arteriography, electroencephalographic studies, and cerebral spinal fluid analyses were not routinely done in that they gave little diagnostic assistance as to the extent of tumor invasion.

Cranial nerve involvement usually indicated incurability, but protopsis, skin fixation, or ulceration only indicated the possibility of more extensive resection being necessary. No patients underwent the operation who had pathologically proven evidence, previous to cranial facial exenteration, of metastatic disease in the neck or below the clavicle. Nine patients refused the operation; six of these had received no previous treatment. Radiation failed to control the disease in five of these six patients. Eight of the nine patients refusing operation were dead within 14 months. One patient is alive at four years after receiving radiation for epidermoid carcinoma. He required four subsequent operations to control bone sequestration and infection.

Six patients not included in this series underwent only the intracranial portion of the operation. Tumor was found extending posteriorly into the optic chiasma, and total resection was not thought possible. All died of local disease within six months in spite of either radiotherapy or chemotherapy.

Surgical Procedure

Less than a complete discussion of the operative technique is reported since this is previously covered in detail (Ketcham, Wilkins, Van Buren, and Smith, 1963; Van Buren, Ommaya, and Ketcham, 1968; Ketcham, Hammond, Chretien, and Van Buren, 1969). It has been found distinctly advantageous to use pre-, intra-, and postoperative antibiotics. Chloramphenicol was the drug of choice in 42 of the 48 patients studied. It was judged that the potential contraindications of this agent were outweighed, in this critically aggressive operation, by the value that it specifically had in controlling the organisms ordinarily encountered in our postoperative complications. It was given only for a restricted 10-day interval at a dosage of 1 or 2 gm. every six hours (Ketcham, Lieberman, and West, 1963; Ketcham, Bloch, Crawford, Lieberman, and Smith, 1962).

The preoperative placement of a lumbar subarachnoid catheter allows adequate decompression of the dura at the time of the intracranial portion of this operation. Figure 1 depicts the location of the frontal skin and bone flap which is elevated to allow retraction of the frontal lobe of the brain and exposure and mobilization of the cribriform area. This portion of the procedure now requires only a relatively small (enlarged burr hole) frontal bone defect through which one can adequately elevate the frontal lobe and explore the floor of the anterior cranial fossa. If tumor is found extending through the cribriform plate, then the adjacent dura is incised and this portion of dura is left attached to the tumor, protruding through the floor of the anterior fossa. Grafting of this defect is carried out using temporalis fascia obtained through the same frontal scalp flap exposure. The defects in the dura which inevitably occur as a result of elevating the dura off the cribriform plate must be meticulously closed. Osteotome dissection about the cribriform plate, as indicated in Figure 1A, frees the roof of the ethmoid from its circumferential bony attachment. The frontal sinus is opened and

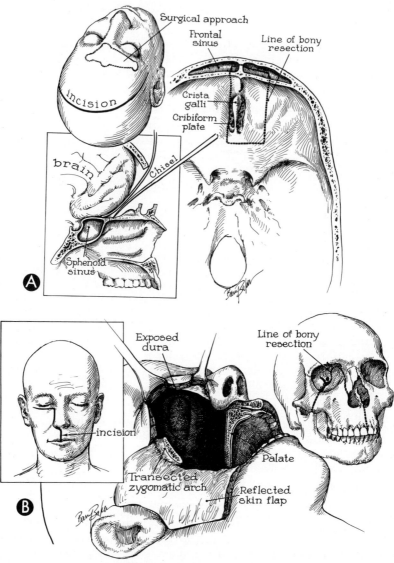

Fig. 1.—A combined resection of malignant tumor involving the paranasal sinuses. *A*, artist's conception of the intracranial approach to the cribriform plate area by reflection of a frontal bone flap and reflection of the frontal lobe. The area of usual osteotome resection is outlined, a procedure which frees the bony roof of the ethmoids from its adjacent attachments and affords adequate intranasal drainage of the frontal sinuses. The lateral view demonstrates how the frontal lobe is retracted and the osteotome dissection may be used either to avoid or include the anterior wall of the sphenoid sinus. *B*, artist's conception of the result of the combined intracranial facial resection showing the defect in the floor of the anterior cranial fossa. The exposed dura is covered by a skin graft

adequate intranasal drainage established. Imbrication of the dural defects is facilitated through the transfacial exposure rather than through the small burr hole frontal bone defect. Through this defect one is also able to determine whether the tumor has extended posteriorly over the sphenoid ridge into the middle fossa. In six such circumstances, the procedure was terminated at this stage.

The modified Weber Ferguson incision (Fig. 1B) is the preliminary step in facilitating the resection of the facial, maxillary, nasal, orbital, bony confinements of the maxillary ethmoid area. Meticulous care must be taken to mobilize the entire specimen from this intrafacial approach, particularly posteriorly where difficulty is often encountered at the level of the pterygoid plates (Terz, Alksne, and Lawrence, 1969).

The medial walls of either or both orbits can be mobilized using a combined dissection from both the intracranial and the transfacial approach. With finger pressure then being directed through the intracranial defect upon the mobilized cribriform plate area, the specimen can ideally be delivered en bloc out through the transfacial exposure. After curettement of any remaining paranasal sinus mucosa, and leveling of sharp bony protuberances, a split-thickness skin graft is taken from the leg and applied to all the denuded areas. Meticulous care must be taken to cover the inferior and medial aspect of the orbital contents in those instances where tumor invasion was limited to the extent that orbital exenteration was not felt necessary. The two hospital deaths in this series occurred early, the first following the use of fascia lata grafting of a dural defect and the second after inadequate closure of a dural rent. Fascia from the temporalis muscle has now been successfully used to close the dural defect in six patients.

Previous to placement of the intrafacial split-thickness graft taken from the leg, it is necessary to carefully and meticulously close all dural tears. These can be readily identified as the spinal fluid, which had previously been aspirated from the translumbar catheter, is reinjected. Cornish wool packing which assists in holding the graft in place is in turn supported by a previously molded dental prosthesis. The packing is ordinarily removed on the fifth to the seventh day, following which frequent saline irrigations are done. Immediately, or within 14 days, a prosthesis is fitted into the maxillary defect. This keeps the skin of the face in its normal contour. If no facial support is offered, it is common for the skin of the cheek to contract, resulting in facial asymmetry and an unpleasing cosmetic result. It has been found absolutely mandatory to have a cooperative dental prosthetic service closely involved in the over-all management of these patients.

---

which lines the entire defect. The two insets outline the facial flap that is elevated and the facial bone that is removed.

Results

The information listed in Table 2 indicates survival by pathological classification. There was a median survival of eight years. Of 27 deaths recorded, two were hospital deaths resulting from complications of the operation. Four patients died free of disease and two patients died of unrelated second primary cancers 19 months to 11 years after operation. Eight patients, therefore, were considered as failures who, in a different method of analysis, would not be considered in the survival evaluation; the reader is reminded that these are included in the survival statistics. Such inclusion, of course, results in a less favorable percentage of survival. In spite of this, the success in the remaining 21 patients indicates an over-all 44 per cent three-year survival. Those patients who have gone more than five years free of recurrent cancer have a 41 per cent survival rate (exclusion of the eight patients mentioned above would have afforded a 53 per cent survival rate). Fifty-one per cent of the patients with carcinoma were alive and free of disease at the time of this evaluation and 43 per cent of those with sarcoma showed no evidence of cancer.

Trying to determine retrospectively the criteria which indicate a poor prognosis is most difficult. Despite the en bloc nature of this surgical procedure, all wounds were irrigated at the end of the resection and the aspirate analyzed for tumor cells. Tumor cells were cytologically identified in 85 per cent of these wounds. There was a slight, but statistically insignificant, trend toward patients with positive cytological wound washings subsequently developing local recurrence. It also was very common for the pathologist to identify positive margins in the operative specimen, or at least for the pathologist to state that the tumor was identified within a millimeter of one of several margins. This is understandable for, in spite of the encompassing nature of this operation and the relatively adequate mobilization of the tumor mass which is obtained, bony margins are often thin, friable, or nonexistent. Manipulation of such a tumor mass predisposes to tumor exposure, particularly when the surgeon is at times restricted in his dissection by the inadvertent failure to transect the anterior wall of the sphenoid adequately or when he has left intact the medial wall of the orbit on the side opposite the bulk of the tumor mass. Actually, the best criteria of complete tumor resection lie in the judgment of the surgeon and in his taking separate pieces of tissue from the operative defect following tumor specimen removal. If such added margins are positive by frozen section, an attempt at immediate further resection is required. If these added fragments are positive for tumor by permanent sections, then postoperative radiation should be considered. Suffice it to say, however, that there has been little correlation between the histiopathological adequacy of margins on the major specimen and our survival data. There is a distressing correlation, however, when the small fragments removed subsequent to the removal of the en bloc tumor specimen are found to be positive for tumor.

The presence of cancer invasion required the removal of the orbital contents in 26 patients (15, or 57 per cent, are now living and free of disease). Twenty-two had neither eye removed even though it was routine to remove a significant portion of the medial as well as the inferior supporting bony structures of the orbit, particularly on the side of the tumor mass (six of these patients, or 27 per cent, are now living and free of disease). Dyplopia was a common feature postoperatively, but surprisingly enough, in no instance was it debilitating. The dyplopia was usually in one field of vision and no patient found wearing an eye patch a necessity. Patients apparently accommodate rapidly to a one-field dyplopia. When one considers that the medial and lateral supporting bony structures of the orbit are removed at surgery, the only explanation for lack of significant eye morbidity lies in the apparent fact that the skin graft applied to the denuded orbital contents must serve as adequate support.

Complications

Table 3 classifies the complications into major and minor categories. There was a significant increase in postoperative morbidity in those patients who have been previous failures to radiotherapy (Table 4).

Table 5 lists the specific complications which produced most postoperative problems. A comprehensive evaluation of complications in this procedure has been previously reported (Ketcham, Hoye, Van Buren, Johnson, and Smith, 1966). The complications listed were all treated aggressively and symptomatically. Edema subsided with head elevation and freedom of infection. The time-consuming and death-threatening complication of meningitis did, of course, require intensive, around-the-clock manage-

TABLE 3.—CLASSIFICATION OF POSTOPERATIVE COMPLICATIONS IN 48 PATIENTS
WHO HAD INTRACRANIAL FACIAL RESECTION OF PARANASAL SINUSES

None	Uneventful convalescence and follow-up	14 patients
Minor	Transient complications resulting in little or no morbidity and not preceding or predisposing to a more serious problem.	19 patients
Major	Life-endangering complications requiring intensive care and prolonged hospitalization.	15 patients

TABLE 4.–Surgical Complications of Intracranial Facial Resection
of the Ethmoid Sinuses in Relation to Previous Treatment

	COMPLICATIONS		
	None	Minor	Major
No treatment	4	3	5*
Surgery	5	3	0
Radiation	1	6	5*
Both	4	7	5

*Postoperative death (2).

ment. All spinal fluid leaks closed within two weeks without treatment
other than keeping the facial defect clean by frequent irrigations. Less
than optimum graft take on the exposed intrafacial surfaces was alarming,
but with frequent cleansing there was rapid regranulation and coverage.
Intrathecal, systemic, and local antibiotics, sometimes administered by the
hour for several days, brought about success in all but two of the eight
instances of clinically recognized meningitis.

As with all surgical procedures, as more experience is gained the complications become less burdensome and the salvage more favorable (Hoye,
Ketcham, and Henkin, 1970). This, of course, must be critically considered in view of the possibility that with experience often comes the ten-

TABLE 5.–Complications Occurring in 48 Patients Who Underwent
Cranial Facial Resection of Ethmoid Sinuses
and Adjacent Structures

	COMPLICATION WAS	
COMPLICATION OF	Minor	Major
Infection		
Graft slough	8	2
Incisional	9	1
Serous otitis	9	–
Removal of burr hole button	4	2
Meningitis	–	6*
Removal of bone plate	–	4*
Subdural abscess	–	2*
Edema, orbital facial	18	4*
Cerebrospinal leak	12	5*
Mental confusion	8	3*
Dyplopia	8	1
Bleeding	4	2*
Hepatitis	5	1
Pituitary insufficiency	4	1*

*There were isolated incidences of gastric hemorrhage, subdural hematoma, renal in-
sufficiency, and hemiplegia, associated with two hospital deaths.

dency to extend the operative indications to larger tumors and poor-risk patients. This has been true in our series in that we continue to accept patients of high medical liability for surgery. There is also a tendency to proceed with surgery even if the pterygoid plates indicate tumor involvement, but not complete bony dissolution, or to include as surgical candidates patients in whom sphenoid sinus involvement is suspected.

Both hospital deaths in this series were directly related to meningitis in patients who had dura resected. Eight patients have required dura grafting. In two, fascia lata was used and one of these died; in six, temporalis fascia grafts were used. The second death occurred in a patient whose dural defect was closed under tension without grafting, resulting in a severe cerebral spinal leak. Graft on graft has, therefore, been satisfactorily done in seven of eight patients in a manner which has previously been shown feasible in unreported animal studies.

There is only one patient in the survival group who received adjuvant therapy postoperatively. This is the youngest patient in the series, a six-year-old boy who had embryonal rhabdomyosarcoma involving the orbit, maxillary antrum, and ethmoid, and extending into the cribriform plate. Local recurrence developed eight months postoperatively. This was successfully treated by definitive radiotherapy. The appearance of ipsilateral neck node involvement 14 months postoperatively was treated by surgical resection and subsequent administration of chemotherapy. He is now past the eight-year interval and remains free of disease.

Comments

There are distinct advantages to this combined procedure: (1) The presence of intracranial tumor extension into the anterior fossae can be established with certainty, (2) the brain can be adequately protected during tumor mobilization, (3) the resection is technically much easier, (4) en bloc tumor removal is possible and (5) cerebral fluid fistula can be avoided.

Preoperative radiotherapy has not been used as an adjuvant to surgical resection. The morbidity in this series of patients, who were previous radiation failures, was significantly greater than that in untreated patients who had received only surgical treatment. This experience, together with a previously reported (Ketcham, Hoye, Chretien, and Brace, 1969) controlled preoperative radiation experience in patients with head and neck cancer, suggests that in our particular environment, preoperative radiation has not adequately improved survival results to the extent of justifying the additional morbidity which our patients have experienced.

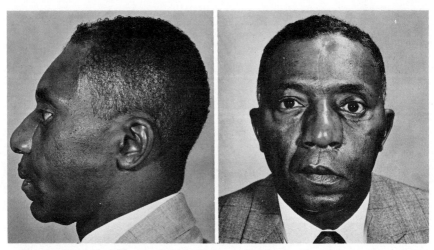

Fig. 2.—A 36-year-old patient with epidermoid carcinoma apparently arising in the ethmoid sinus and grossly involving the cribriform plate area. Tumor resection did not require removal of the orbital contents; however, the entire medial wall and floor of the orbit were removed. This patient has been free of disease for 12 years without symptomatic dyplopia.

Fig. 3.—A 26-year-old patient with orbital invasion of a fibrosarcoma primarily located in the ethmoid sinus. There has been no local recurrence in an eight-year follow-up period, although at three years postoperatively, a pulmonary metastasis and then rib metastasis were resected. A protruding palatal prosthesis restores facial contour despite the loss of the maxillae and zygomatic arch.

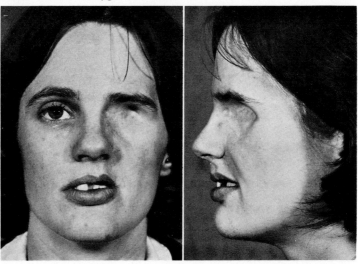

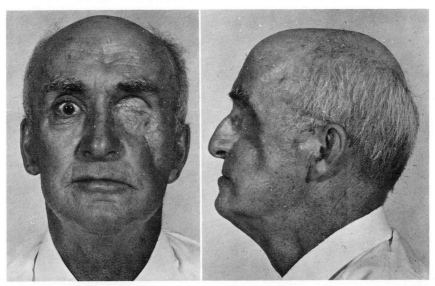

Fig. 4.—A craniofacial exenteration was required to remove an undifferentiated carcinoma in this 60-year-old male patient. Tumor had apparently arisen in the ethmoid sinus and involved the cribriform plate with direct extension into the orbital contents and inferiorly into the maxillary sinus. Satisfactory facial contour restoration was obtained by the immediate fitting of an intraoral palatal prosthesis which held the skin of the face in its usual contour. The observed skin depression in the frontal bone caused by the burr hole resulted at one year postsurgery from the spontaneous, uncomplicated, transnasal expulsion of his frontal burr-hole tantalum prosthetic button. The patient is living and free of disease at seven years.

As shown in the photographs of the male patient with his orbital contents left intact following resection of an epidermoid carcinoma of the ethmoid (Fig. 2), and that of the female patient with fibrosarcoma resected from the ethmoid area (Fig. 3), the cosmetic results, while not ideal, are judged to be acceptable. If the cooperative assistance of the dental prosthodontist and the healing of the intrafacial wound allows, rapid restoration of the facial contour may be achieved by the intrapalatal prosthesis being put in place immediately after pack removal, even if wound healing is not complete (Fig. 4).

While this procedure appears to be a formidable surgical approach, it must be emphasized that it is actually much less radical, in its encompassing nature, than many of the procedures required to bring neoplastic disease under control in other anatomical regions of the body. Our three-year survival rate of 44 per cent and five-year survival of 41 per cent includes two patients who died as a result of the operation and six who died free of the disease for which they were surgically treated. If those eight patients had been eliminated from the series, there would have been an even more acceptable 53 per cent survival rate for a group of patients who all had cancer arising in or grossly extending into the ethmoid sinuses. The fact that only 26 per cent of the surviving patients had both orbital contents preserved while 57 per cent of the surviving patients had a unilateral resection suggests that attempts to preserve both eyes may be fraught with a less than favorable survival.

Summary

Using the expertise of the neurosurgeon and the oncological orientation of the surgeon interested in cancer of the paranasal sinus area, a combined intracranial, transfacial, separate incision approach to cancers of this diffi-cult anatomical area has been performed in 48 patients. Two postopera-tive deaths occurred, resulting from meningitis. Without excluding two patients who died as a result of the operation and six additional patients who subsequently died free of the cancer for which they were treated, there is an alive and free of disease five-year survival of 41 per cent. If the procedure is carried out with meticulous attention to good surgical tech-nique and the principles of en bloc tumor resection, this combined proce-dure has the advantage of (1) allowing accurate evaluation of intra-cranial tumor extension, (2) protection of the brain, (3) avoidance of cerebral spinal fistulization, (4) providing adequate hemostasis, and (5) facilitation of the en bloc tumor resection.

REFERENCES

Ashley, F. L., and Schwartz, A. N.: Malignant tumors of the maxilla. In Converse, J. M., and Littler, J. W., Eds.: *Reconstructive Plastic Surgery.* Philadelphia, Pennsylvania, W. B. Saunders Co., 1964, Vol. III, pp. 1038-1052.
Coleman, C. C., and Ruffin, W., Jr.: Cancers invading the bones of the face and skull. *Annals of Surgery,* 156:129-137, 1962.
Dalley, V. M.: Cancer of the antrum and ethmoid: Classification and treatment. *Proceedings of the Royal Society of Medicine,* 50:533-534, 1957.
Dandy, W. E.: Orbital tumor. *Results following the Transcranial Operative At-tack.* New York, New York, Oskar Piest, 1941, 168 pp.
Devine, K. D., Scanlon, P. W., and Figi, F. A.: Malignant tumors of the nose and paranasal sinuses. *Journal of the American Medical Association,* 163:617-621, 1957.
Dodd, G. D., Collins, L. C., Egan, R. L., and Herrera, J. R.: The systematic use of tomography in the diagnosis of carcinoma of the paranasal sinuses. *Radiology,* 72:379-393, 1959.

Frazell, E. L., and Lewis, J. S.: Cancer of the nasal cavity and accessory sinuses. A report of the management of 416 patients. *Cancer*, 16:1293-1301, 1963.

Gibb, R.: The treatment of carcinoma of the maxillary antrum and ethmoid by radium. *Proceedings of the Royal Society of Medicine*, 50:534-537, 1957.

Hoye, R. C., Ketcham, A. S., and Henkin, R. I.: Hyposmia after paranasal sinus exenteration or laryngectomy. *American Journal of Surgery*, 120:485-491, 1970.

Ketcham, A. S., Bloch, J. H., Crawford, D. T., Lieberman, J. E., and Smith, R. R.: The role of prophylactic antibiotic therapy in control of staphylococcal infections following cancer surgery. *Surgery, Gynecology and Obstetrics*, 114:345-352, 1962.

Ketcham, A. S., Chretien, P. B., and Pilch, Y. F.: Sarcomas of the head and neck. In Gaisford, J. C., Ed.: *Symposium on Cancer of the Head and Neck*. St. Louis, Missouri, C. V. Mosby Co., 1969, Vol. II, pp. 337-342.

Ketcham, A. S., Hammond, W. G., Chretien, P., and Van Buren, J. M.: Treatment of advanced cancer of the ethmoid sinuses. In Hamburger, C. A., and Wersäll, J., Eds.: *Nobel Symposium 10: Disorders of the Skull Base Region*. Stockholm, Almqvist and Wiksell; New York, New York, Wiley Interscience Division, John Wiley and Sons, Inc., 1969, pp. 327-334.

Ketcham, A. S., Hoye, R. C., Chretien, P. B., and Brace, K. C.: Irradiation twenty-four hours preoperatively. *American Journal of Surgery*, 118:691-697, 1969.

Ketcham, A. S., Hoye, R. C., Van Buren, J. M., Johnson, R. H., and Smith, R. R.: Complications of intracranial facial resection for tumors of the paranasal sinuses. *American Journal of Surgery*, 112:591-596, 1966.

Ketcham, A. S., Lieberman, J. E., and West, J. T.: Antibiotic prophylaxis in cancer surgery and its value in staphylococcal carrier patients. *Surgery, Gynecology and Obstetrics*, 117:1-6, 1963.

Ketcham, A. S., Wilkins, R. H., Van Buren, J. M., and Smith, R. R.: A combined intracranial facial approach to the paranasal sinuses. *American Journal of Surgery*, 106:698-703, 1963.

MacComb, W. S., and Martin, H. E.: Cancer of nasal cavity. *The American Journal of Roentgenology, Radium Therapy and Nuclear Medicine*, 47:11-23, 1942.

Malecki, J.: New trends in frontal sinus surgery. *Acta oto-laryngologica*, 50:137-140, 1959.

Martin, H.: Cancer of the head and neck. *Journal of the American Medical Association*, 137:1306-1315; 1366-1376, 1948.

Pool, J. L., Potanos, J. N., and Krueger, E. G.: Osteomas and mucoceles of the frontal paranasal sinuses. *Journal of Neurosurgery*, 19:130-135, 1962.

Salem, L. E., Zaharia, M., and Travezan, R.: Carcinoma of the paranasal sinuses. *American Journal of Surgery*, 106:826-830, 1963.

Schall, L. A.: Malignant tumors of the nose and nasal accessory sinuses. *Journal of the American Medical Association*, 137:1273-1276, 1948.

Smith, R. R.: Discussion: Management of tumors of the nasopharynx and accessory sinuses. *Symposium on Cancer of the Head and Neck*. Annual Scientific Session, New York, New York, American Cancer Society, Inc., 1957, pp. 141-143.

Smith, R. R., Klopp, C. T., and Williams, J. M.: Surgical treatment of cancer of the frontal sinus and adjacent areas. *Cancer*, 7:991-994, 1954.

Snelling, M. D.: Discussion on the radiation treatment of cancer of the antrum and ethmoid. *Proceedings of the Royal Society of Medicine*, 50:529-531, 1957.

Tabah, E. J.: Cancer of the paranasal sinuses. A study of the results of various methods of treatment in fifty-four patients. *American Journal of Surgery*, 104: 741-745, 1962.

Terz, J. J., Alksne, J. F., and Lawrence, W., Jr.: Craniofacial resection for tumors invading the pterygoid fossa. *American Journal of Surgery*, 118:732-740, 1969.

Tym, R.: Piloid gliomas of the anterior optic pathways. *British Journal of Surgery*, 49:322-331, 1961.

Van Buren, J. M., Ommaya, A. K., and Ketcham, A. S.: Ten years' experience with radical combined craniofacial resection of malignant tumors of the paranasal sinuses. *Journal of Neurosurgery*, 28:341-350, 1968.

Watson, W. L.: Cancer of paranasal sinuses. *Laryngoscope*, 52:22-42, 1942.

Wilkins, S. A., Jr.: Surgery in the treatment of cancer of the maxillary antrum. *Journal of the Medical Association of Georgia*, 41:9-14, January 1952.

Treatment of Extensive Cancer of Nasal Cavity and Paranasal Sinuses by Intra-arterial Infusion and Radiotherapy

HELMUTH GOEPFERT, M.D.,
RICHARD H. JESSE, M.D., AND
ROBERT D. LINDBERG, M.D.

*Department of Otolaryngology, Baylor College of Medicine, Houston,
Texas, and Departments of Surgery and Radiotherapy, The
University of Texas System Cancer Center, M. D.
Anderson Hospital and Tumor Institute,
Houston, Texas*

THE SURVIVAL RATE of patients with carcinoma of the nasal cavity and paranasal sinuses is very low. The majority of cancers in this location are very large when the patient is first observed. The local disease is often so extensive that the patient is beyond reasonable hope of cure when treated by surgical procedures, radiation therapy, or a combination of the two. Residual or recurrent cancer at the local site is the main cause of failure, even in patients who are treated for cure (Ketcham, Wilkins, Van Buren, and Smith, 1963; Lederman, 1970; MacComb and Fletcher, 1967).

Surgical resection of the involved area is the mainstay of conventional treatment, and the administration of radiation pre- or postoperatively is thought by some to be of benefit (Jesse, 1965; Shukovsky and Fletcher, 1972). The surgical procedures necessary to eradicate the local disease produce an immediate and lasting morbidity and an aesthetic deformity (Fairbanks-Barbosa, 1961; Ketcham, Wilkins, Van Buren, and Smith, 1963; MacComb and Fletcher, 1967).

Recently, some authors have reported encouraging results in treating patients with cancers of the head and neck by combining intra-arterial chemotherapy with radiation therapy (Nervi *et al.*, 1970; Sato *et al.*, 1970). In a previous report, we presented our experience utilizing this technique for a number of primary sites within the head and neck area (Jesse, Goepfert, Lindberg, and Johnson, 1969). The present report analyzes the results in patients with cancer of the paranasal sinuses and nasal cavity because more patients have been added and the follow-up period is longer.

Materials and Methods

The charts of 25 patients with advanced carcinoma of the nasal cavity and paranasal sinuses treated at The University of Texas M. D. Anderson Hospital between February 1963 and December 1969 were analyzed. Only those patients with extensive lesions (T_3 and T_4 by current staging methods [Sisson, Johnson, and Ammiri, 1963]) were included. With one exception, the 25 patients had no previous therapy. All were considered to have only a remote chance of cure by surgical resection, radiotherapy, or a combination of the two. All patients had histologic confirmation of their disease and all had preoperative sinus tomography.

The chemotherapeutic drug was administered by placing a polyvinyl or Teflon catheter in one or both external carotid arteries. The superficial temporal artery was the usual route of insertion of the catheter, and the procedure was usually performed under local anesthesia. The majority of patients had a simultaneous drainage procedure by opening the canine fossa or by producing a large nasal-antral window. Twenty per cent fluorescin dye was injected while the catheter was being placed, and the area of stain was determined with a Wood's lamp. The final position of the catheter was satisfactory when all visible tumor was stained (Jesse, Goepfert, Lindberg, and Johnson, 1969).

Twenty-one patients received 5-fluorouracil alone, an average dose of 6 mg./kg. in 500 cc. of one-fourth strength saline being administered in 24 hours. If bilateral catheters were used, each side received this dose. Three patients received methotrexate, 50 mg. in 500 cc. of one-fourth strength saline daily, until some type of systemic toxicity developed, at which time they were placed on the 5-fluorouracil regimen. One patient received methotrexate alone during 15 days. While on methotrexate, the patient received systemic leucovorin, 6 mg. every six hours intramuscularly. Except for the last patient, the radiation therapy was given in concomitance with the 5-fluorouracil infusion.

Radiation therapy was administered daily, commencing on the second infusion day. The radiotherapy was continued at a rate of 1,000 rads weekly on a five-day week schedule, to a total dose of 6,000 to 7,000 rads in six to seven weeks. The patient received the chemotherapeutic agent during the first ten radiotherapy treatments.

Results

Of the 25 patients, 22 (21 with squamous carcinoma and one with adeno-carcinoma) completed the therapy according to the protocol (Table 1). The remaining three patients could not tolerate a full course of therapy and all died of cancer within 11 months of their first observation. Of the 22 patients who completed therapy, 11 had no local recurrence from 24 to 84 months (median 44 months). Nine of these 11 patients are still alive free of sinus cancer; two patients died at 50 and 63 months, respectively, of unrelated causes.

Eleven patients did not have a disease-free interval of 24 months. Seven of these 11 patients, three with residual disease and five with recurrent disease, had failure in the primary site. One of these patients is living with disease at 48 months, following multiple excisions of recurrences within the skin of the face. The local treatment in the other three patients was successful until their death from regional or distant metastasis. Because these three patients did not live to be at risk for 24 months, they are counted as failures of local treatment, as is one case lost to follow-up.

Table 2 summarizes, by position and extension, the ability to control the local cancer. The denominator in the table reflects the number of times an area was involved, not the number of patients. There was less ability to control lesions extending to the ethmoid, sphenoid, and orbit since these areas receive a portion of their blood supply from the internal carotid artery which was not included in the infusion.

The absolute two- and five-year survival figures are 50 per cent (11 of 22 patients) and 28 per cent (4 of 14 patients), respectively. Thus far,

TABLE 1.—STATUS AT 24 MONTHS OF 22 OF 25
PATIENTS COMPLETING THERAPY

No local recurrence		11
Treatment failure		11
Local failure	7	
Regional or distant metastasis	3	
Lost to follow-up	1	

TABLE 2.—CONTROL BY SITE OF
EXTENSION* AT 24+ MONTHS

Ethmoid and sphenoid	3/7
Orbit	4/14
Pterygoid	5/11
Infrastructure	4/9
Nasal cavity	5/10

*More than one site involved in many patients.

these results are not greatly dissimilar from the ones obtained at this institution with conventional means of treatment (Jesse, Goepfert, and Lindberg, 1973).

Complications

The technical difficulty of the infusion procedures discussed in one of our previous papers (Stehlin, Goepfert, Jesse, and Smith, 1970) are less of a problem in patients with sinus cancer, since the tip of the catheter needs only to be below the take-off of the internal maxillary artery and rarely below the take-off of the facial artery.

All patients developed an early, severe, dry and moist desquamation of the skin (Jesse, Goepfert, Lindberg, and Johnson, 1969). A fibrinoid mucositis of the mucous membrane within the fields receiving both the infusion and the radiation was usually severe with ulceration. The areas receiving both the infusion and the radiation therapy showed a much higher degree of reaction than did the areas outside the infusion field but within the radiation portal. When the eye was included in the radiation portal, a keratoconjunctivitis of variable degree developed. The keratoconjunctivitis was usually easy to control by topical anti-inflammatory medication, but in a few patients required extensive procedures such as closure of the lids and extensive local treatment.

The late complications included soft tissue and bone necrosis, which was an important side effect in three patients. Only one of these patients required major surgical therapy in which resection of the zygoma, part of the mandible, the eye, and total maxillary resection was necessary to control the pain incident to the necrosis of bone.

Twelve patients had various degrees of problems related to the eye. These were transitory in six patients, but four patients had permanent damage to the anterior portion of the eye and two had damage to the retina and optic nerve (Shukovsky and Fletcher, 1972). Four of these latter six patients became blind on the ipsilateral side, and two of these four patients suffered total blindness by developing an optic neuritis in the opposite eye, 11 and 20 months, respectively, after treatment.

Conclusions

The rate of local control ability varies in different reports, depending upon the extent of the primary disease within the sinus area. A uniform staging of sinus cancer is not available, although various methods have been advocated (Ketcham, Wilkins, Van Buren, and Smith, 1963; Lederman, 1970; MacComb and Fletcher, 1967; Sisson, Johnson, and Ammiri, 1963). In a nonsurgical series, the determination of the extent of the disease prior to treatment is even more difficult and depends largely upon the roentgenological diagnosis (Dodd, Collins, Egan, and Herrera, 1959). Lesions which are small to moderate in size with minimal bone destruction lying in front of Ohngren's line have a good prognosis when treated by radiation and surgical therapy alone or in combination. Superior, posterior, and superior-medial extension of the cancer is the most difficult to control by conventional therapy (Jesse, Goepfert, and Lindberg, 1973; Lederman, 1970; MacComb and Fletcher, 1967; Shukovsky and Fletcher, 1972). Nervi *et al.* (1970) and Sato *et al.* (1970) have recently reported a series on combined intra-arterial chemotherapy and irradiation for lesions of the sinuses. The results in Sato's series are roughly equivalent to the series herein reported, although comparisons are difficult because the numbers of patients are small and his series includes some patients with early lesions. Sato's series, however, employs 5-fluorouracil intra-arterially with radiation therapy in a somewhat different regimen.

Unanswered questions remain. Since three patients in the present series died of distant metastasis with local control of the cancer, one wonders whether the chemotherapeutic agent may be affecting the host tumor relationship systemically (Jesse, Goepfert, Lindberg, and Johnson, 1969; Nervi *et al.*, 1970). Would combinations of chemotherapeutic agents be superior to sensitizing the tumor to irradiation than one agent alone? 5-Fluorouracil has been the drug used in this series because since it does not give systemic toxicity in this dose, radiation therapy does not need to be interrupted.

We are disturbed by the two patients in the series who have become blind on the side opposite to that of the major involvement. Whether the 5-fluorouracil sensitizes the optic nerve and/or retina to the radiation therapy or whether a change in radiotherapeutic technique in moving the field away from the retina on the opposite side is necessary (Shukovsky and Fletcher, 1972) has not been answered.

Whether to include the ipsilateral internal carotid artery to infuse those portions of the tumor which are provided with blood from the ophthalmic and anterior ethmoidal branches of the internal carotid is also unanswered. The neurotoxic effect of combined 5-fluorouracil and irradiation on that portion of the brain in the irradiation field has not been studied.

The over-all result of this small series of patients with advanced cancer of the paranasal sinuses has been encouraging and should continue. To obtain this result with only two patients in the series having a maxillary resection has been aesthetically and functionally of benefit to the patients.

REFERENCES

Ballantyne, J., Groves, J., and Scott-Brown, W. G., Editors: *Diseases of the Ear, Nose and Throat*. Philadelphia, Pennsylvania, J. B. Lippincott Co., 1971, 792 pp.

Dodd, G. D., Collins, L. C., Egan, R. L., and Herrera, J. R.: The systematic use of tomography in the diagnosis of carcinoma of the paranasal sinuses. *Radiology*, 72:379-393, March 1959.

Fairbanks-Barbosa, J.: Surgery of extensive cancer of paranasal sinuses. Presentation of a new technique. *Archives of Otolaryngology*, 73:129-138, February 1961.

Jesse, R. H.: Preoperative versus postoperative radiation in the treatment of squamous carcinoma of the paranasal sinuses. *American Journal of Surgery*, 110: 552-556, October 1965.

Jesse, R. H., Goepfert, H., and Lindberg, R. D.: Squamous carcinoma of maxillary and ethmoid sinuses. In *Seventh National Cancer Conference Proceedings*. Philadelphia, Pennsylvania, J. B. Lippincott Co., 1973, pp. 193-197.

Jesse, R. H., Goepfert, H., Lindberg, R. D., and Johnson, R. H.: Combined intra-arterial infusion and radiotherapy for the treatment of advanced cancer of the head and neck. *The American Journal of Roentgenology, Radium Therapy and Nuclear Medicine*, 105:20-25, January 1969.

Ketcham, A. S., Wilkins, R. H., Van Buren, J. M., and Smith, R. R.: A combined intracranial facial approach to the paranasal sinuses. *American Journal of Surgery*, 106:698-703, November 1963.

Lederman, M.: Tumours of the upper jaw: Natural history and treatment. *Journal of Laryngology and Otology*, 84:369-401, April 1970.

MacComb, W. S., and Fletcher, G. H.: *Cancer of the Head and Neck*. Baltimore, Maryland, Williams and Wilkins, 1967, 598 pp.

Nervi, C., Arcangeli, G., Casale, C., Cortese, M., Guadagni, A., and LePera, V.: A reappraisal of intra-arterial chemotherapy. Results obtained in 145 patients with head and neck cancer treated during 1963-1966 with intra-arterial chemotherapy followed by radical radiotherapy. *Cancer*, 26:577-582, September 1970.

Sato, Y., Morita, M., Takahashi, H., Watanabe, N., and Kirikae, I.: Combined surgery, radiotherapy, and regional chemotherapy in carcinoma of the paranasal sinuses. *Cancer,* 25:571-579, March 1970.

Shukovsky, L. J., and Fletcher, G. H.: Retinal optic nerve complications in a high dose technique of ethmoid sinus and nasal cavity irradiation. *Radiology,* 104: 629-634, September 1972.

Sisson, G. A., Johnson, N. E., and Ammiri, C. S.: Cancer of the maxillary sinus. Clinical classification and management. *Annals of Otology, Rhinology and Laryngology,* 72:1050-1059, September 1963.

Stehlin, J. S., Goepfert, H., Jesse, R. H., Jr., and Smith, J. P.: Regional chemotherapy by continuous intra-arterial infusion. In Cole, W. H., Ed.: *Chemotherapy of Cancer.* Philadelphia, Pennsylvania, Lea & Febiger, 1970, pp. 248-276.

Correlation of Immunologic Reactivity and Clinical Course in Patients with Solid Neoplasms

FREDERICK R. EILBER, M.D.,
DONALD L. MORTON, M.D., AND
ALFRED S. KETCHAM, M.D.

*Department of Surgery, The University of Texas System Cancer
Center, M. D. Anderson Hospital and Tumor Institute,
Houston, Texas, and National Cancer Institute,
National Institutes of Health,
Bethesda, Maryland*

IT HAS BEEN SPECULATED that "immunologic" factors may be important determinants in the progression of malignant diseases in human beings. The clinical documentation of "spontaneous" regression of human neoplasms (Everson and Cole, 1966) indicates that under certain circumstances, without definitive medical treatment, control of malignant tumors may be achieved by the host. Additionally, evidence is accumulating from patients with congenitally defective immune systems that the "spontaneous" development of malignant disease is inordinately prevalent (Peterson, Kelley, and Good, 1964). Finally, another clinical suggestion of the importance of the "immune" system comes from the increased incidence of spontaneous neoplasms in patients chronically immunosuppressed for renal homograft prolongation (Penn and Starzl, 1970).

With the recent experimental evidence suggesting that tumor-specific antigens do in fact exist in human malignant disease (Morton, Malmgren, Holmes, and Ketcham, 1968; Eilber and Morton, 1970b; Hellstrom, Hellstrom, Pierce, and Yang, 1968; Klein *et al.*, 1967), it is logical to assume that a patient's immune competence, or ability to react against a foreign

211

antigen, may be a very important determinant for both the spontaneous development and further progression of established malignant disease.

Previous investigations of the immunologic competence of patients with malignant disease have generally shown no impairment of the capacity for humoral antibody production (Hoffman and Rottino, 1950; Larson and Tomlinson, 1953). However, examinations of the cellular immune response have shown a notable impairment of this important immune function (Sokal, 1966; Solowey and Rapaport, 1965; Krant, Manskopf, Brandrup, and Madoff, 1968; Lamb, Pilney, Kelley, and Good, 1962). This impairment has been manifested by an inability to display delayed cutaneous hypersensitivity to known antigenic substances such as purified protein derivative and mumps as well as by prolonged survival of histoincompatible skin grafts (Kelley, Good, and Varco, 1958). The majority of these prior studies has been of patients with malignant diseases of the lymphoreticular system or far-advanced solid neoplasms.

The purpose of this study was to evaluate preoperative cancer patients with potentially localized and surgically resectable solid neoplasms in terms of their ability to display delayed cutaneous hypersensitivity to a known antigenic substance. A correlation between this immune reactivity, or lack thereof, was then made with the subsequent clinical course of their disease.

Materials and Methods

One hundred and fifty-four patients were studied preoperatively and all were considered operable for cure on clinical grounds. Excluded from evaluation were patients greater than 70 years of age and those who had received immunosuppressive agents such as steroids or chemotherapeutic drugs within four months of testing. The patients ranged in age from 14 to 70 years (Waldorf, Wilkens, and Decker, 1968) and the majority had squamous cell diseases of the head and neck area (31) or uterine cervix (32); some patients with sarcomas, melanomas, and adenocarcinomas were also included. Twenty normal persons served as controls. Also evaluated were ten patients with benign neoplasms and 14 patients who survived free of disease more than eight years following total pelvic exenteration for carcinoma of the cervix. A more detailed analysis of the patients with malignant diseases of the head and neck was made, as these patients initially had the more localized disease and a more definitive determination of local or regional recurrence could be made.

The ability of these patients to display delayed cutaneous hypersensitivity was evaluated using a topically potent skin sensitizing agent, 2,4-dinitrochlorobenzene (DNCB) (Brown *et al.*, 1967; Eilber and Morton, 1970A). Briefly, this involved cleansing the skin of the right arm and forearm with acetone. The sensitizing dose of 2,000 mg. of DNCB dissolved in 0.1 ml. of acetone was then applied to the medial aspect of the right arm to an area confined by a plastic ring 2.2 cm. in diameter. The acetone was then evaporated and the test site occluded with a dressing for 48 hours. Doses of 100 and 50 mg. were similarly applied to the right forearm to test for prior sensitization.

Challenge doses of 100 and 50 mg. of DNCB were reapplied to the right forearm 14 days following sensitization, occluded with a dressing for 24 hours, and the reactions recorded at 48 and 72 hours. Reactions were considered positive only if induration was present in an area of erythema in at least one half of the test site.

No systemic reactions or evidence of prior sensitization were encountered. However, erythema, itching, and mild vesiculation were common reactions, often persisting for two to three weeks. Severe vesiculation and mild ulceration were observed in two patients; these responded with complete healing after the application of topical steroid cream.

The clinical course of these patients was evaluated at intervals of six months and one year, with an additional evaluation of the patients with head and neck cancer at the four-year interval from initial treatment.

Results

The relationship between delayed cutaneous hypersensitivity to DNCB and subsequent clinical course of the entire group of patients evaluated is shown in Table 1. Of the control group of normal individuals, 95 per cent had the capacity to manifest a delayed cutaneous reaction to DNCB. Those with benign disease and those with long-term survival from previously treated malignant disease had an incidence of reactivity that did not differ significantly from the controls.

Of the 110 patients studied preoperatively, 70 (65 per cent) had a positive delayed reactivity whereas 40 (35 per cent) were incapable of reaction to this very potent antigen. Those patients who were DNCB-positive preoperatively were all operable, and 63 of 70 (90 per cent) were free of disease at six months. Only seven developed local recurrence or metastasis within this interval. However, of the 40 patients incapable of reacting to DNCB, only one was free of disease at six months and 39 of 40 had recurrence or metastasis. Of the 39, 12 were found at laparotomy to be inoper-

TABLE 1.—INCIDENCE OF DELAYED CUTANEOUS HYPERSENSITIVITY
TO DNCB IN PATIENTS TESTED

	DNCB-POSITIVE		DNCB-NEGATIVE	
TYPE OF PATIENTS	No. Pos./No. Tested	% Pos.	No. Neg./No. Tested	% Pos.
Control	19/20	95	1/20	5
Benign	10/10	100	0/10	0
Long-term survival (<5 years)	14/14	100	0/14	0
All patients preoperatively	70/110	65	40/110	35
Free of disease (<6 months)	63/70*	90	1/40*	3
Local recurrence or inoperable	7/70	10	39/40	97
Free of disease at 1 year	53/70†	75	1/40†	3
Local recurrence or metastasis	7/70	10	39/40	97

*Numbers significantly differ (p < .01) by × 2.
†Numbers significantly differ (p < .01) by × 2.

able because of periaortic involvement with carcinoma of the cervix. The remaining 27 were operated upon for cure but subsequently developed recurrence or metastasis.

One year following surgery, 53 of the 70 patients who were DNCB-positive preoperatively (75 per cent) remained free of disease. Seventeen developed local recurrence or metastasis and 10 of these retained a positive skin test. Seven patients initially DNCB-positive reverted to negative with the development of recurrence. Again at one year, only one patient who was DNCB-negative was free of disease, and 97 per cent of such patients had developed recurrence; 70 per cent of these patients had died.

Of this group of 110 patients, 16 (14 per cent) had a second primary neoplasm. Because all of these 16 patients were initially treated for cancer of the head and neck, and because these patients at initial evaluation had the most systemically localized disease, a closer evaluation of this group seemed warranted.

Table 2 depicts the histologic type of malignancy in those patients with neoplasms of the head and neck region. No patient had a clinical stage T_1-N_0 lesion but none had evidence of distant metastasis or locally unresectable disease.

Table 3 correlates the clinical course of these patients with the histologic cell type of the primary tumor and the occurrence of a second primary lesion. Since the majority of patients had squamous cell cancer, no

TABLE 2.—Histologic Type of Neoplasm
in Patients Studied

Histology	No. Patients
Squamous cell (oral, pharyngeal, laryngeal)	31
Melanoma	2
Basal cell	3
Squamous cell of skin	4
Sarcoma	2
Adenocarcinoma	2
Total	44

correlation could be drawn between the histology, survival rates, and development of a second neoplasm. All four of the patients with squamous cell carcinoma of the skin died at four years, of locally recurrent lesions involving the central face and brain.

If these same patients with head and neck neoplasms are grouped according to their ability to display delayed cutaneous hypersensitivity to DNCB (Table 4), the results are similar to the over-all group of cancer patients studied. Of the 44 patients studied preoperatively, 27 (61 per cent) were DNCB-positive and 17 (39 per cent) were DNCB-negative. Of those patients free of disease at six months, 24 (92 per cent) were DNCB-positive; two DNCB-negative patients were apparently free of disease. At one year, 22 of 27 (81 per cent) of the DNCB-positive patients remained free of disease, whereas no DNCB-negative patient was free of recurrent disease.

TABLE 3.—Relationship between Histology
and Clinical Course

Histology	Alive and NED 6 Months	Alive and NED 4 Years	Second Primary
Squamous cell, (oral, pharyngeal, laryngeal)	14/31	11/31	11
Melanoma	2/2	1/2	0
Basal cell	3/3	1/3	1
Squamous cell (skin)	2/4	0/4	0
Sarcoma	2/2	1/2	1
Adenocarcinoma	2/2	1/2	0
Total	25/44 (57%)	15/44 (34%)	13 (29%)

NED = no evidence of disease.

TABLE 4.—INCIDENCE OF DELAYED CUTANEOUS HYPERSENSITIVITY
TO DNCB IN PATIENTS WITH HEAD AND NECK NEOPLASMS

TYPE OF PATIENTS	DNCB-POSITIVE		DNCB-NEGATIVE	
	No. Pos./No. Tested	% Pos.	No. Neg./No. Tested	% Pos.
Control	19/20	95	1/20	5
All patients preoperatively	27/44	61	17/44	39
Free of disease (6 months)	24/27*	92	2/27*	8
Free of disease (1 year)	22/27†	81	0/27†	0

*Numbers significantly differ (p < .01) by × 2.
†Numbers significantly differ (p < .01) by × 2.

Of the initial group of 44 patients, 17 were living four years following surgery (Table 5). Those that were free of disease all had been DNCB-positive preoperatively, and the one patient who was DNCB-negative preoperatively was living but with widespread metastatic disease.

Three patients died of unrelated causes during this four-year interval, and although clinically free of disease were excluded from analysis. Of the 24 patients who died, 18 (75 per cent) were DNCB-negative preoperatively and only six were DNCB-positive. Additionally, the mean survival of those who died was 27 months for the DNCB-positive patients and only 13 months for the DNCB-negative patients.

Table 6 shows the results of delayed cutaneous hypersensitivity in those patients in whom a second primary tumor was discovered. The second primary of two patients was the neoplasm for which they received treatment at the time of testing. Both were DNCB-positive and both were free of clinical disease at four years. In 11 patients, a second primary neoplasm was discovered at the time of initial evaluation or at intervals thereafter.

TABLE 5.—STATUS AT FOUR-YEAR INTERVAL OF PATIENTS STUDIED

	DNCB-POSITIVE		DNCB-NEGATIVE	
	No. Pos./No. Tested	% Pos.	No. Neg./No. Tested	% Pos.
Free of disease	15/15	100	0/0	0
Local recurrence or metastasis	2/3	66	1/3	33
Living	17/18	94	1/18	6
Dead	6/24	25	18/24	75
Median survival of those who died	27 months		13 months	

TABLE 6.—Occurrence of Second Primary Neoplasm in Patients Studied

	No. Patients	%	DNCB+	DNCB−	Alive at 4 Years
Discovered prior to surgery	2	15	2	0	2
Discovered following surgery:					
(A) 0–1 year	8	62	0	8	0
(B) 1–3 years	3	23	0	3	0
Total	13	100	2	11	2

All of these patients died of malignant disease by four years and six of the 11 died as a result of their second primary or its metastasis, with apparent control of their primary tumor.

Conclusion

The results of this study indicate that the inability to display delayed cutaneous hypersensitivity to DNCB is correlated with an extremely poor prognosis.

The existence of anergy in malignant diseases of the lymphoreticular system and its correlation with the extent of systemic involvement is understandable, since the cells responsible for delayed cutaneous hypersensitivity are involved with malignant disease. The explanation for the existence of anergy in malignant solid neoplastic disease is unknown. But it seems evident that it is closely associated with persistent or metastatic disease. This observation is apparently consistent in patients with squamous cell carcinoma of the head and neck and those with cancer of the uterine cervix, as these tumors comprise the majority of the malignant diseases in the group studied. Whether this correlation exists for other histologic types of cancer in other anatomic locations must await further evaluation. Additionally, anergy is not always present with metastasis, even with severe debilitation; we have observed 10 patients with extensive metastasis and cachexia from malignant melanoma and osteosarcoma who retained positive delayed cutaneous reactivity to DNCB until they died. These few observations indicate that there must be additional mechanisms to explain cutaneous anergy other than the presence of metastatic disease per se.

The occurrence of a second primary neoplasm also appears to be correlated with anergy in this study. Again, the relationship is unknown, but a search for a second primary neoplasm in anergic patients who have achieved control of their primary disease seems warranted.

The increasing evidence that human malignant diseases do contain detectable tumor-specific antigens provides a firm theoretical basis for the observed relationship between immunologic reactivity and the progression of human neoplasia. These results also suggest that immunologic reactivity plays an important role in the host defense mechanism against the progression of human malignant disease.

REFERENCES

Brown, R. S., Haynes, H. A., Foley, H. T., Godwin, H. A., Berard, C. W., and Carbone, P. P.: Hodgkin's disease: Immunologic, clinical, and histologic features of 50 untreated patients. *Annals of Internal Medicine*, 67:291-302, August 1967.

Eilber, F. R., and Morton, D. L.: Impaired immunologic reactivity and recurrence following cancer surgery. *Cancer*, 25:362-367, February 1970A.

————: Immunologic studies of human sarcomas: Additional evidence suggesting an associated sarcoma virus. *Cancer*, 26:588-596, September 1970b.

Everson, T. C., and Cole, W. H.: *Spontaneous Regression of Cancer*. Philadelphia, Pennsylvania, W. B. Saunders Co., 1966, 560 pp.

Hellstrom, I., Hellstrom, K. E., Pierce, G. E., and Yang, J. P. S.: Cellular and humoral immunity to different types of human neoplasms. *Nature*, 220:1352-1354, December 28, 1968.

Hoffman, G. T., and Rottino, A.: Studies of immunologic reactions of patients with Hodgkin's disease: Antibody reaction to typhoid immunization. *Archives of Internal Medicine*, 86:872-876, December 1950.

Kelley, W. D., Good, R. A., and Varco, R. L.: Anergy and skin homograft survival in Hodgkin's disease. *Surgery, Gynecology and Obstetrics*, 107:565-570, November 1958.

Klein, G., Clifford, P., Klein, E., Smith, R. T., Minowada, J., Kourilsky, F. M., and Burchenal, J. H.: Membrane immunofluorescence reactions of Burkitt lymphoma cells from biopsy specimens and tissue cultures. *Journal of the National Cancer Institute*, 39:1027-1044, November 1967.

Krant, M. J., Manskopf, G., Brandrup, C. S., and Madoff, M. A.: Immunologic alterations in bronchogenic cancer. *Cancer*, 21:623-631, April 1968.

Lamb, D., Pilney, F., Kelley, W. D., and Good, R. A.: A comparative study of the incidence of anergy in patients with carcinoma, leukemia, Hodgkin's disease and other lymphomas. *The Journal of Immunology*, 89:555-558, October 1962.

Larson, D. L., and Tomlinson, L. J.: Quantitative antibody studies in man; antibody response in leukemia and other malignant lymphomata. *Journal of Clinical Investigation*, 32:317-321, April 1953.

Morton, D. L., Malmgren, R. A., Holmes, E. C., and Ketcham, A. S.: Demonstration of antibodies against human malignant melanoma by immunofluorescence. *Surgery*, 64:233-240, July 1968.

Penn, I., and Starzl, T. E.: Malignant lymphomas in transplantation patients: A review of the world experience. *Internationale Zeitschrift für Klinische Pharmakologie, Therapie und Toxikologie*, 3:49-54, January 1970.

Peterson, R. D. A., Kelley, W. D., and Good, R. A.: Ataxia-telangiectasia. Its association with a defective thymus, immunological-deficiency disease, and malignancy. *Lancet,* 1:1189-1193, May 30, 1964.

Sokal, J. E.: Discussion on manifestations of immunologic unresponsiveness in Hodgkin's disease. *Cancer Research,* 26:1161-1164, June 1966.

Solowey, A. C., and Rapaport, F. T.: Immunologic responses in cancer patients. *Surgery, Gynecology and Obstetrics,* 121:756-760, October 1965.

Waldorf, D. S., Wilkins, R. F., and Decker, J. L.: Impaired delayed hypersensitivity in an aging population. Association with antinuclear reactivity and rheumatoid factor. *Journal of the American Medical Association,* 203:831-834, March 1968.

Role of the Oral Surgeon in the Diagnosis of Head and Neck Cancer

JOHN E. PLEASANTS, D.D.S.

Department of Surgery, The University of Texas at Houston Dental Branch, Houston, Texas

IN TODAY'S SOCIETY of specialization in medical fields, there might be some confusion as to exactly what an oral surgeon does. Since today, in dentistry, there are eight recognized specialties with corresponding specialty certifying boards, a definition of oral surgery seems apropos. Oral surgery is defined as that part of dental practice which deals with the diagnosis, surgical and adjunctive treatment for the disease, and injuries and defects of the human jaws and associated structures. This definition has been further classified into seven categories: (1) Extraction of teeth, (2) treatment for abnormalities and diseases of oral tissues, (3) treatment for facial trauma and jaw fractures, (4) treatment for cysts and benign tumors of the mouth and jaws, (5) surgical preparation of the mouth for dentures, (6) treatment for temporomandibular joint diseases and problems, and (7) treatment for jaw deformities.

In the role of diagnosing head and neck cancer, the oral surgeon is probably the best qualified to early recognize and diagnose any suspect lesion of the mouth and jaws. This is not to infer that he is better qualified than is the head and neck surgeon, but he is more likely to have an earlier opportunity because usually such patients are not seen by the head and neck surgeon until there is an obvious cancer or it has already been diagnosed. There have been many instances of early lesions being discovered by the oral surgeon who then referred the patient to a cancer institution for treatment, thereby reducing morbidity and mortality. Lesions at the periphery of dentures, and small fibrous lesions often are early carcinoma, and the oral surgeon is much more likely to see patients with these lesions than is the head and neck surgeon.

In spite of attempts to teach the general practitioner of dentistry to do a thorough and complete examination of the oral cavity, he is primarily interested in teeth and usually cannot see the "forest for the trees." Likewise members of the medical profession usually look "through" the mouth but not "at it" to view the pharynx. The oral surgeon's training programs insist on a complete and detailed history and a thorough and complete examination of the oral cavity and associated structures. This examination includes everything one can learn by the use of his own senses. These avenues of perception have been modified into: Inspection, Palpation, Percussion, and Auscultation, or Look, Feel, Tap, and Listen.

All "lumps" and "bumps" are routinely investigated by the oral surgeon. By investigating all of these lumps and bumps and arriving at a diagnosis, many valuable hours are saved for the head and neck surgeon. Another aid that is routinely used today is the panoramic X-ray examination. This is not to be considered a definitive diagnostic tool, but it is an excellent screening device, and many unsuspected lesions have been discovered with its use.

Oral exfoliative cytology also has a place in the diagnosis of oral lesions but it is not a panacea, nor is it intended to take the place of biopsy. It is very simple to perform, however, and can be done with almost any instrument, without anesthesia. Some patients will refuse to have a biopsy but will submit to a "scraping." In our experience, it has served a very useful purpose at times, but also at other times it has been detrimental to the welfare of the patient. False-positive as well as false-negative results have been obtained and in instances of false-negative results some patients have been dismissed and not followed—with disastrous consequences. It is imperative that these patients have adequate follow-up.

It is not intended that the oral surgeon treat the head and neck cancer patient, but it is intended that he do a thorough and complete examination, including all X-ray studies and biopsy procedures, and arrive at a diagnosis. Regarding the biopsy, there is an important point to make here. Unless it is done by the person who will ultimately treat the patient and who is qualified to manage the possible sequelae, an excisional biopsy is to be condemned. Attempting an excisional biopsy and then referring the patient for treatment is unfair to the patient and to the doctor who must give the treatment. An incisional biopsy for a definitive diagnosis is the procedure of choice in this case.

Salivary gland problems have long been neglected in diagnosis. This is evidenced by the fact that the average duration of tumors of these glands before surgical treatment is seven years. To the average general practitioner of medicine, these glands represent the site of mumps; to the average general practitioner of dentistry, they represent a problem of xerostomia or ptyalism; and to the head and neck specialist, they represent a site of neoplasm. The oral surgeon with a careful and detailed history, properly exposed X-ray films and sialography can arrive at a diagnosis and either treat the patient or, in the case of tumors, refer the patient to the head and neck specialist.

Salivary gland disorders, swellings, or masses may be developmental, functional, infectious, or traumatic as well as neoplastic. A good diagnostic work-up with X-ray films and sialography will show foreign bodies, stricture of ducts, filling defects, and any other irregularities.

In summary, the oral surgeon can and should play an important and integral role in the diagnosis of head and neck cancer. His diagnosis of and treatment for benign conditions should relieve the cancer surgeon of many long hours of tedious diagnostic procedures and, most importantly, bring about the early recognition and referral of the malignant tumors.

Dental Care for Irradiated Patients

THOMAS E. DALY, D.D.S., AND
JOE B. DRANE, D.D.S.

*The University of Texas System Cancer Center, M. D. Anderson
Hospital and Tumor Institute, and The University of Texas
at Houston Dental Branch, Houston, Texas*

MANY TREATMENT SEQUELAE are encountered when treating head and neck cancer patients by means of radiation therapy. In many cases, these sequelae are compounded by various nutritional and other medical problems. Many sequelae can eventually result in severe complications of the jaws and teeth.

The radiotherapist needs to utilize help of the dentist as well as the surgeon to prevent many of these complications from occurring, to maintain and manage those that do occur, and to contribute to the over-all care of head and neck cancer patients.

For years, problems of the jaws and teeth, such as osteoradionecrosis and postirradiation caries of the teeth, were thought to be an end product of aggressive radiotherapy. When treatment is less aggressive, fewer complications, as well as less-than-optimal survivals, are evident.

Dental Care Program

Many complications which were once thought merely to be an end product of therapy are now being prevented. Prevention of some of the complications has come about as a result of an intensified dental care program which was first established in 1966 at M. D. Anderson Hospital.

Results of the new, integrated dental program have shown that there can be a lowering of the incidence and severity of postirradiation complications. This is particularly true in the cases of osteoradionecrosis of the jaws and postirradiation caries of the teeth. The new dental program has shown that various dental procedures performed before, during, or after therapy can directly contribute to the presence or absence of posttherapy complications.

Dental procedures should be carried out according to multiple medical and dental findings. Contributing factors that should influence one's choice of procedures in the phases before, during, and after therapy include: (1) the stage of the disease, (2) the primary site, (3) the histology of the tumor, (4) the age of the patient, (5) the modality of treatment, (6) the presence or absence of major medical problems such as diabetes, negative nitrogen balance, alcoholism, etc., (7) the staging of neck disease, and (8) the presence or absence of distant metastasis.

All of the above clinical problems can and should influence the extent of dental procedures performed for the patient. When the above factors are less important, then one can become somewhat more aggressive or definitive in his dental treatment. Conservative management of dental tissues should be recommended when the above factors are of such magnitude that they influence prognosis, tissue tolerance, normal healing, etc.

Objectives

The major objectives of an integrated dental program for the head and neck cancer patient should be: (1) To improve, where possible, the oral hygiene of the patient, (2) to eliminate or control pain and/or irritation in the oral cavity, (3) to eliminate sources of infection where possible and maintain those sources that cannot be totally eliminated, (4) to maintain and/or improve function, (5) to maintain and/or improve aesthetics, (6) to lower treatment complications, and (7) to lessen the need for costly and extended rehabilitation of the patient.

Between January 1, 1966, and July 1, 1969, 304 patients were examined to study the cause and course of osteoradionercosis as well as the problems of the teeth such as postirradiation caries.

Bone Necrosis

Cause

Of the 304 head and neck cancer patients studied over a period of six and one half years, 67 developed bone necrosis. These 67 patients had 74 incidents of necrosis. Table 1 shows the total number of necroses by major cause to be as follows: Spontaneous or unknown (29), trauma other than extractions after radiation therapy (2), prosthesis after radiation therapy (5), extractions before radiation therapy (22), extractions after radiation therapy (3), and jaw surgery for disease in an irradiated area (13).

TABLE 1.—CAUSE OF NECROSIS, NUMBER AND PERCENTAGE:
JANUARY 1966 TO JUNE 1972

CAUSE	RATIO	PER CENT
Spontaneous and/or unknown	29/74	39%
Trauma other than extractions	2/74	3%
Prosthesis (Post-XRT)	5/74	7%
Extractions before XRT	22/74	30%
Extractions after XRT	3/74	4%
Jaw surgery for disease in irradiated area	13/74	17%

NOTE: Of 304 patients studied, 67 had 74 incidents of necrosis.
Abbreviation: XRT, radiation treatment.

It was found that osteoradionecrosis could have multiple causes and that the predisposing factors could be in the pre- or posttherapy phases. It was also found, however, that surgical treatment or trauma before radiation often resulted in conditions which predisposed to subsequent bone exposure and necrosis. Patients who have surgical therapy before radiation therapy must have adequate healing prior to the start of radiation, as should those patients who have preirradiation tooth extractions. A high percentage of the patients with inadequate healing will have tissue breakdown at the site of extraction or operation. Patients who are most prone to bone necrosis are those who have impacted teeth removed or multiple difficult extractions, or those where much bone contouring is necessary to obtain primary closure. In these patients, it is necessary to allow time for adequate healing, otherwise bone exposure and/or necrosis is likely. Other preradiation treatment factors accounting for increased necrosis include the nutrition, age, and over-all health of the irradiated patient. Patients having severe alcoholism, diabetes, negative nitrogen balance, and other medical problems, where delayed healing is expected, should be restored to as good a state of health as possible before starting radiation treatment.

The second major cause of osteoradionecrosis was found in the extraction sites of those patients who had extraction of teeth prior to radiation therapy. It was thought that either longer healing would be needed if teeth were to continue to be extracted prior to therapy, or one would have to become more conservative in caring for these teeth before radiation treatment.

EXTRACTIONS BEFORE THERAPY

In cases where teeth extraction is done before radiation therapy, gingival tissues must be approximated to eliminate socket openings and underlying bone must be contoured so that primary closure is possible in the extraction site. All loose spicules and sharp projections of bone must be removed so that eventual puncture or erosion of bone to the gingival tissues will not occur. Closure should be neither too loose nor too tight. Looseness of closure site allows entrance of debris; closures that are too tight often tear gingival tissues, allowing bone exposure.

Sufficient time must be allowed not only for the gingival tissues to heal but also for adequate clotting organization in the socket itself. It is from this original clot formation that all subsequent bone formation and healing will take place. Healing usually cannot be achieved in less than 10 days, and in many cases three to four weeks or longer will be necessary, depending on the amount of trauma caused by removal of the teeth and contouring of the bone. In many cases where a traumatic procedure, such as removal of impacted teeth or multiple difficult extractions, is performed several weeks of healing are necessary, or bone exposure and eventual bone necrosis develop without adequate healing of dental tissues.

One must be cautious in recommending extractions before therapy. Only teeth which are completely unsalvageable and which would require extraction shortly after treatment or those which if left in place would be the source of severe postirradiation complications, such as the creation of soft tissue necrosis by friction, should be considered for removal. If great difficulty in the extraction of teeth is contemplated or if it is thought that healing will be inadequate, or in cases where there is a problem of tumor growth, size, or contiguity to the teeth to be extracted, the teeth should not be considered for elective removal.

Many patients had extractions before radiation therapy; 22 of the 74 necroses which occurred were in the extraction site, giving a total of 30 per cent of total bone necrosis of the 304 patients. The total number of days healing for these patients shows an average healing of 11.1 days. It should be noted that 13 of the 20 patients had 10 or more days healing prior to the start of therapy and that five (25%) of the patients had two weeks or more. It is thought that either a longer healing time will be necessary before the start of therapy, which is not possible in many cases, or more caution should be used in recommending extractions.

EXTRACTIONS DURING THERAPY

With regard to extractions of teeth during radiation therapy, we would like to say that teeth should not be extracted during the course of treatment except perhaps in the case of a tooth which is outside the direct field of radiation and which presents a problem that cannot be managed in any other way. All available conservative dental procedures should be considered in order to eliminate the necessity of extractions during radiation therapy before elective removal. Careful preirradiation evaluation and treatment can almost completely eliminate the necessity for any type of extraction during therapy.

EXTRACTIONS AFTER THERAPY

Elective extraction of teeth after radiation therapy should not be considered. A number of patients at our institution have had extractions after radiation therapy which led to creation of bone necrosis and, in many cases, loss of the jaw. Conservative measures such as root canal therapy, fillings, analgesics, antibiotics, etc., should be tried first before decision is made to remove a tooth in an irradiated field. Even when there is severe periodontal breakdown or severe mobility of the tooth, there is no guarantee that healing difficulties will not occur and lead to osteoradionecrosis.

In our study group of 304 patients, three patients had extractions after radiation therapy and all three developed bone necrosis. Two of the three had hemimandibulectomies, and in one necrosis is still present. Even though the three patients who had extractions after therapy all developed necrosis, it is believed that with good patient education and cooperation between the dentists and physicians of the community, and by the use of conservative dental procedures, the need for extractions of teeth in the posttreatment phase can be almost completely eliminated.

Management of Necrosis

In the management of necrosis, the first aim is conservatism. It was found that different onset, clinical appearance, and prognosis are noted in osteoradionecrosis. When the patient has had a radium implant alone, for example, the adjacent aspect of the mandible receives an appreciable dose of radiation, yet the fall-off is such that there are areas of little damage. If bone exposure occurs, the chance of healing is better than it is in those patients receiving external irradiation alone or external irradiation combined with an implant, because a larger volume of bone will be irradiated.

The initial management of necrosis should be conservative. No surgical intervention should be attempted unless there has been a continuous failure using conservative procedures. Surgical intervention in irradiated bone may extend the necrotic site to include areas that clinically were not necrotic, because of the inability of bone to repair properly after radiation damage. Healing of bone exposure and bone necrosis is promoted if infection is brought under control. If gross infection is not present and the area of bone necrosis is not too great, the body will treat bone fragments as foreign bodies and seek to sequestrate them. This process may take months or even years. Conservative treatment, such as zinc peroxide packs, topical 1 per cent neomycin solutions, or systemic antibiotics, etc., is indicated for limited necroses. Other conservative procedures include gentle removal of loose spicules of bone above the gingival crest to keep them from irritating surrounding tissues. Good oral hygiene is imperative. Food debris must be carefully flushed from the area to lower the total bacterial count. The patient must be cognizant of the importance of his total involvement in caring for the area if conservative procedures are to be beneficial.

Postirradiation Tooth Decay

It has been found that the postirradiation caries of the teeth are an end product of reduction of normal salivary gland activity resulting from the effect of radiation on the major salivary glands. This, combined with inadequate dental hygiene, predisposes to conditions that cause postirradiation caries of the teeth. The end result of unchecked postirradiation caries is complete amputation of the teeth.

PREVENTION

With a preventive program, it has been found that postirradiation caries of the teeth can be almost completely eliminated. In our original study of 304 patients, 134 had teeth remaining after completion of radiation therapy. These patients were randomized into groups that did or did not receive daily topical applications of 1 per cent sodium fluoride dental gel. Of those who received the daily applications of the fluoride only 30.7 per cent developed postirradiation decay, whereas of those who were in the control group, not receiving the fluoride, 68 per cent developed decay (Table 2).

TABLE 2.—RADIATION COMPLICATIONS STUDY, CONTROL
vs. FLUORIDES: JANUARY 1966 TO JUNE 1972

GROUP	RANDOMIZED	TOTAL NUMBER PATIENTS	PATIENTS' RADIATION DECAY
Group III	Control	43	30 (69%)
Fair	Fluoride	38	13 (34%)
Group IV	Control	26	17 (65%)
Good	Fluoride	27	7 (25%)

It was thought that with better patient cooperation, even those of the fluoride group who developed the caries would have had a considerably lower incidence of this decay process. This fluoride is worn in custom-made mouth guards for five minutes each day, indefinitely. Any patient who has major salivary gland radiation is now put on a preventive program of this 1 per cent sodium fluoride each day. As long as the patient wears the fluoride and demonstrates good oral hygiene, he has no problems with the decay or extreme sensitivity of the teeth. It is now believed that with adequate patient education and cooperation and the use of fluoride, radiation caries of the teeth and postirradiation sensitivity can be almost completely eliminated.

Conclusion

In conclusion, it may be said that when the patient and the local dentist become an integral part of the head and neck cancer treatment team, and when preventive dentistry is employed to the fullest, the desired goal of minimum complications will be achieved. A good dental follow-up program, utilizing conservative procedures for irradiated tissues, will minimize the complications that do occur and diminish the need for extensive rehabilitation procedures for these patients.

Acknowledgments

This project was initially partially sponsored and supported by the Cancer Control Branch, Division of Chronic Diseases, USPHS Grant No. 4614, through The University of Texas at Houston Dental Branch and in cooperation with The University of Texas M. D. Anderson Hospital and Tumor Institute at Houston. Continuation of the dissemination of the results was partly supported by the Regional Medical Program, Grant Project 1020. Biomedical computation and biomathematical consultation was supported by USPHS Grant No. 11430 from the National Cancer Institute.

Role of the Maxillofacial Prosthodontist in Rehabilitation of the Head and Neck Cancer Patient

JOE B. DRANE, D.D.S.

Department of Surgery, The University of Texas System Cancer Center, M. D. Anderson Hospital and Tumor Institute; Director, Regional Maxillofacial Restorative Center; and The University of Texas at Houston Dental Branch, Houston, Texas

THE MAXILLOFACIAL PROSTHODONTIST'S ACTIVITIES related to the care of cancer patients have increased greatly in the past several years. As recently as 20 years ago, there were very few dentists who had the training and background to be able to assist the physician in both treatment for the primary disease and the rehabilitative stages of the patient's care. Dr. Andrew Ackerman developed a dental internship training program at Memorial Hospital in New York City, which included rotation through the Head and Neck Section, and this was probably the first formal training program in maxillofacial prosthetics in this country. From this modest but important beginning, a core group of partially trained maxillofacial prosthodontists developed and migrated to various medical centers throughout the country.

There are now several institutions, such as Memorial Hospital, Roswell Park in Buffalo, N. Y., Indiana University School of Dentistry, and The University of Texas Dental Branch and M. D. Anderson Hospital here in Houston, which offer advanced training in this field. Our program includes all phases of maxillofacial prosthetics: design, construction, and insertion of treatment prostheses, interim prostheses, and rehabilitative prostheses.

233

These may be intraoral removable prostheses, such as obturators, splints, resection appliances, etc.; implant prostheses, such as mandibular or facial bone replacements; or extraoral or facial prostheses, used to replace facial features lost because of surgical treatment, disease, or trauma.

We try to include preplanning the rehabilitation of the cancer patient in planning the total treatment for the patient's primary disease. By doing this, we have the opportunity to choose the method that is best for the individual patient, whether it be surgical reconstruction, prosthetic reconstruction, or a combination of both. Such preplanning also precludes the development of certain problems which may result from the primary treatment. This is illustrated by the use of protective prostheses during the administration of radiation therapy. These types of prostheses protect the uninvolved tissues and allow them to develop normally, thus eliminating the need later for rehabilitative procedures.

Even with such planning of the patient's total care, we cannot of course prevent the occurrence of defects after certain types of resections. One of the most disabling defects, and one that is being seen more frequently, is the midthird of the face resection. A defect of this type is both functionally and cosmetically disabling. It is also very difficult to correct surgically. Prosthetically, this type of patient is treated in two stages. The first stage is to correct the functional disability by replacing the missing palate, alveolar ridge, and, in some instances, the teeth, in order to restore the patient's ability to swallow normally and speak intelligibly. The second stage is the replacement by prosthetic means of the missing facial features to correct the cosmetic disability. As previous speakers have stated, it is imperative that the patient not only be "cured" of his disease, but also that he be returned to as near normal in his function and appearance as possible.

Some of the rehabilitative prostheses necessarily become very involved and complex. These are demonstrated by such types as those that require chrome-cobalt metal castings, those that require special retention features, or those that have to cover or be based on abnormal soft tissues.

Most prostheses, however, are comparatively simple to construct and require a very short time in their fabrication. Immediate obturators are in this category. They require only a preoperative visit by the patient for an impression of the upper jaw. Following the taking of this impression and a consultation with the surgeon to determine, as nearly as possible, where the lines of resection will be, an acrylic palate, utilizing either autopolymerizing or heat-cure material, can be made any time before the operation and then inserted during the surgical procedure.

These comparatively simple prostheses have many advantages and some disadvantages. The main disadvantage is the necessity for the prosthodontist to be present during the surgical procedure. I believe, however, that the time spent in the operating room is more than compensated for later by the time saved in eliminating the need for postoperative impression techniques prior to adequate healing.

Some of the advantages of the use of immediate obturators are that they aid the surgeon in placing and retaining the packing in the defect; they allow the patient to take food by mouth, eliminating the need for the nasogastric feeding tube; they allow the patient to speak normally; and they prevent the forming of compensatory speech habits that need to be corrected at a later time. I believe that the main advantage, however, is that those patients on whom immediate obturators are used are able to be discharged from the hospital one-third sooner than those on whom they are not used. This was shown by a review by Dr. Nakamoto of the charts of 120 maxillary resection patients at M. D. Anderson Hospital in 1971.

The rehabilitation of the head and neck cancer patient can be either a very simple procedure, a very complicated procedure, or at times an almost impossible procedure. For this reason, all available modalities of prevention, treatment, and rehabilitation should be utilized. The maxillofacial prosthodontist should be formally trained in all procedures, should be capable of utilizing this training, and should involve himself as a participating member of the cancer treatment team.

Flaps in Repair of Oral Defects

MARGA H. SINCLAIR, M.D.

*Plastic Surgery Service, Department of Surgery, The University of
Texas System Cancer Center, M. D. Anderson Hospital and
Tumor Institute, Houston, Texas*

THIS DISCUSSION WILL CONCERN ITSELF only with the method of repair after the resection of the tumor. I hope to show that restoration of function to the oral cavity can justify the often extremely destructive procedures which are necessary to completely remove the cancer, even if later a local recurrence or distant metastasis occurs. I shall present the history of 10 patients, divided into four groups, according to the method of repair.

Group 1 consists of three patients with similar lesions involving tongue, floor of the mouth, and mandible. The defects were repaired by a forehead flap.

CASE 1.—(Fig. 1). This was a 60-year-old woman, who had had two separate lesions in the past: a squamous cell carcinoma in the right retromolar triangle which was treated by irradiation in 1962, and a squamous cell cancer in the mucosa of the left soft palate treated by excision and grafting in 1968. In 1970, she had two new lesions: a squamous cell carcinoma in the left lower gum with X-ray findings of bone involvement, and a spindle cell carcinoma of the left side of the tongue. Hemiglossectomy, hemimandibulectomy (from the midline at the chin and disarticulation), removal of the old graft and remaining mucosa of the left half of the soft palate, and the total mucosa of the left cheek from close to the commissure to the pharynx, were done. To cover this large defect, a wide forehead flap with the pedicle on the left side was tunneled through a low cheek incision and sutured to all mucosal defect borders as far as possible. Five weeks later, after primary healing, the pedicle of the flap was separated and returned to the forehead. The patient returned to a normal life; she was able to eat and speak. She had upper dentures made for cosmetic appearance.

237

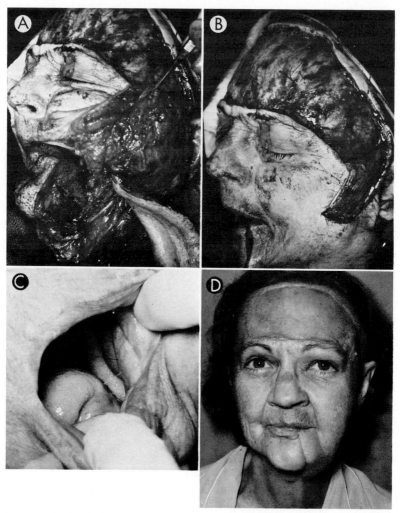

Fig 1.—*A,* forehead flap tunneled through a cheek incision to replace lining of cheek, left half of tongue, left buccal sulcus. *B,* forehead flap sutured to defect in oral cavity and cheek flap returned. *C,* forehead flap well healed on inside of oral cavity. *D,* patient after separation and returning of unused part of forehead flap.

Eight months later, large nodes in the left side of the neck appeared; the patient refused further surgical treatment. She died, outside the hospital, 17 months after her last operation.

CASE 2.—(Fig. 2). A 72-year-old woman had a large exophytic squamous cell carcinoma in the right buccal mucosa from the right retromolar tri-

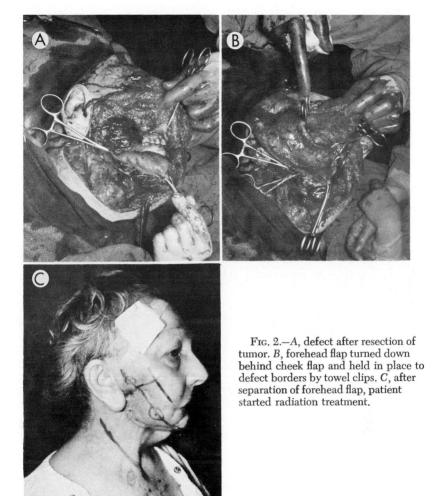

Fig. 2.—*A*, defect after resection of tumor. *B*, forehead flap turned down behind cheek flap and held in place to defect borders by towel clips. *C*, after separation of forehead flap, patient started radiation treatment.

angle to about 1 cm. distant from the commissure, with infiltration of the masseter muscle and involvement of the mandible visible on X-ray films. The operation included a right upper neck dissection, superficial right parotidectomy, right hemimandibulectomy, partial maxillectomy, and resection of the floor of the mouth and buccal mucosa. A large forehead flap was tunneled into the oral cavity behind and subcutaneously to the cheek flap and sutured intraorally to all defect borders. The forehead flap inside the mouth healed primarily, but at the lower border of the cheek-neck flap a superficial necrosis occurred. At the time of the separation of the forehead flap, the necrotic part was replaced by a skin graft. The patient underwent postoperative radiation treatment without difficulties. She is free of disease and doing well.

CASE 3.—(Fig. 3). A 58-year-old man had right radical neck dissection, right hemimandibulectomy, and resection of the buccal mucosa, soft palate, and right tonsillar and pterygoid area. The repair was accomplished by a forehead flap turned in subcutaneously and sutured to all defect borders. The flap healed without difficulties. Since the resection was not

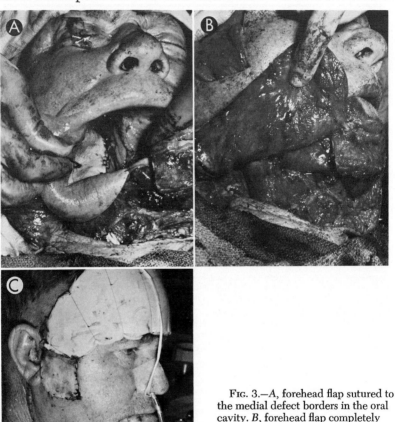

FIG. 3.—*A*, forehead flap sutured to the medial defect borders in the oral cavity. *B*, forehead flap completely sutured into the oral defect. *C*, patient at the completion of the operation.

considered adequate, irradiation was started soon after the operation. The separation of the flap was postponed for seven months until all reaction had disappeared.

Ten months later, a large mass appeared in the neck; because of pain, surgical removal was attempted, but the patient died several months later, one and one half years after his first operation.

Group 2 consists of two patients who demonstrate the versatility of the medially based deltopectoral flap, described by Bakamjian.

CASE 4.—(Fig. 4). A 67-year-old man had recurrent disease after radia-

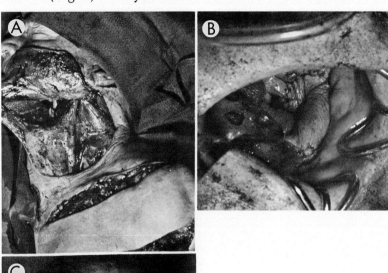

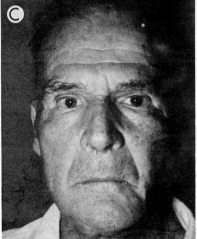

FIG. 4.—*A,* defect of floor of mouth, left half of tongue after resection of squamous cell cancer, deltopectoral flap elevated. *B,* flap sutured in place. *C,* patient after healing of flap.

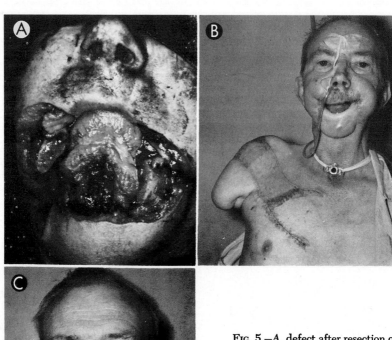

FIG. 5.—*A*, defect after resection of recurrent tumor. *B*, patient showing partially returned deltopectoral flap on chest wall and reconstructed chin and lower lip. *C*, flap in place and after insertion of fascia sling.

tion treatment for squamous cell carcinoma in the left retromolar triangle and margin of the tongue. A left commando, including the left half of the tongue, left mandible, and retromolar triangle was performed. A medially based upper chest flap was used to cover the intraoral defect. After separation of the flap and closure of the fistula, the patient could eat and talk.

CASE 5.—(Fig. 5). The patient had a wide resection of the anterior lower lip, chin, anterior mandible, and floor of the mouth to the root of the tongue for an extensive recurrent squamous cell cancer after previous surgical treatment and radiation. Repair was done by a folded deltopectoral flap. At the time of separation of the flap, a fascia sling was inserted and fastened to the zygomatic arch on both sides to hold the lip up. The patient can eat well by mouth, although he still has some problem with drooling.

There is no evidence of local recurrence, but in September 1972 lung metastases were found.

Fig. 6.—*A*, medially based deltopectoral flap used to form new pharynx and cervical esophagus. *B*, bipedicle forehead flap replaces resected neck skin. *C*, pedicles of flaps are tube during healing time. *D*, after separation of pedicles and complete healing of flaps.

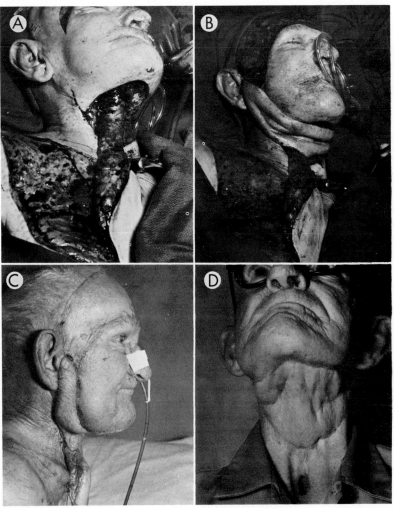

In Group 3, forehead and medially based deltopectoral flaps were used to accomplish reconstruction.

CASE 6.—(Fig. 6). A 67-year-old man had had a laryngectomy followed by radiation 15 years ago. In 1968, he underwent total pharyngectomy, resection of the base of the tongue, and excision of the heavily radiated skin of the lower chin and upper neck for squamous cell carcinoma of pharynx and base of the tongue. Repair of the pharynx was accomplished by a medially based deltopectoral flap while the skin defect was covered with a bipedicled forehead flap. After separation of both flaps, the patient was able to eat by mouth.

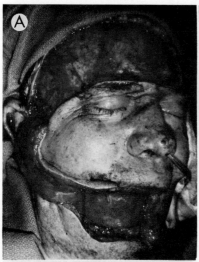
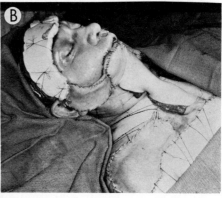
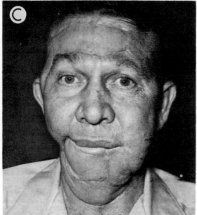

FIG. 7.—*A*, forehead flap used for lining. *B*, deltopectoral flap covers the forehead flap and forms the new chin. *C*, after separation of both flaps.

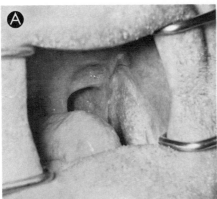

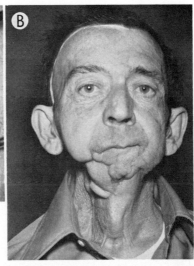

Fig. 8.—*A*, forehead flap healed in oral cavity. *B*, deltopectoral flap provides outside cover.

He had one good year, then a local recurrence in the upper posterior pharynx was removed by cautery; later a massive recurrence in the sub-mental area was treated with methotrexate. The patient died, outside our hospital, 17 months after his last operation.

CASE 7.—(Fig. 7). A 50-year-old man had resection of the lip and chin and hemimandibulectomy, including the gingivo-buccal mucosa up to the anterior pillar, for a massive recurrence four years postoperatively. A large forehead flap was used for the lining, while a deltopectoral flap, 10 × 25 cm., covered the outside defect. Both flaps healed well and were separated four weeks later. The patient started radiation treatment soon afterward because the mandibular nerve contained tumor up to the foramen ovale and radiation treatment was considered necessary. No difficulties were encountered during the radiation treatment. The patient is free of disease and doing well.

CASE 8.—(Fig. 8). A 57-year-old man had a wide resection of the right mandible, floor of the mouth, and inferior surface of the tongue for a re-current squamous cell carcinoma after previous radiation and surgical therapy. A forehead flap with the pedicle on the right side was tunneled through a cheek incision and sutured to the mucosal defect borders; the anterior two thirds of the undersurface of the tongue was grafted to give the tongue good mobility. A medially based deltopectoral flap was used to cover the outside defect. The patient is doing well, eating, and talking.

In Group 4, consisting of two patients, we encountered difficulties with

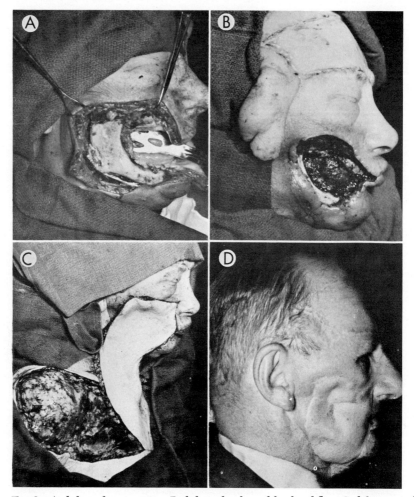

Fig. 9.—*A*, defect after resection. *B*, defect after loss of forehead flap. *C*, deltopectoral flap used to cover defect on cheek. *D*, patient two and one-half years after start of his treatment.

the immediate reconstructive procedure, but we succeeded in rehabilitating both of them by secondary procedures. Both are free of disease and doing well.

CASE 9.—(Fig. 9). A 68-year-old man had wide resection of the right cheek for an extensive squamous cell carcinoma of the buccal mucosa after preoperative radiation. A tongue flap was used to close the mucosal defect and a forehead flap was used for the skin defect. For unknown reasons, most of the forehead flap and part of the tongue flap became necrotic. One month after the first operation, the necrotic part of the tongue flap was removed and the remnants used to close the mucosal defect. After resection of the necrotic part of the forehead flap, the large outer defect was covered by a deltopectoral flap. Healing was satisfactory, although the patient had a tremendous amount of edema lasting for a long time. Now he is free of disease and doing well. Figure 9 D is a photograph taken two years after his first operation.

CASE 10.—(Fig. 10) A 46-year-old man had received planned preoperative radiation for a squamous cell carcinoma of the anterior floor of the mouth with bilateral neck nodes, but without involvement of the mandible. After bilateral upper neck dissection, resection of the floor of the mouth and inner gingival mucosa, and partial resection of the inner surface of the mandible anteriorly, an upper neck flap was wrapped around the mandible and a split thickness skin graft was used to cover the undersurface of the tongue and the upper neck. Several weeks later, the mandible became exposed after partial loss of the neck flap and the tongue dropped out through the floor of the mouth.

A bipedicled forehead flap was used to cover the exposed mandible completely on the right side and up to 1 cm. on the left side. The tongue was freed, pulled upward inside the mouth, and the lower border of the forehead flap was sutured to the mucosal edge of the tongue. Five weeks

FIG. 10.—*A*, deltopectoral flap covers defect below chin and on upper neck. *B*, after separation of flap and complete healing.

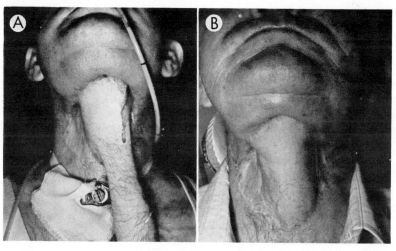

later, the forehead flap was divided and the left pedicle was used to completely cover the mandible. At the same time, a deltopectoral flap was elevated to cover the defect on the anterior neck after removal of the skin graft. Six weeks later, the deltopectoral flap was divided. The patient can eat and drink by mouth, feels fine, and shows no evidence of recurrence. Three years have elapsed since the start of his treatment.

Summary

The histories of ten patients are discussed. All had advanced disease, several had recurrence after previous treatment by surgery and/or radiation, and several had a second cancer. Most of the patients were of poor general health. Three were heavy drinkers and had damaged livers.

All underwent reconstruction procedures immediately at the time of the ablative cancer operation. Two needed a second procedure because of partial failure of the first operation. The other eight patients healed satisfactorily within a short time so that radiation therapy, where it was indicated, could be started soon. In all ten patients, the oral function was restored. While three are dead from recurrent disease and/or metastasis, they did enjoy a fairly normal life for one to one and one-half years because of the reconstructive procedure.

REFERENCES

Bakamjian, V. Y.: A two-stage method for pharyngoesophageal reconstruction with a primary pectoral skin flap. *Plastic and Reconstructive Surgery*, 36:173-184, 1965.
————: Total reconstruction of pharynx with medially based deltopectoral skin flap. *New York State Journal of Medicine*, 68:2771-2778, 1968.
Bakamjian, V. Y., Culf, N. K., and Bales, H. W.: Versatility of the deltopectoral flap in reconstructions following head and neck cancer surgery. In *Transactions of the Fourth International Congress of Plastic and Reconstructive Surgery*, Amsterdam, The Netherlands, Excerpta Medica Foundation, 1969, pp. 808-815.
Bakamjian, V. Y., and Littlewood, M.: Cervical skin flaps for intraoral and pharyngeal repair following cancer surgery. *British Journal of Plastic Surgery*, 17:191-210, 1964.
Bakamjian, V. Y., Long, M., and Rigg, B.: Experience with the medially based deltopectoral flap in reconstructive surgery of the head and neck. *British Journal of Plastic Surgery*, 24:174-183, April 1971.
Conley, J.: *Concepts in Head and Neck Surgery*. Stuttgart, Germany, Georg Thieme Verlag, 1970, 292 pp.
DesPrez, J. D., and Kiehn, C. L.: Methods of reconstruction following resection

of anterior oral cavity and mandible for malignancy. *Plastic and Reconstructive Surgery,* 24:238-249, 1959.

Edgerton, M. T., Jr.: Replacement of lining to oral cavity following surgery. *Cancer,* 4:110-119, 1951.

Edgerton, M. T., and DesPrez, J. D.: Reconstruction of the oral cavity in the treatment of cancer. *Plastic and Reconstructive Surgery,* 19:89-113, 1957.

Harrold, C. C.: Management of cancer of the floor of the mouth. *American Journal of Surgery,* 122:487-493, 1971.

McGregor, I. A.: The temporal flap in intra-oral cancer; its use in repairing the post-excisional defect. *British Journal of Plastic Surgery,* 16:318-335, 1963.

————: The temporal flap in faucial cancer. A method of repair. (Abstract) In *Transactions of the Third International Congress of Plastic Surgery.* Amsterdam, The Netherlands, Excerpta Medica Foundation, 1963, pp. 178-179.

————: The temporal flap in intraoral reconstruction. In Gaisford, J. C., Ed.: *Symposium on Cancer of the Head and Neck.* Total Treatment and Reconstructive Rehabilitation. St. Louis, Missouri, The C. V. Mosby Co., 1969, Vol. II, pp. 72-88.

McGregor, I. A., and Jackson, I. T.: The extended role of the delto-pectoral flap. *British Journal of Plastic Surgery,* 23:173-185, 1970.

McGregor, I. A., and Reid, W. H.: The use of the temporal flap in the primary repair of full-thickness defects of the cheek. *Plastic and Reconstructive Surgery,* 38:1-9, 1966.

McLaren, L. R.: Reconstructive surgery in the treatment of malignant disease of of the mouth. *British Journal of Plastic Surgery,* 16:305-317, October 1963.

Repair of the Pharynx following Total Laryngopharyngectomy

VAHRAM Y. BAKAMJIAN, M.D.

*Roswell Park Memorial Institute, New York State
Department of Health, Buffalo, New York*

RECONSTRUCTION of the pharynx and cervical esophagus following resection for cancer has been one of the more intriguing problems challenging surgical ingenuity in the management of head and neck tumors. Attesting to its difficulties are the great numbers of solutions that have been proposed over the years since Czerny performed the first cervical esophagectomy in 1877. For clarity of discussion they may be categorized into four principal groups, as follows:

I. Experimentally tried methods
  A. Autografts
    1. Dermis (Rob and Bateman, 1949; Connar *et al.*, 1956)
    2. Fascia lata (Baronofsky and Hilger, 1951)
  B. Homograft of lyophilized aorta (Javid, 1952)
  C. Foreign body implants, as of nylon, Teflon, etc. (Berman, 1952; Morfit *et al.*, 1962)
II. Methods of laryngotracheal substitution for the pharynx (Asherson, 1954; Wilkins, 1955; Som, 1956)
III. Gastrointestinal methods
  A. Pedicled segments
    1. Jejunum (Wullstein, 1904; Roux, 1907; Harrison, 1949)
    2. Tube fashioned from the greater curvature of the stomach (Beck and Carrell, 1905; Gavriliu, 1959)
    3. The stomach (Sweet, 1948; Shefts and Fischer, 1949)
    4. Right colon (Roith, 1924)
    5. Left colon (Goligher and Robin, 1954)

    B. Free segments revascularized at the recipient site
       1. Jejunum (Seidenberg *et al.*, 1959)
       2. Gastric antrum (Hiebert and Cummings, 1961)
       3. Colon (Nakayama *et al.*, 1962)
IV. Cutaneous methods
    A. Pedicle flaps
       1. Secondary inversion of local flaps (Mikulicz, 1886; Conley, 1956)
       2. Primary inversion of a transverse cervical flap (von Hacker, 1908; Lane, 1911; Trotter, 1913; Wookey, 1942)
       3. Secondary reconstruction with distant flaps (Watson and Converse, 1953; Erdeyli, 1956)
       4. Primary inversion of a deltopectoral flap (Bakamjian, 1965)
    B. Free grafts
       1. Split-thickness (Negus, 1950; Edgerton, 1952)
       2. Full-thickness skin of penis (Kaplan and Markowicz, 1964)

The group of miscellaneous techniques in the experimental category can be dismissed simply by saying that none has proved of value for clinical application. Likewise, we may dismiss Asherson's laryngotracheal substitution for the pharynx as having little, if any, application since early enough detection of a small and suitably located cancer to allow use of this technique is so very uncommon. Besides, if adequate removal of such a cancer permits the larynx to be retained, it would be more logical to save it for speech rather than as a passageway for food.

Gastrointestinal techniques were developed primarily for bypassing or replacing obstructed intrathoracic portions of the esophagus. Later, they were extended boldly into the neck for replacing also the cervical esophagus and even the hypopharynx. More recently, with the advent of techniques for anastomosing vessels of small caliber, free gut segments have been transplanted into the neck with revascularization by such anastomoses. Despite the obvious advantage of using a mucosa-lined and ready-made tubular substitute, these gastrointestinal methods cannot be warranted for routine application, particularly when the reparative problem is limited strictly to the confines of the neck. Not only do the required abdominal, and sometimes thoracic, interventions greatly compound the ablational cancer operation (in itself a formidable undertaking in patients who usually are elderly and often ill), but, in addition, the uncertainties of vascular sufficiency in the transplanted segment of gut greatly augment the risks of serious complications.

Beginning with Mikulicz's (1886) secondary closure of an established pharyngostoma by means of a turnover skin flap from the immediate vicinity of the opening, cutaneous methods have been the oldest and most commonly employed approach to pharyngeal reconstruction. A horizontal primary neck flap, used variously by von Hacker (1908), Lane (1911), and Trotter (1913), was rediscovered by Wookey in 1942 to become and remain a standard technique for many years, despite some real shortcomings. The method aims to reconstitute the gullet continuity in two stages, with the first stage accompanying the excisional operation. A transverse primary neck flap, intended for the reconstruction, is elevated at the start of the excision to expose the field of dissection. The width of this flap predetermines the length of the pharynx it will replace. Once the excision is completed, the flap is laid across the prevertebral fascia in the defect. Its end is folded first forward, then toward the base, and then backward again to form a skin-lined gutter between the pharyngostoma above and the esophagostoma below (Fig. 1). Subsequently, this gutter is secondarily converted into a full tube several weeks after the first-stage operation.

The luxuriant hairiness of neck skin in male patients is obviously an objectionable feature in the case of the Wookey operation. Viability of the flap is easily jeopardized by an accompanying radical lymph node dissection, and the technique is definitely precluded by previous irradiation to the neck. If, for any reason, the excision needs to be extended any higher than the hyoid level and/or much below the immediate subcricoid level, the width chosen for the flap at the start of the operation may well prove inadequate for the length of pharynx to be restored. Profuse leakage of

Fig. 1.—First stage of the Wookey operation for pharyngeal reconstruction using Trotter's transverse cervical skin flap.

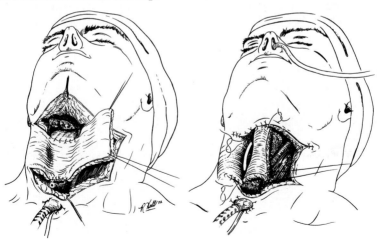

saliva down the front of the neck, in the interim between the two stages of reconstruction, requires attentive nursing care if serious pulmonary complications resulting from aspiration are to be avoided in geriatric patients. And, if nothing else, stricture formation at the esophageal junction to the skin tube is reported to be an unduly common complication of the method.

Skin pedicles from outside the neck may be used to overcome or avoid some of the disadvantages of the Wookey operation, or free inlay skin grafting techniques may be used with temporary support from a Portex tube (Negus, 1950) or a tubular stent of tantalum gauze (Edgerton, 1952). Proverbially, however, the migration of flaps from outside has heretofore required multiple stages, thus prolonging costly hospitalization and the period in which the patient has to suffer the considerable annoyances of a salivary fistula. It may also incur the tragic possibility of not ever completing the reconstruction before a local recurrence of disease dooms the patient to a miserable end. As for inlay free-skin grafting techniques, their apparent simplicity and expediency belie the very high rate of failures in many surgeons' hands that result in losses of graft, fistulae, strictures, and serious infections which pose the threat of a rupture of the carotid artery.

Deltopectoral Flap Technique

Like the Wookey method, this is a two-stage procedure, with the first stage immediately following the resection. It differs, however, in using a primary skin flap from outside the neck to form a completely tubular replacement for the missing pharynx at the first stage, leaving only a small, fistulous outlet for closure in the second stage (Fig. 2). This fistula is located just to one side and a little below the tracheostomal opening and does not incur the problem of saliva trickling into the trachea.

I routinely perform the excisional operation through a pair of transverse incisions modified after MacFee's (1960) parallel incisions for neck dissection. I place the upper incision in a prominent skin crease at the hyoid level. My second incision differs from MacFee's in being considerably lower, at a level with the inferior border of the clavicle on the side of the neck dissection. This second incision also marks the upper border of the deltopectoral flap intended for use in the reconstruction. Although, for a novice, this approach to neck dissection and laryngopharyngectomy may seem somewhat more tedious and difficult than ordinary, the advantages that accrue from it, in terms of safety and aesthetically better results, are definitely worth the negligible inconvenience. The deltopectoral flap is

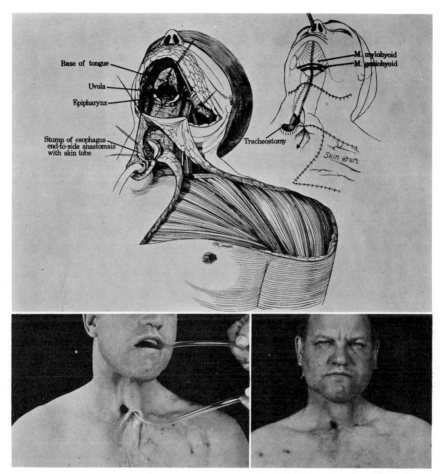

Fig. 2.—The author's operation for pharyngeal reconstruction using a medially based deltopectoral skin flap.

based parasternally over the first three or four intercostal spaces. Its lower border runs two or three fingerbreadths above the nipple (in the recumbent male) and passes to the deltoid region of the arm just above the apex of the anterior axillary fold. Its curvilinear distal end may be marked at varying distances from the base on the anterior, lateral, or even posterolateral aspect of the shoulder, depending on the length needed for the flap to reach its destination. Because of the excellent blood supply through the perforating branches of the internal mammary vessels, the flap is safe, in most instances, to use without delay. If for any reason, however, trouble can be anticipated (such as when a patient is extremely old, diabetic, arteriosclerotic, malnourished, anemic, etc.), delaying the flap 10 to 15 days ahead of the resection and first-stage reconstruction may be wise. This can be done satisfactorily simply by incising the outline of the flap and undermining minimally through the lateral half of its upper border, enough only to find and divide the cutaneous branch from the thoracoacromial axis which enters the undersurface of the flap a little medial to the deltopectoral groove.

The flap is raised in the almost avascular plane of the deep fascia over the deltoid and pectoralis major muscles. As its base is approached, care is exercised not to injure the perforating branches of the internal mammary vessels. It is then introduced into the area of the pharyngeal defect beneath the bipedicled flap of neck skin raised at the beginning of neck dissection. Starting above, the tip of the flap is sutured to the excision lines in the oropharynx and at the base of the tongue, so that the lateral edges begin to meet somewhat anterolaterally away from the side of the neck dissection. The suturing is then continued to convert the flap into a hollow epidermal tube with a longitudinal seam that spirals gently backwards in its downward course to meet the cut end of the esophagus in the lower neck. Here, a small marginal slit enlarges the end opening of the esophagus which is then anastomosed in end-to-side fashion to the skin tube a few suture points above the lower termination in the latter's longitudinal seam. Before completion of the anastomosis, however, a nasal tube is passed via the skin tube and esophagus into the stomach for feeding during the interim between the two stages of the reconstruction. Closure of the neck, and finally resurfacing the flap donor area on the chest with split-thickness skin grafts from the abdomen completes the first stage, leaving the above-mentioned temporary fistulous outlet at the base of the neck.

The second operation, which is minor, is performed approximately four or five weeks after the first. The esophageal connection to the skin tube is exposed by reopening the medial half of the lower neck incision. The deltopectoral skin tube is divided at an appropriate level, and the anastomosis between skin tube and esophagus is revised to a better fit in end-to-end manner. Any stricture that may have formed at this site is easily corrected at this time. The remainder of the flap is returned to its original site on the anterior chest wall after removing a corresponding area of the previously applied skin graft. In a matter of 8 to 10 days after this stage, the patient is usually ready to eat by mouth again.

Summary

A relatively expeditious and safe method for pharyngoesophageal reconstruction in two stages is presented. The first stage immediately follows a total laryngopharyngeal resection for cancer. A primary flap from outside the operative area in the neck is used and offers several advantages over the classical Wookey operation. In many ways, the deltopectoral flap is better suited for pharyngeal reconstruction than is Trotter's transverse cervical flap used in the Wookey operation. It provides more plentiful skin that is much less often objectionably hairy. It also has a thicker subcutaneous padding of fat that helps, partially at least, to fill the large void left by the excision in the neck. In no way does the magnitude of the excisional operation, whether it includes a unilateral or bilateral radical neck node dissection, adversely influence the vitality of the flap. Nor can preoperative irradiation to the neck affect it, although the latter may cause healing problems of the flap into the irradiated recipient bed. Nonetheless, when the flap is used in conjunction with the pair of transverse incisions described for neck dissection, the chances for success are much better than with a cervical flap or with free inlay skin grafts. The well-vascularized and healthy deltopectoral flap also provides protection for the carotid artery which it overlaps in passing into position in the dissected neck. Furthermore, with its easy reach high into the epipharynx, the length of pharynx it can replace is not limited or predetermined as in the Wookey technique. Neither is there a need to assume from the start that the entire circumference of the pharynx is to be resected, since the deltopectoral flap can replace any part or all of the pharyngeal circumference. The temporary fistula just to one side and a little below the tracheostoma eliminates the dangers of aspiration and greatly simplifies the nursing care of the patient in the interim. Finally, the technique does not rob the neck of its natural covering, and hence produces better end results, both aesthetically and functionally.

REFERENCES

Asherson, N.: Pharyngectomy for post-cricoid carcinoma: one stage operation with reconstruction of pharynx using larynx as auto graft. *Journal of Laryngology and Otology*, 68:550-559, August 1954.

Bakamjian, V. Y.: A two-stage method for pharyngoesophageal reconstruction with a primary pectoral skin flap. *Plastic and Reconstructive Surgery*, 36:173-184, August 1965.

Baronofsky, I. D., and Hilger, J. A.: Fascia lata transplants for resected cervical esophagus. *Surgery*, 30:355-360, August 1951.

Beck, C., and Carrell, A.: Demonstration of specimens illustrating a method of formation of aprethoracic esophagus. *Illinois Medical Journal*, 7:463, 1905.

Berman, E. F.: The experimental replacement of portions of the esophagus by a plastic tube. *Annals of Surgery*, 135:337-343, March 1952.

Conley, J. J.: Management of pharyngostome, esophagostome and associated fistulae. *Annals of Otology, Rhinology and Laryngology*, 65:76-91, March 1956.

Connar, R. G., Campbell, F. H., and Pickrell, K. L.: Esophageal reconstruction with free autogenous dermal grafts: An experimental study. *Surgery*, 39:459-469, March 1956.

Czerny, V.: Resektion des oesophagus. *Centralblatt für Chirurgie*, 4:433-450, 1877.

Edgerton, M. T.: One-stage reconstruction of the cervical esophagus or trachea. *Surgery*, 31:239-250, February 1952.

Erdeyli, R.: Tubular flap procedure for closure of large pharyngeal fistula. *The British Journal of Plastic Surgery*, 9:72-76, April 1956.

Gavriliu, D., as cited by Heimlich, H. J.: Postcricoid carcinoma and obstructing lesions of the thoracic esophagus: a new operation for replacement of the esophagus. *A.M.A. Archives of Otolaryngology*, 69:570-576, May 1959.

Goligher, J. C., and Robin, I. G.: Use of left colon for reconstruction of pharynx and oesophagus after pharyngectomy. *The British Journal of Surgery*, 42:283-296, November 1954.

Harrison, A. W.: Transthoracic small bowel substitution in high stricture of esophagus. *The Journal of Thoracic and Cardiovascular Surgery*, 18:316-326, June 1949.

Hiebert, C. A., and Cummings, G. O., Jr.: Successful replacement of the cervical esophagus by transplantation and revascularization of a free graft of gastric antrum. *Annals of Surgery*, 154:103-106, July 1961.

Javid, H.: Bridging of esophageal defects with fresh and preserved aorta grafts. *Surgical Forum*, 3:83-86, 1952.

Kaplan, I., and Markowicz, H.: One-stage primary reconstruction of the cervical oesophagus by means of a free tubular graft of penile skin. *British Journal of Plastic Surgery*, 17:314-319, July 1964.

Lane, W. A.: Excision of a cancerous segment of the oesophagus; restoration of the oesophagus by means of skin flap. *British Medical Journal*, 1:16, 1911.

MacFee, W. F.: Transverse incisions for neck dissection. *Annals of Surgery*, 151:279-284, February 1960.

Mikulicz, J.: Ein fall von resektion des carcinomatösen oesophagus mit plastischem ersatz des excidirten stückes. *Prager Medizinische Wochenschrift*, 11:93, 1886.

Morfit, H. M., and Kramish, D.: Long-term end results in bridging esophageal defects in human beings with Teflon prostheses. *The American Journal of Surgery*, 104:756-760, November 1962.

Nakayama, K., Tamiya, T., Yamamoto, K., and Akimoto, S.: A simple new apparatus for small vessel anastomosis. (Free autograft of sigmoid included.) *Surgery*, 52:918-931, December 1962.

Negus, V. E.: The problem of hypopharyngeal carcinoma. *Proceedings of the Royal Society of Medicine*, 43:168-169, 1950.

Rob, C. G., and Bateman, G. H.: Reconstruction of trachea and cervical oesophagus; preliminary report. *The British Journal of Surgery,* 37:202-205, October 1949.

Roith, O.: Die einzeitige antethorakale oesophagoplastik aus dem Dickdarm. *Deutsche Zeitschrift für Chirurgie,* 183:419-423, 1924.

Roux: L'oesophago-jéjuno-gastrostomose, nouvelle opération pour rétrécissement infranchissable de l'oesophage. *La Semaine Médicale,* 27:37-40, 1907.

Seidenberg, B., Rosenak, S. S., Hurwitt, E. S., and Som, M. L.: Immediate reconstruction of the cervical esophagus by a revascularized isolated jejunal segment. *Annals of Surgery,* 149:162-171, February 1959.

Shefts, L. M., and Fischer, A.: Carcinoma of the cervical esophagus with one-stage total esophageal resection and pharyngogastrostomy. *Surgery,* 25:849-861, June 1949.

Som, M. L.: Laryngoesophagectomy; primary closure with laryngotracheal autograft. *A.M.A. Archives of Otolaryngology,* 63:474-480, May 1956.

Sweet, R. H.: Carcinoma of superior mediastinal segment of the esophagus; technique for resection with restoration of continuity of the alimentary canal. *Surgery,* 24:929-938, December 1948.

Trotter, W.: The Hunterian Lectures on the principles and technique of the operative treatment of malignant disease of the mouth and pharynx. *The Lancet,* 1:1075, 1913.

von Hacker: Ueber resektion und plastik am halsabschnitt der speiserohre, insbesondere beim carcinom. *Archiv für Klinische Chirurgie,* 82:257-323, April 1908.

Watson, W. L., and Converse, J. M.: Reconstruction of the cervical esophagus. *Plastic and Reconstructive Surgery,* 11:183-196, March 1953.

Wilkins, S. A., Jr.: Immediate reconstruction of the cervical esophagus: A new method. *Cancer,* 8:1189-1197, November-December 1955.

Wookey, H.: Surgical treatment of carcinoma of the pharynx and upper esophagus. *Surgery, Gynecology and Obstetrics,* 75:499-506, October 1942.

Wullstein, L.: Ueber antethorakale oesophago-jejunostomie und operationen nach gleichem prinzip. *Deutsche Medizinische Wochenschrift,* 31:734-736, 1904.

Sensory Rhizotomy (Cranial and Spinal) and Gasserian Ganglionectomy in Pain of the Head and Neck Resulting from Cancer

MILAM E. LEAVENS, M.D., AND
J. MARTIN BARRASH, M.D.

*Department of Surgery, The University of Texas System Cancer Center,
M. D. Anderson Hospital and Tumor Institute, and Division of
Neurosurgery, Baylor College of Medicine, Houston, Texas*

PAIN IN THE HEAD AND NECK resulting from cancer can be relieved in many instances if the cranial or spinal nerves innervating the painful area are interrupted. The trigeminal, the nervus intermedius portion of the facial nerve, the glossopharyngeal, the vagus, and cervical sensory roots innervate the pain ending containing structures of the head and neck. The ophthalmic, maxillary, and mandibular branches of the trigeminal nerve, and the second cervical root supply most of the head with pain endings. The nervus intermedius (White and Sweet, 1969), the sensory branch of the facial nerve, supplies deep structures of the face and head, the facial muscles, a portion of the ear, the palate, and the tongue. The glossopharyngeal nerve innervates a portion of the pharynx, tonsil, posterior third of the tongue, posterior epiglottis, and pyriform recess. The tympanic branch of the glossopharyngeal supplies the middle ear, mastoid air cells, and eustachian tube. The superior laryngeal branch of the vagus supplies the somatic innervation of the larynx and vocal cords. The vagus also innervates part of the ear. Dividing only the rostral one or two filaments of the vagus is done to stop pain from vagus-innervated structures. Dividing all of the vagus nerve on one side is dangerous because of the resulting disabling

TABLE 1.—Sex—Age

Male	28 Patients
Female	5 "
Age 25—87 Years	
Average Age—53 Years	

dysphagia and the risk of aspiration of food and liquids into the trachea and lungs. At M. D. Anderson Hospital, the operative cranial and cervical spinal rhizotomy has been utilized in an attempt to relieve head and neck pain of cancer origin in a number of patients. A discussion of the treatment given these patients and the results will be presented.

From 1961 through 1972, 33 patients were treated. Table 1 shows the sex and age of these patients; most were males and middle-aged.

The sites of origin of cancer in these patients are listed in Table 2. The nasopharynx, tongue, tonsil, mouth, palate, and ear were the sites of origin in over half of the patients. Pain from these sites and immediately adjacent areas is transmitted over more than one cranial nerve. In such patients, multiple cranial nerve sensory division is indicated.

The pathology of the head and neck tumors in these patients is given in Table 3. The majority were squamous cell carcinomas. In most patients referred for treatment for pain, the head and neck surgeons could demonstrate by examination or X-ray studies the obvious presence of cancer. In some, the pain resulted from an ulcer with exposed necrotic bone. In a few patients, especially those with pain in the nasopharynx or ear, recurrence of tumor may not be proven until postmortem examination. Also, in a few, the pain is apparently the result of fibrosis resulting from surgical and/or radiation therapy.

It is not uncommon for the head and neck surgeon to find direct invasion by the tumor into branches of the trigeminal and other cranial nerves.

TABLE 2.—Sites of Origin of the Cancer (33 Patients)

Nasopharynx	5	Soft Palate	1
Tongue	5	Nasal Cavity	1
Tonsil	4	Lacrimal Gland	1
Antrum	3	Submaxillary	
Middle Ear	2	Gland	1
Orbit	2	Parotid Gland	1
Skin of Face	2	Maxilla	1
Lip	1	Mandible	1
Floor of Mouth	1	Unknown	1

TABLE 3.—Pathology

Squamous Carcinoma	27
Adenocarcinoma	3
Cylindroma	1
Adenocystic Carcinoma	1
Rhabdomyosarcoma	1

These tumors may reach an intracranial location by spreading along these nerves. We have seen in one patient, with squamous cell carcinoma of the antrum, diffuse involvement (50 to 75 per cent) of the cross section of the maxillary nerve anterior to, at, and a few millimeters posterior to, the foramen rotundum. Microscopically there was tumor spreading along the central one or two filaments of the middle and posterior third of the intracranial maxillary nerve. The more vascular gasserian ganglion was diffusely involved by tumor. In other patients, the tumor invasion can be beyond the trigeminal nerve and involve the cavernous sinus, floor of the middle fossa, dura, and other adjacent structures.

Of 18 patients who had trigeminal rhizotomies via the transtemporal approach, four had tumor involving the fifth cranial nerve in the middle fossa. One patient with squamous carcinoma of the lower lip had tumor in the mandibular nerve in and anterior, but not posterior, to the foramen ovale. A patient with squamous carcinoma of the antrum had tumor in both the maxillary and mandibular nerves in the middle fossa. Another patient with squamous carcinoma of the tonsillar fossa had tumor in the gasserian ganglion and mandibular nerves. A fourth patient with squamous carcinoma originating in the cheek had tumor in the maxillary and mandibular nerves, gasserian ganglion, and trigeminal posterior root fibers.

In Table 4, in the middle left vertical column, are indicated the various sensory roots or ganglion divided or removed. The V 1-2-3 refers to the fifth cranial nerve posterior (posterior to the gasserian ganglion) root ophthalmic, maxillary, and mandibular fibers. Ganglion refers to gasserian ganglion. N7 refers to the sensory nervus intermedius portion of the facial nerve. N10 indicates that the upper one or two filaments of the vagus nerve were divided and, finally, C indicates that one or more cervical posterior sensory roots were divided. The upper horizontal portion of Table 4 shows how many times a particular operation was done and whether it was a first, second, or third operation. The bottom horizontal portion of Table 4 may be used to determine which operation patients 1 to 33 had. The figure 2 or 3 above the patient's number indicates that the operation was a second or third operation for that patient.

TABLE 4.—SENSORY RHIZOTOMY IN 33 HEAD AND NECK CANCER PATIENTS

	C1	C2	C3	C4	C5	C6	C7	C8	C9	C10	C11	C12	C13	C14	C15	C16	C17	C18	C19
No. Patients—1st op.	8	1	2	1	2	4	1	1	1	4	1	3	1	1	2	1	1	1	1
No. Patients—2nd op.					1			1		1			1						1
No. Patients—3rd op.			1			1										1			
Cranial and/or Cervical Root Rhizotomy																			
V 1-2-3	*	*																	
V 1-2-Part 3			*																
V 2-3						*													
Maxillary and Mandibulary Nerve and Total Ganglion				*															
Maxillary and Mandibulary Nerve and Adjacent Ganglion							*												
N 7					*	*	*	*	*	*	*	*	*		*		*	*	*
N 9					*	*	*	*	*	*	*	*	*		*	*	*	*	*
N 10					*	*	*	*	*	*	*	*	*		*	*	*	*	*
C 2					*	*	*	*	*	*	*	*	*	*	*		*	*	*
C 3					*	*	*	*	*	*		*	*	*	*		*	*	*
C 4					*	*	*	*	*	*				*			*		*
C 5						*	*		*	*									*
Patients 1–33	4, 5, 6, 12, 18, 22, 24, 32	9	19	3, 23	16, 19², 29	2, 14, 15, 21	4	18², 33	1	7, 15², 30, 31	10	25, 26, 28	6²	10	11, 27	8, 18³	20	17	23²

The operations done may be divided into three groups for the purpose of analysis. In the first group, the operation was directed toward division of the fifth nerve posterior root fibers or removal of the maxillary or mandibular nerve and gasserian ganglion. In the second group, multiple cranial sensory root rhizotomies were done, usually with cervical sensory root division. In the third group, cervical root rhizotomies were done. All operations were done under general endotracheal anesthesia. A number of patients had tracheostomies because that procedure had been required at a previous head and neck surgical procedure.

These patients generally were considered for an operative procedure to relieve pain which had become severe enough to interfere with enjoyment of life, work, play, and sleep, and which, in a number of instances, had an indirect, adverse effect on other members of the family. They required daily codeine or stronger narcotics. Additional irradiation and/or head and neck surgery to relieve pain in these patients in most instances was considered impossible or not indicated.

These patients complained of an aching, burning, boring, and, at times, sharp pain which often eventually became constant except when relieved by narcotics. The pain in these patients was unilateral on the side of their disease and located in the eye, ear, suboccipital region, nasopharynx, jaw or neck, or in a combination of these areas.

In the first group of patients, 19 operations were done in 18 patients. In 12, fifth nerve posterior root rhizotomies were done for pain which seemed to be confined to fifth nerve distribution in the upper, mid-, or lower part of the face, and did not include the nasopharynx or ear. In one patient, the fifth nerve rhizotomy was done in combination with a C2 rhizotomy via the posterior fossa to relieve pain in the jaw and upper neck. All others in this group were operated upon by the transtemporal approach. The seven patients who had gasserian ganglionectomies and maxillary and mandibular nerve excision had tumor in the trigeminal nerve. They had this particular operation to remove intracranial tumor and to relieve pain. Other patients without pain, not included in this study, have had this same operation to eradicate intracranial tumor.

In four patients in the first group, the operation on the trigeminal nerve was inadequate to relieve the pain and eventually multiple cranial nerve rhizotomies were done. In one patient, a subtotal posterior trigeminal root section was inadequate. A total gasserian ganglionectomy and excision of the maxillary and mandibular nerve was done two months after the first operation. Tumor was found in the maxillary and mandibular nerves. Gross total removal was accomplished and relieved his pain. This was followed by 4,000 rads irradiation to the middle fossa. In this, as in other similar cases, the head and neck surgeon removes the tumor anterior to the middle fossa, usually during a separate operation before, and sometimes after, the neurosurgical procedure.

Four grades of postoperative pain relief or improvement were used in evaluating the effectiveness of surgical therapy in these 33 patients. In Grade 1, there was no, or little, relief of pain or the patient could not be evaluated or died postoperatively. In Grade 2, there was mild to moderate pain relief with the patient taking considerably less pain medication but still requiring some narcotics, usually codeine. In Grade 3, there was moderate to excellent pain relief with analgesics but no narcotics required. In Grade 4, there was complete, or almost complete, pain relief, and analgesics were no longer required.

Table 5 shows the grade and duration of improvement in 18 patients with trigeminal rhizotomy or ganglionectomy. All the patients were improved somewhat. Of the two Grade 2 patients, one obtained relief by having a second, more complete (ganglionectomy) trigeminal operation. The second Grade 2 patient was not benefited by a later multiple cranial

TABLE 5.—TRIGEMINAL RHIZOTOMY OR
GANGLIONECTOMY IN 18 PATIENTS

PATIENT NUMBER	GRADE 1–4 IMPROVEMENT	DURATION—RELIEF		
		Years	Months	Days
2	4	7	—	—
3	4	1	1	—
4	4	2	6	—
5	4	—	11	—
6*	3	—	3	—
9	4	—	4	—
12	4	—	6	—
14	3	—	2	—
15*	3	—	7	—
16	4	—	1	—
18*	2	—	—	20
19[1]	2	—	—	21
19[2]	4	—	1	—
21	4	—	3	—
22	3	—	1	—
23*	3	—	2	21
24	4	—	7	—
29	4	1	2	—
32	4	—	8.5	—
Total of 18 Pts. had 19 Operations	4 = 12 3 = 5 2 = 2	20 Days to 7 Years Average 10.5 months		

*Patients Later Had Multiple Cranial Nerve Rhizotomies.

nerve root rhizotomy. Satisfactory relief was obtained in the Grades 3 and 4 patients for a number of months to a few years. One of these patients survived with excellent relief of pain for seven years and three others survived with relief for one to two years. There were 12 Grade 4, five Grade 3, and two Grade 2 patients. The duration of relief was 20 days to seven years, averaging 10.5 months.

Table 6 lists the morbidity and operative mortality (none) in these 18 patients. Generally, the transtemporal approach to the trigeminal nerve is tolerated well by the patient. The temporal lobe does have to be retracted and can be bruised during the operation. This can eventually result in a convulsive disorder in the patient. One patient developed temporal lobe epilepsy but this was controlled with anticonvulsant medication. This was the only significant complication in these 18 patients.

Both the transtemporal approach to the trigeminal nerve and the posterior fossa approach for multiple rhizotomy are done best with the patient in the sitting position. The actual nerve dissections and divisions are more accurately done with such aids as a loupe or dissecting microscope, bipolar coagulators, and microinstruments.

In Table 4 it will be seen that 18 patients had multiple cranial sensory rhizotomies. In most of these, a trigeminal rhizotomy was combined with rhizotomy of the nervus intermedius, glossopharyngeal, upper fibers of the vagus, and two or more of the upper cervical sensory roots. In one patient in this group (No. 23), the trigeminal rhizotomy which had been done in a prior transtemporal fifth nerve rhizotomy was not repeated. This patient, with squamous carcinoma of the tongue, had good relief from the original trigeminal rhizotomy for almost three months. When pain returned, the nervus intermedius, glossopharyngeal, upper vagal fibers, and upper two cervical sensory roots were divided, relieving this patient's pain for another five years and three months. The patient required Darvon compound for pain during the remaining two years of his life. Patient No. 17, with pain mainly in the deep ear and throat as a result of carcinoma of the tongue, had a cranial nerve 7, 9, and upper 10 rhizotomy. Pain was relieved for a year. Pain then returned and narcotics were required before

TABLE 6.—18 TRIGEMINAL RHIZOTOMY AND
GANGLIONECTOMY PATIENTS

MORBIDITY	No.	MORTALITY
Exposure Keratitis—Transient	1	
Dilutional Hyponatremia	1	None
Temporal Epilepsy	1	

he died. We believe that relief in this patient, in which the fifth nerve was left intact, is an exception and we would not exclude sectioning the fifth nerve in other similar cases.

Sectioning of the nervus intermedius was excluded from the multiple cranial nerve and cervical rhizotomies in three patients either because they did not have ear pain or because the technical separation of the nervus intermedius was difficult or impossible with the limited help of a three-power loupe. This dissection is greatly facilitated now with 16× to 40× magnification of the dissecting microscope. One of these three patients died postoperatively. Patient No. 10, with squamous carcinoma of unknown origin, had face and neck pain; he was relieved of pain and lived for three months following rhizotomy. Patient No. 8 had squamous carcinoma of the tonsil with pain in the throat on swallowing and some ache in the ear. A complete fifth nerve posterior root, ninth nerve, and upper fibers of the tenth cranial nerve were sectioned. This patient continues to do well, and was tumor- and pain-free when last seen in September, 1972, eight years after surgical treatment. The original treatment consisted of

TABLE 7.—MULTIPLE CRANIAL NERVE AND CERVICAL
ROOT RHIZOTOMY IN 18 PATIENTS

PATIENT NUMBER	GRADE 1–4 IMPROVEMENT	DURATION—RELIEF Years	Months	Days
1	3	—	3.5	—
6*	3	1	5	—
7	4	1	—	—
8	4	8	—	—
10	3	—	8	—
11	1	—	—	8
13	4	—	1	—
15*	3	—	3	—
17	4	1	—	—
18*	1	—	—	0
20	1	—	—	8
23*	4	5	3	—
25	1	—	—	2
26	2	1	6	—
27	4	—	4	—
28	1	—	—	6
30	4	1	6	—
31	4	—	1	—

Total 18 Pts.   4 = 8   3 = 4   None To 8 Years
2 = 1   Average 1 Year 2 Months
1 = 5

*Patients Previously Had Trigeminal Rhizotomy.

TABLE 8.—18 MULTIPLE CRANIAL NERVE AND
CERVICAL ROOT RHIZOTOMIES

MORBIDITY		MORTALITY
Exposure Keratitis—		
Transient	3	
Dysphagia—		
Transient in 3	5	
Confusion—Transient	2	4 Patients
Hoarseness	2	2—8 Postoperative Day
CSF Leak	2	1 Wound Hematoma
Pneumonia	2	
Paresthesias—Head	1	
None	5	

6,000 rads irradiation to the carcinoma of the tonsil in September, 1964.

Table 7 indicates the grade and duration of improvement in these 18 patients with multiple cranial and cervical root rhizotomies. Eight were Grade 4, four Grade 3, one Grade 2, and five Grade 1. The duration of relief was none to eight years, with an average of one year and two months. Four patients had previously had trigeminal rhizotomy.

The posterior fossa and cervical laminectomy exposure for multiple cranial and cervical root rhizotomy is a larger, longer, and more difficult operation than the transtemporal trigeminal rhizotomy, which will result in more postoperative problems and a greater operative mortality than in the former procedure. Table 8 outlines the morbidity and mortality in these 18 patients. Two thirds of these patients had postoperative complications or disabilities which, in most, were transient or corrected by treatment. Some dysphagia and hoarseness were permanent in two. Four patients died within the first eight postoperative days. One had a wound hematoma removed but did not survive. Another probably died of a wound hematoma. The other deaths may well have been the result of poor selection of a debilitated patient, unable to tolerate such a major operative procedure. There was an operative mortality of 22 per cent in the 18 patients with multiple cranial rhizotomy, zero in the patients with trigeminal rhizotomy alone, and zero in the patients with laminectomy alone. The operative mortality for the 33 patients who had 39 rhizotomy operations was 10 per cent. Cervical root rhizotomy to relieve neck pain in head and neck cancer patients was done in two patients (Table 9).

One patient (No. 18) with squamous carcinoma of the tonsil had transtemporal trigeminal rhizotomy for face pain. Three weeks later severe neck pain developed. Two months after the original operation, a C2,4 uni-

TABLE 9.—MULTIPLE CERVICAL ROOT RHIZOTOMY

PATIENT No.	GRADE 1–4 IMPROVEMENT	Yrs.	DURATION RELIEF Mos.	Days
18[2]	1	—	—	0
33	4	—	6	—

C_{2-3-4} In Each—Bilateral In Patient No. 33.

lateral sensory rhizotomy was done. This may have helped the neck pain but improvement, if any, was difficult to evaluate because of the rapid onset of severe throat and ear pain.

The second patient (No. 33), a 42-year-old man, had nasopharyngeal carcinoma at the time he was seen for pain. This patient had had his tumor for two and one-half years and had been treated with cobalt irradiation to the nasopharynx and with methotrexate. For five months, he had had severe pain deep in the cervical paraspinal muscles. Extension and lateral rotation of the neck were limited and painful. There was tenderness of the paraspinal cervical muscles. Occasionally there was some suboccipital pain. There were no cord or cervical root findings. X-ray films of the sinus showed probable tumor in the ethmoid sinuses. X-ray films of the cervical spine showed no evidence of metastatic disease. Degenerative changes in the lower cervical spine were present. Results of myelography were essentially normal. No masses were felt in the neck. It was believed that the nasopharyngeal tumor was involving the upper cervical vertebrae or soft tissue paraspinal structures and accounted for his pain. A C1-4 laminectomy and bilateral C2-4 sensory root rhizotomy were done. The laminae and spinal canal anatomy were normal. No tumor was seen. This patient has been relieved of his neck pain but has developed two complications following the surgical procedure. A small pseudomeningocele has developed in the wound because the dural wound, made at the time of the laminectomy, failed to heal. This small meningocele is of little consequence and surgical correction is not indicated. Postoperatively, this patient has a sensory loss in C2-4 dermatomes bilaterally. Since surgery, he has complained of tightness in his neck and has a tendency to hold his neck in a forward flexed position. He is able to extend his neck somewhat, but is not able to hold his head and neck in a vertical position for very long. Additional X-ray films of the cervical spine have shown only osteoporosis. We believe at least part of his difficulty in maintaining his head in an upright posture is hypotonia and loss of position and joint sense as a result of the bilateral cervical sensory rhizotomy. This complication has been dealt with by having him wear a cervical collar. He has been essentially free from his preoperative neck pain for six months following surgical treatment.

Discussion

A number of authors have reported the results of their attempts to relieve pain in patients with head and neck cancer. Grant (1943) reported a series of patients treated by sectioning of the trigeminal nerve. Relief from pain was obtained in 70 per cent of his patients. Fifteen patients were treated by Grant with combined sectioning of the trigeminal and glossopharyngeal nerve; 86 per cent obtained relief. There was a 14 per cent operative mortality. Parsons (1961) reported good relief from pain in 70 per cent of 120 patients who had cranial nerve rhizotomies in various combinations for pain in the head and neck caused by cancer. In 1961, Botterell reported his series of 31 cases of rhizotomy for head and neck cancer pain. His conclusion was that dividing the trigeminal nerve alone was too conservative. However, some patients with a painful mouth or jaw ulceration after irradiation could be maintained for three to six months with alcohol injection of the appropriate trigeminal nerve branch. White and Sweet (1969) found that pain recurred in over 50 per cent of their 36 patients who had trigeminal rhizotomy for cancer pain. They recommended dividing, during the first operation, multiple cranial nerves if the lesion is situated so that other cranial nerves would soon be involved in pain transmission.

In our own experience with 18 patients, trigeminal rhizotomy was worthwhile in 17 of the 19 operations done. The average duration of relief was 10.5 months. In four patients, or about one fifth of the patients, pain again became a problem in a few days to a few months, and multiple cranial nerve rhizotomies were done. There was no operative mortality in this series. We would reserve trigeminal rhizotomy for those selected cases in which the pain seemed to be superficial in the jaw, cheek, or forehead and eye. Those patients who have pain in the ear, nasopharynx, or tonsil should have multiple cranial nerve rhizotomies. Eighteen of our patients had this latter procedure. About two-thirds had satisfactory relief of pain which lasted an average of one year and two months. The average duration of relief was four months longer in the patients with multiple cranial nerve rhizotomy than in those with trigeminal rhizotomy. Pain relief can be as long as seven years in trigeminal rhizotomy and eight years in multiple cranial rhizotomy, as seen in two patients in our series. Morbidity and mortality are understandably greater in patients with multiple cranial nerve rhizotomies because of their more complex nature. Two thirds of the patients had postoperative complications, most of which were transient. There was a 22 per cent operative mortality. This should be less with better selection of patients and avoidance of postoperative hematoma. The mortality rate of the whole rhizotomy series was 10 per cent.

Cervical root rhizotomy is indicated if the pain is in the neck, ear, mastoid, or suboccipital region. It is combined with cranial nerve rhizotomy unless the pain is confined to the neck.

REFERENCES

Botterell, E. H.: Discussion of: Parsons, H., Operation on the cranial nerves and posterior cervical roots for other forms of neuralgia and pain in malignant disease. In *Second International Congress of Neurological Surgery*, International Congress Series #36, Washington, D.C., Excerpta Medica Foundation, 1961, S16, p. E26.

Grant, F. C.: Surgical methods for relief of pain. *Bulletin of the New York Academy of Medicine*, 19:373-385, 1943.

Parsons, H.: Operation on the cranial nerves and posterior cervical roots for other forms of neuralgia and pain in malignant disease. In *Second International Congress of Neurological Surgery*. International Congress Series #36, Washington, D.C., Excerpta Medica Foundation, 1961, S16, p. E25.

White, J. C., and Sweet, W. H.: *Pain and the Neurosurgeon. A Forty-Year Experience*. Springfield, Illinois, Charles C Thomas, 1969, pp. 306-434.

Changing Concepts in Surgical Treatment for Malignant Salivary Gland Cancers

OSCAR M. GUILLAMONDEGUI, M.D.

Department of Surgery, The University of Texas System Cancer Center, M. D. Anderson Hospital and Tumor Institute, Houston, Texas

MALIGNANT SALIVARY GLAND tumors have been reported originating in all sites within the upper respiratory and upper digestive tracts, as well as in the major salivary glands (parotid, submaxillary, and sublingual).

In the past, the therapeutic approach to these tumors has been generally accepted as primarily surgical. With the recent advent of megavoltage radiation, the previous beliefs concerning the radioresistance of these cancers have been challenged. In addition, the concept of managing microscopic residual or subclinical disease with postoperative irradiation therapy has broadened our therapeutic approach and integrated the combined modalities of treatment for local control of malignant salivary gland tumors.

Materials and Methods

The clinical records of 125 patients with malignant parotid gland tumors definitively treated at M. D. Anderson Hospital from 1944 to 1965 were studied and analyzed. In a similar manner, the records of 36 patients with malignant submaxillary gland tumors also were studied and analyzed during the same period of time. The 125 patients with malignant parotid tumors were so selected that the analysis would reflect a homogeneous group of patients treated by surgeons of the Head and Neck Service, using similar criteria for therapy and similar surgical expertise. The small number of patients with primary malignant submaxillary gland tumors pre-

273

TABLE 1.—PAROTID CANCER (1944–1965):
125 SELECTED PATIENTS

Mucoepidermoid	43	34%
Malignant Mixed	30	24%
Adenocarcinoma	12	
Undifferentiated	12	
Acinic Cell	12	
Adenoid Cystic	10	
Squamous Cell	6	

cluded any similar selectivity. All available histopathological material was critically studied.

HISTOLOGIC CLASSIFICATION

Most tumors of salivary gland origin occur in the parotid; however, only about 30 per cent of these are malignant. In contrast to the parotid, however, the proportion of malignant diseases originating in the submaxillary gland and minor salivary glands is much greater.

In this study, the malignant tumors were divided into seven histological categories:

1. Mucoepidermoid carcinomas of high and low grade
2. Malignant mixed tumors
3. Adenocarcinomas
4. Adenoid cystic carcinomas
5. Acinic cell carcinomas
6. Undifferentiated carcinomas
7. Squamous carcinomas

Tumors of mesenchymal and lymphomatous origin were not included. Squamous carcinoma, though undeniably originating at times in the sali-

TABLE 2.—MALIGNANT SUBMAXILLARY GLAND
TUMORS (1944–1965)

Adenoid Cystic Carcinoma	21	60%
Mucoepidermoid Carcinoma	8	22%
High Grade 5		
Low Grade 3		
Malignant Mixed	5	14%
Adenocarcinoma	1	
Squamous Carcinoma	1	
Total	36	

vary glands, far more commonly represents a metastasis to the parotid or submaxillary gland from a primary tumor elsewhere, usually from the skin of the head or face.

The relative frequency of the various types of malignant parotid tumors is shown in Table 1. The experience at M. D. Anderson Hospital with submaxillary gland tumors is shown in Table 2. No significant correlation was found between the cellular type of the tumor and the sex, age, or race of the patient.

CLINICAL CLASSIFICATION

The prognosis of patients with malignant salivary gland tumors is affected not only by the histological classification, but also greatly by the factors of site of origin, behavior, rate of growth, and aggressiveness. Site of origin is important since an adenoid cystic carcinoma, originating in the ethmoids, is indeed quite different from the same type of tumor originating in the hard palate. The findings of nodal metastasis and invasion of connective tissue, bone, and particularly nerves are pertinent criteria in predicting the tumor's histologic behavior. This is especially true as it relates to submaxillary gland tumors.

Low grade mucoepidermoid carcinomas and acinic cell carcinomas can be grouped together in a moderately malignant category whereas high grade mucoepidermoid carcinomas, the undifferentiated carcinomas, the malignant mixed tumors, the poorly differentiated adenocarcinomas, and the adenoid cystic carcinomas, fall into a category of virulent cancers with a clinical course which is sometimes rapid and sometimes moderate but in either case indicates a poor ultimate prognosis for the patient.

DIAGNOSIS AND TREATMENT

The differential diagnosis between benign and malignant tumors through clinical symptoms and findings is usually difficult except in the most aggressive and rapidly growing tumors. Rapid growth, invasion of other anatomical structures, pain, facial paralysis, numbness in the area of the lingual nerve, a weakness of the tongue, and enlarged regional lymph nodes are typical of malignant salivary gland tumors. Vim Silverman or aspiration needle biopsies are inadequate and misleading for diagnostic purposes, because many of these tumors are notoriously nonhomogeneous. More than 90 per cent of the malignant parotid tumors appear in the superficial portion of the parotid gland.

A superficial parotidectomy was the minimally recommended surgical procedure for biopsy. A superficial parotidectomy was also therapeutic if the lesion was found upon frozen histology section to be benign, or one of the low grade malignant tumors, and was found at operation to be confined to the superficial lobe of the gland. If the histology section revealed a low grade malignant tumor and the facial nerve was grossly involved, the involved portion of the nerve was removed. If frozen section revealed a moderate to high grade lesion, the surgeon performed a total parotidectomy, resected the facial nerve, and also resected any other structures, such as the skin, masseter muscle, and ascending ramus of the mandible, which were involved with the tumor. When the lesion was moderate to high grade, the subdigastric nodes in the neck were resected. If these first level nodes were pathologically negative, no neck dissection was done; if they were positive, a radical neck dissection was performed. In the absence of a recurrent primary tumor, cervical node metastasis rarely developed later if the first echelon of nodes was negative.

The patients in this study were treated by surgical methods; radiation therapy was used almost exclusively in treatment for recurrent disease or, in a few instances, in the immediate postoperative period for treating suspected or known residual cancer.

The proper diagnosis and treatment of submaxillary gland tumors required a high index of suspicion on the part of the surgeons. Any painless, hard mass was considered cancer until proved otherwise by biopsy of the mass. Most of these masses were lymphadenitis or an inflammatory process in the submaxillary gland. A thorough head and neck examination, routine diagnostic studies, and X-ray study of the mandible were performed. In order to avoid an incomplete excision of a malignant tumor, a complete submaxillary triangle dissection was performed as a biopsy. A gross and histological study of the contents of the submaxillary triangle supplied information regarding the histological diagnosis, the degree of differentiation, and the presence or absence of nodal metastasis and/or nerve or mandible invasion. If any of these adverse clinical criteria were present, the surgical procedure included a radical neck dissection, removal of the myelohyoid, digastric, geniohyoid, and hypoglossus muscles and often a portion of the oral mucosa in the floor of the mouth. The lingual nerve was usually resected and, less often, the hypoglossal nerve. Other structures such as the mandible, parotid gland, pterygoid muscles, and masseter muscle were resected as indicated by the extent of tumor invasion. In the later years of the series, the patients with moderate to high grade lesions were given irradiation in the immediate postoperative period.

TABLE 3.—PAROTID GLAND CANCER—FIVE-YEAR
SURVIVAL OF 125 SELECTED PATIENTS

Acinic Cell	92%
Mucoepidermoid, Low Grade	76%
Adenocarcinoma	66%
Malignant Mixed	50%
Adenoid Cystic	50%
Squamous Cell	50%
Mucoepidermoid, High Grade	46%
Undifferentiated	33%

Results

PAROTID

The results of treatment of the 125 patients with malignant parotid gland tumors are shown in Table 3. The patients with acinic cell carcinomas had a five-year survival of 92 per cent, whereas the patients with undifferentiated carcinomas, at the bottom of the prognostic scale, had a 33 per cent five-year survival.

Of the patients with low grade mucoepidermoid carcinoma, 76 per cent survived five years, as contrasted to only a 46 per cent survival of patients with high grade mucoepidermoid tumors.

Only five of the 18 patients who died with distant metastasis from primary parotid cancers had control at the local site. This appears to indicate that complete local control reduces the patient's chance of developing distant metastasis (Table 4).

TABLE 4.—ANALYSIS OF 18 PATIENTS WITH
DISTANT METASTASIS

125 PATIENTS	DM WITH LOCAL CONTROL	DM WITHOUT LOCAL CONTROL
Mucoepidermoid	1	1
Malignant Mixed	3	2
Adenoid Cystic	1	2
Adenocarcinoma	–	3
Undifferentiated	–	3
Acinic Cell	–	1
Squamous Cell	–	1
Total	5	13 (72%)

SUBMAXILLARY GLAND

Adenoid cystic carcinoma was the histological diagnosis in 21 of the 36 patients with malignant submaxillary gland cancers. Six of the 21 patients were free of cancer when results were tabulated seven or more years after the day of diagnosis. Fourteen patients died of the disease and one was living with disease three years after treatment. Two of eight patients having mucoepidermoid carcinoma survived seven or more years free of cancer; the remaining six died of their disease. Only one of five patients with malignant mixed carcinoma was disease-free at seven years.

Discussion

One of the most distressing decisions for a surgeon treating patients with a malignant parotid lesion is to recommend sacrifice of the facial nerve. Any combination of modalities of treatment which enables the surgeon to eradicate the cancer while preserving the facial nerve is better for both the surgeon and patient. Thus, the most important change in the concept of managing malignant salivary gland tumors is the use of irradiation, postoperatively, to sterilize obvious or suspected residual disease in the operative site. In this series, we did not purposely leave gross tumor that was invading the facial nerve. Often, however, the tumor was dissected off the nerve—a procedure which is likely to leave residual microscopic disease. In these instances, we followed the surgical procedure with postoperative irradiation, and our results seem to show that this is beneficial in controlling the local disease. Our treatment policy in the future will include postoperative irradiation, not only for patients in whom microscopic disease is in the facial nerve, but also for all patients in whom the lesion is of aggressive or high grade malignant potential. This hypothesis will be tested by the accession of more patients into the study and by time as well, since the natural history of recurrence of many of these tumors is often prolonged.

Malignant submaxillary gland tumors behave in a much more virulent way than do their equivalent histologic tumors in the parotid. Also, there is a much larger proportion of adenoid cystic carcinomas in the submaxillary group. The adenoid cystic lesion has a definite propensity for invading nerves. Since nerve invasion greatly influences both therapy and prognosis, it is looked for diligently, both grossly when the surgical procedure is performed and microscopically in the removed specimen.

One might theorize why a given malignant tumor of the submaxillary gland may generally carry a worse prognosis than a similar malignant tumor of the parotid. Delay in diagnosis may play a role, but perhaps more important is the fact that many of these tumors are removed with a clinical impression of chronic sialadenitis and it is some days later that the pathologist notifies the surgeon that the mass he removed was, indeed, malignant. The surgeon mistakenly believes that because the submaxillary gland shelled out easily, the margin of resection is adequate. Our experience indicates that if the gland only is removed, the tumor will recur locally, sometimes at a considerable distance from the operative site.

Great stress has been placed herein upon the availability of a confident and competent frozen section evaluation by the pathologist. If this service is not available to a surgeon, he should not perform major resections of the salivary glands in patients in whom a high probability of cancer exists. Invasion of the nerves, mandible, or cervical nodes all carry a poor prognosis in patients with submaxillary cancer and if any of these are present, all of the gross tumor should be resected and the entire surgical field given 6,000 rads of irradiation as soon as the wound is healed. The value of immediate postoperative irradiation in patients with malignant submaxillary tumors has not been well tested, but in view of the rather bleak pronosis, it is well worth trial.

The Changing Treatment of Rhabdomyosarcoma in Children, Particularly in Treatment for Inoperable Rhabdomyosarcoma of the Nasopharynx and Oropharynx

J. R. WILBUR, M.D., W. W. SUTOW, M.D., AND
M. P. SULLIVAN, M.D.

Department of Pediatrics, The University of Texas System Cancer Center, M. D. Anderson Hospital and Tumor Institute, Houston, Texas

RHABDOMYOSARCOMA is the most common soft tissue sarcoma in children. It frequently occurs in the head and neck region (Grosfeld, Clatworthy, and Newton, 1969; Mahour, Soule, Mills, and Lynn, 1967; Sutow *et al.,* 1970). Children who have rhabdomyosarcoma of the head and neck with the disease localized in the scalp or the orbit have frequently been long-term survivors (Jones, Reese, and Kraut, 1966; Sagerman, Tretter, and Ellsworth, 1972; Sutow *et al.,* 1970). This has been achieved with surgical or radiation therapy. With few exceptions (Conte and Sagerman, 1971; Cunningham and Kung, 1972; Fish, Koch, and Canales, 1972; Ragab, Vietti, Kissane, and Sessions, 1972), patients with inoperable rhabdomyosarcoma in the nasopharynx or oropharynx or with disease in the middle ear have died in less than two years (Sutow *et al.,* 1970; Jaffe, Fox, and Batsakis, 1971; Mahour, Soule, Mills, and Lynn, 1967; Potter, 1966). This report includes children with inoperable rhabdomyosarcoma in the nasopharynx or oropharynx, including patients with middle ear involvement, treated at M. D. Anderson Hospital between January 1967 and June 1970.

281

TABLE 1.—CLINICAL STAGING OF HEAD AND NECK RHABDOMYOSARCOMA*

T-1 Tumor localized to one region or site, *i.e.*, orbit, scalp.
T-2 Tumor extension to neighboring structures or two or more sites, *i.e.*, cheek → tonsillar area, nasopharynx, soft palate.
T-3 Radiographic evidence of bone destruction, or cranial nerve involvement.
N-0 No clinical evidence of lymph node metastasis.
N-1 Single clinically positive lymph node less than 3 cm. in diameter.
N-2 Single lymph node more than 3 cm. in diameter, or multiple ipsilateral palpable nodes.
N-3 Fixed lymph nodes or bilateral palpable nodes.

*Modification of American Joint Committee for Cancer Staging and the U.I.C.C. classification.

The patients included are limited to those who had not had previous chemotherapy or radiation therapy and, at the time they were first treated, were without evidence of distant metastases. Four of them had apparent metastases in regional neck nodes. The group consisted of 11 children, ages 3 to 15 years, with a median age of 8 years; there were five boys and six girls. A more complete summary of children with head and neck rhabdomyosarcoma treated during this period was reported elsewhere (Donaldson, Castro, Wilbur, and Jesse, 1973).

The clinical staging nomenclature utilized is indicated in Table 1. Two of the patients had T-2 lesions with tumor extending to neighboring structures; both had regional lymph node involvement. Nine patients had T-3 lesions with either bone or cranial nerve involvement. The amount of bone destruction was often extensive, including invasion of tumor into the middle cranial fossa. Pathologic study of the tumor biopsy specimens indicated that ten were embryonal rhabdomyosarcoma and one was alveolar rhabdomyosarcoma.

Therapy

An important factor in treatment for this group of patients is that the therapy was coordinated and planned in advance in a cooperative effort involving pediatricians, radiotherapists, surgeons, and dentists.

Following completion of studies to determine if distant metastases were present, the standard approach consisted of surgical biopsy and tracheotomy if indicated. Subsequently, combination therapy consisting of radiation therapy and VAC chemotherapy (vincristine, actinomycin D, and cyclophosphamide) was initiated. The radiation therapy usually consisted of high-dose irradiation given at tumor doses of 5,000 rads in five weeks to

TABLE 2.—VAC Combination Chemotherapy

Vincristine:	2 mg./M² I.V. weekly × 12 weeks (max. 2 mg.)
Actinomycin D:	.075 mg./kg./course I.V. over 5–8 days
	(max. 0.5 mg./day) every 3 months × 5 courses
Cyclophosphamide:	2.5 mg./kg./day P.O. for 2 years

6,500 rads in eight weeks to the primary tumor using ^{60}Co irradiation, and in some instances electron beam irradiation with energies ranging from 6 to 18 MeV. Adjacent neck nodes were included in the radiation field. Three of the 11 patients had a split course of irradiation therapy. This consisted of 3,000 to 3,500 rads in three to four weeks, a two- to four-week rest period, followed by 2,000 to 3,000 rads in three weeks.

The VAC combination chemotherapy given simultaneously with irradiation is indicated in Table 2.

The maximum individual dose of vincristine utilized was 2 mg. I.V. weekly. Actinomycin D at 75 gamma/kilo intravenously per course of therapy was given over five to eight days with a usual maximum of 0.5 mg. (500 micrograms) each day. The actinomycin D was routinely given every three months for a total of five or six courses, usually for a total of 15 months. The cyclophosphamide was usually not begun until completion of radiation therapy to minimize the extent of the blood count suppression during irradiation.

Results

All patients were evaluated recently or had current follow-up reports. All had completed their chemotherapy within two years after initiation of treatment. Of the 11 children, nine are alive with no evidence of disease from 28 to 62 months from the beginning of treatment. The median disease-free survival at this point is 41 months. The two deaths that have occurred, occurred at 12 months. None of the nine patients who are still alive have shown evidence of disease since the start of their treatment, and none are still receiving chemotherapy. The therapy was complex and very toxic. Complications during therapy included severe mucositis in every patient. This is caused primarily by the combination of radiation to the oropharynx and actinomycin D given simultaneously. Meticulous care of the mouth during this period of time is required. Blood count suppression frequently occurred; however, only one patient developed a bacterial septicemia which was successfully treated. Vincristine toxicity consisted primarily of neurotoxicity and adynamic ileus which usually developed in association with severe constipation. Both of these problems require close observation, but a significant amount of toxicity is considered acceptable in order to deliver an adequate dose of chemotherapy to the patient. Weight loss and malnutrition are major problems. A feeding tube is almost routinely required to maintain adequate nutrition. Eye complications occur both during therapy (keratoconjunctivitis) and over the long term (keratoconjunctivitis and cataract). When the eye is included in the treatment field, usually because of involvement of the lower portion of the orbit with bony invasion of the tumor, some ophthalmologic problems can be anticipated. One of the 11 patients subsequently has had enucleation of the eye because of radiation keratitis, iritis, and conjunctivitis. One patient was blind before starting therapy as a result of the tumor growth. Two patients have no useful vision in the affected eye; one of these had a cataract which has been successfully removed, but the eye still does not have useful vision. One patient currently has fairly severe radiation keratitis and conjunctivitis and is being treated conservatively at this point.

Secondary problems in the mouth also occur frequently. Four patients had severe trismus; one of these had severe trismus, secondary to the tumor, at the start of therapy and it has continued posttreatment. Tooth decay can also be a major problem. It has been prevented to a large extent by the administration of careful dental care, including the use of fluoride carriers, under the direction of our Dentistry Service. One patient has possible osteoradionecrosis of part of the mandible. Problems of mouth dryness and thick mucus production are a regular postradiation complication. Infections have occurred in the radiation treatment area following completion of therapy in a majority of the patients. Some patients have had recurrent episodes of cellulitis, conjunctivitis, or sinusitis; all, however, have been responsive to antibiotic therapy. On each occasion where swelling in the treatment area caused the suspicion of recurrent disease, the swelling was the result of infection.

Case Examples

CASE 1.—This boy was 14 years old at the time he was initially seen at M. D. Anderson Hospital in December 1968. He had notable trismus which was secondary to an embryonic rhabdomyosarcoma involving the left tonsillar area extending to the base of the tongue and up into the soft palate. He also had a left submandibular 6 × 5 cm. node. The soft palate was pushed down by the tumor mass and his airway was partially obstructed. He required tracheotomy as did two of the other patients in this treatment series.

The local actinomycin D and radiation toxicity was relatively severe.

The neck in this instance received a tumor dose of 4,000 rads/four weeks, and the primary tumor 6,000 rads/six weeks. A relatively severe skin reaction subsequently cleared. Following completion of the chemotherapy, the patient has done well with the exception of residual trismus.

CASE 2.—This 15-year-old girl was initially diagnosed and treated in September 1969. The primary tumor was apparently arising in the right tonsillar area, but extended into the pharynx to the level of the vocal cords, up into the nasopharynx involving the uvula, and crossing over to the left side in the nasopharynx.

This tumor was growing very rapidly and within six days it had massively filled almost the entire oropharynx. She required an emergency tracheotomy and partial surgical removal of the mass in her mouth which had become necrotic. She subsequently received radiation therapy, 6,000 rads over six weeks, with VAC chemotherapy. The radiation field on the right side included the lower neck because of a palpable hard lymph node, suggestive of metastatic disease. She developed very severe oral mucositis which occurred secondary to the combination of actinomycin D mucositis and radiation mucositis. She required very careful mouth care with repeated mouth irrigation and gentle suctioning. Nasogastric feeding was required for several weeks. There was great concern near the end of her radiation treatment program because of the poor condition of the mouth, with continuing thick, tenacious mucus production. Because of this severe reaction, she received only one course of actinomycin D. Subsequent courses of actinomycin D were withheld in order to prevent the possible reactivation of her mucositis resulting from the recall phenomenon that occurs with actinomycin D. She had already developed apparent maximum tolerable radiation effects on the oral mucosa. Following completion of her therapy, she has continued to do well. She graduated from high school in June 1972.

Chemotherapy

For patients with metastatic disease or large inoperable disease, pulse VAC therapy (VAC_{pu}) may be more effective. It differs from standard VAC therapy in that cyclophosphamide is given simultaneously with vin-

---

TABLE 3.—PULSE VAC (VAC_{pu}) CHEMOTHERAPY

Vincristine:	2 mg./M^2 I.V. weekly × 12 weeks (max. 2 mg.)
Actinomycin D:	.075 mg./kg./course I.V. over 5–8 days (max. 0.5 mg./day) every 3 months × 5 courses
Cyclophosphamide:	10 mg./kg./day for 7 days I.V. or P.O. every 6 weeks

cristine and actinomycin D (Table 3), and at a dose of 10 mg. per kilogram per day for seven days. It is a very effective but a very toxic schedule. It causes severe granulocytopenia lasting several days and should be used in patients with significant metastatic disease or large inoperable disease.

The next case is not one of the eleven reported in this series because of the patient's wide metastatic disease at the time of diagnosis, but is presented to illustrate how effective VAC chemotherapy can be.

CASE 3.—This 21-month-old boy presented with a primary embryonal rhabdomyosarcoma on the face which extended into the maxillary sinus

FIG. 1.—Primary embryonal rhabdomyosarcoma extending into the maxillary sinus in a 21-month-old boy. A, appearance when first seen. B, X-ray film showing multiple lesions in all major bones. C, eight weeks after therapy was initiated. D, X-ray film showing evidence of complete healing of bones three months after initial therapy began.

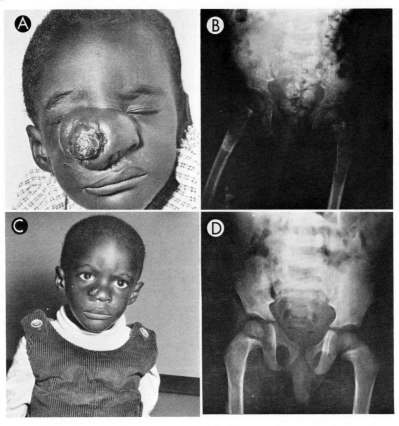

(Fig. 1A). He had widespread extensive disease throughout the body with multiple lesions throughout all major bones (Fig. 1B) and involvement of all of the vertebrae with compression fractures. He also had lung metastases and bone marrow replacement by tumor. He was started on the VAC chemotherapy program. Within two weeks there was regression of the primary tumor and he had relief of his bone pain. He began to eat again. By four weeks after initiation of therapy, he was feeling much better and was walking, which he had not been doing for months. His bone marrow was normal. By eight weeks after initiation of therapy, his primary tumor had almost totally subsided and he was treated as an outpatient (Fig. 1C).

At three months after initiation of therapy, his X-ray films had completely cleared with evidence of complete bone healing throughout (Fig. 1D). Unfortunately, this patient was not one of our successes because he suddenly died from complications of brain metastasis before adequate treatment could be directed to his central nervous system.

At postmortem examination the tumor was absent in the bones, the lung, the bone marrow, or in any other area except the small area of the primary on the face and the brain metastasis that caused his death.

The results of treatment of this child eloquently illustrate the effectiveness of chemotherapy in some patients in helping to reduce extensive disease.

Summary

Inoperable rhabdomyosarcoma of the nasopharynx usually has been considered a fatal disease. A high percentage of patients with it should now be considered potentially curable. So far, in this group of nine surviving patients, no relapses have occurred after discontinuation of chemotherapy at two years. The patients surviving longest are now over three years after discontinuation of chemotherapy. This treatment program requires cooperative intensive combination therapy and excellent supportive care by all the people involved, particularly the physicians and nurses who provide the day-to-day care. It is important to recognize that the successful treatment of these patients has been a team effort which requires involvement and cooperation of all the various members of the treatment team. If approached in this manner, the potential for successful treatment of patients with inoperable nasopharyngeal rhabdomyosarcoma is available now.

Acknowledgments

In giving this type of a report, the major results have been the contribution of many people and I would like to acknowledge the contribution of the various combined staffs who have been involved in this treatment program. M. D. Anderson staff includes Drs. Jesse, Ballantyne, and Mac-Comb, Department of Surgery; Drs. Fletcher, Castro, and Lindberg, Department of Radiation Therapy; and Dr. Daly, Dental Section. In addition to these staff members, without the devoted care of the nursing and house staff in Pediatrics, some of these excellent results would not have been possible.

Dr. Wilbur is currently at Children's Hospital at Stanford, Palo Alto, California.

REFERENCES

Conte, P. J., and Sagerman, R. H.: Embryonal rhabdomyosarcoma of the middle ear with long term survival. *New England Journal of Medicine*, 284:92-93, January 14, 1971.

Cunningham, M. D., and Kung, F. H.: Combined therapy for middle ear rhabdomyosarcoma. *American Journal of Diseases of Children*, 124:401-402, September 1972.

Donaldson, S. S., Castro, J. R., Wilbur, J. R., and Jesse, R. H., Jr.: Rhabdomyosarcoma of head and neck in children: Combination treatment by surgery, irradiation and chemotherapy. *Cancer*, 31:26-35, January 1973.

Fish, C. A., Koch, H. F., and Canales, L.: Survival in rhabdomyosarcoma. *American Journal of Diseases of Children*, 124:408-409, September 1972.

Grosfeld, J. L., Clatworthy, H. W., Jr., and Newton, W. A., Jr.: Combined therapy in childhood rhabdomyosarcoma: An analysis of 42 cases. *Journal of Pediatric Surgery*, 4:637-645, December 1969.

Jaffe, B. F., Fox, J. E., and Batsakis, J. G.: Rhabdomyosarcoma of the middle ear and mastoid. *Cancer*, 27:29-37, January 1971.

Jones, I. S., Reese, A. B., and Kraut, J.: Orbital rhabdomyosarcoma. An analysis of 62 cases. *American Journal of Ophthalmology*, 61:721-736, April 1966.

Mahour, G. H., Soule, E. H., Mills, S. D., and Lynn, H. B.: Rhabdomyosarcoma in infants and children: A clinico-pathologic study of 75 cases. *Journal of Pediatric Surgery*, 2:402-409, October 1967.

Potter, G. D.: Embryonal rhabdomyosarcoma of the middle ear in children. *Cancer*, 19:221-226, February 1966.

Ragab, A. H., Vietti, T. J., Kissane, J. M., and Sessions, D. G.: Rhabdomyosarcoma of the middle ear. A four-year survival. *Cancer*, 30:648-650, September 1972.

Sagerman, R. H., Tretter, P., and Ellsworth, R. M.: The treatment of orbital rhabdomyosarcoma of children with primary radiation therapy. *The American Journal of Roentgenology, Radium Therapy and Nuclear Medicine*, 114:31-34, January 1972.

Sutow, W. W., Sullivan, M. P., Ried, H. L., Taylor, H. G., and Griffith, K. M.: Prognosis in childhood rhabdomyosarcoma. *Cancer*, 25:1384-1390, June 1970.

Metastatic Carcinoma in Cervical Lymph Nodes: Unknown Primary Site

CARLOS A. PEREZ, M.D.,
RICHARD H. JESSE, M.D., AND
GILBERT H. FLETCHER, M.D.

Washington University School of Medicine, St. Louis, Missouri, and
Departments of Surgery and Radiation Therapy, The University
of Texas System Cancer Center, M. D. Anderson Hospital
and Tumor Institute, Houston, Texas

AN ENLARGED CERVICAL LYMPH NODE is not infrequently the first clinical manifestation of a neoplastic process in the head and neck. However, in some instances, despite a thorough search, a primary tumor cannot be found. A radical therapeutic approach has been advocated, since a significant proportion of these patients will be cured (Fletcher, 1966; Jesse and Neff, 1966).

Clinical Material

A retrospective analysis was done of 210 patients treated at M. D. Anderson Hospital and Tumor Institute between July 1948 and July 1968 for metastatic nodes in the neck with undetermined primary site at the time of definitive treatment. An additional 32 patients with far-advanced disease not receiving therapy, and 17 patients treated for palliation (10 with irradiation, seven with chemotherapy) were excluded from the study. Patients with a known diagnosis of thyroid cancer or melanoma, and a few patients with skin cancer thought to be the origin of the lymph node metastases, were not included in the study. All patients have been followed for a minimum of three years.

AGE AND SEX DISTRIBUTION

Of the patients studied, 80 per cent were between the fifth and seventh decade of life at the time of diagnosis. There were 172 men and 48 women (2.8 to 1 ratio).

LOCATION OF LYMPH NODES

The most frequently involved nodes were in the subdigastric or upper jugular chains (55 per cent of the patients). The submaxillary triangle was the site of metastatic nodes in 19 patients (9 per cent). An additional 10 per cent of the patients presented with multiple neck nodes, some of which were in the upper jugular chain. Supraclavicular nodes were present in 26 patients (12.3 per cent). There were 20 patients with bilateral lymph nodes (9.5 per cent). The locations of the nodes are shown in Figure 1.

Fig. 1.—A, location of enlarged single lymph nodes. Forty-three per cent of the patients had involvement of the subdigastric nodes. B, location of lymph nodes on patients with multiple levels of involvement. C, location of lymph nodes on patients with bilateral neck involvement.

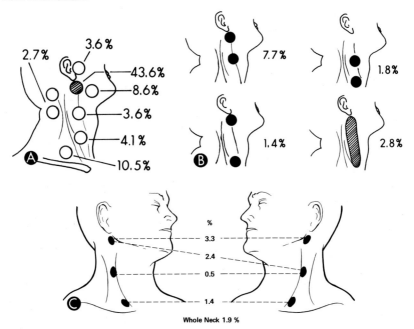

HISTOLOGICAL DIAGNOSIS

In 130 patients (62 per cent), a diagnosis of squamous cell carcinoma was made. In 59 of the patients (28 per cent), the tumor was diagnosed as undifferentiated or unclassified carcinoma, and in 21 (10 per cent) as adenocarcinoma or mucoepidermoid carcinoma. The distribution in the various treatment method groups was approximately the same.

DIAGNOSTIC WORK-UP

All patients received a thorough examination, including the oral cavity, nasopharynx, oropharynx, and larynx. In those patients in whom the histological diagnosis was adenocarcinoma, or in patients with squamous cell carcinoma in low cervical or supraclavicular nodes, a search was made for a primary tumor below the clavicles, and bronchoscopy, esophagoscopy, and even gastroscopy, as well as contrast media radiographic studies, were performed. Pelvic examination was done in women, and in men with supraclavicular adenocarcinoma, rectal examination as well as evaluation of the prostate was mandatory.

Routine radiographic studies of the nasopharynx, paranasal sinuses, and chest were obtained. In addition, tomographic studies of the paranasal sinuses and larynx, as well as a laryngogram, were performed in a significant proportion of the patients.

Although excision or biopsy of a cervical lymph node had been performed before admission in half of the patients, the diagnosis was made in 31 (17 per cent) by needle biopsy. Direct laryngoscopy under anesthesia is an integral part of the evaluation. Random biopsies of apparently normal mucosa (so-called "blind biopsies") of the nasopharynx, base of the tongue, tonsillar area, and pyriform sinuses were recorded in 110 patients (52.3 per cent). Routine biopsies were performed on any mucosal areas which appeared slightly abnormal. If the primary tumor was found before definitive treatment for the cervical nodes was instituted, the patient was excluded from this study.

CLINICAL STAGING

Using the description recorded in the chart, the metastatic lymph nodes were retrospectively staged according to the following classification:

Nx   Node excised prior to admission, with no palpable adenopathy at the initiation of therapy.

N1   Single not fixed node less than 3 cm. in diameter.

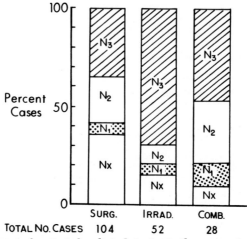

Fig. 2.—Distribution of patients by clinical staging in the various treatment modality groups. There is a large number of patients with early lesions treated by operation, as opposed to most of the patients with large or fixed lymph nodes treated by radiation alone or combined therapy.

N2   Single mobile lymph node, larger than 3 cm. in diameter, or multiple unilateral not fixed lymph nodes.

N3A   Fixed unilateral lymph nodes.

N3B   Bilateral lymphadenopathy, fixed or not fixed.

Approximately 40 per cent of the patients in the surgical group are in the early stages as opposed to 20 per cent in the irradiation and combined therapy groups (Fig. 2). The largest number of N3 lesions is in the irradiation group (70 per cent) as opposed to the surgical or combined groups (approximately 40 to 45 per cent).

Methods of Treatment

SURGICAL PROCEDURES

In about half of the patients, a radical neck dissection was performed. In nine cases, a bilateral neck dissection, usually staged rather than simultaneous, was done. The jugular vein was preserved on one side, if possible. Because of involvement of a parotid node or suspicion of a mass in the parotid, a partial parotidectomy in conjunction with the neck dissection was done in 28 patients. In four patients, a subtotal thyroidectomy was performed because of suspicion of a primary lesion in the thyroid. In a small group of seven patients with a single upper jugular node, a partial

TABLE 1.--METASTATIC CARCINOMA IN CERVICAL
LYMPH NODES: UNKNOWN PRIMARY SITE

SURGICAL PROCEDURES

Radical Neck Dissection (RND)	
Unilateral	51
Bilateral	9*
RND with Parotidectomy	28
RND with Thyroidectomy	4
Wide Local Excision	5
Partial ND Only	4
Partial ND with Parotidectomy	3
	104 patients

*Five patients required resection of the mandible and one
a thyroidectomy.

suprahyoid neck dissection was performed. There were three patients with a small single node who were treated by wide local excision and two with larger lesions on whom this procedure was performed; in one of these, it was for palliative purposes. The types of surgical procedure are listed in Table 1.

Of the 104 patients, 29 had subsequent secondary treatment for recurrences in the treated side of neck or the untreated contralateral side of neck, or for a diagnosed primary site. Radiation therapy was employed as an additional treatment in 22 of these patients, with nine of them surviving longer than three years after the second treatment without evidence of disease. Seven additional patients were treated by a surgical procedure; six of them showed no further cancer three years or longer after the second operation.

RADIATION THERAPY

Forty-three patients were treated with ports covering the nasopharynx, tonsils, and base of the tongue as well as the entire neck and supraclavicular regions (Fletcher, 1966). Megavoltage irradiation has been used since 1954—either ^{60}Co alone or combined with high energy photons.

Irradiation of the upper neck and nasopharynx was done through parallel opposing lateral ports to a minimal midline dose of 5,000 rads (Fig. 3). If the palpable lymph nodes were in the posterior cervical chain, the tumor dose was carried to 6,000 rads because of the possibility of a nasopharyngeal primary. The posterior margin of the ports was moved forward after 4,500 rads to exclude the spinal cord from the irradiation fields. On patients with large posterior cervical nodes, a posterior split field is used

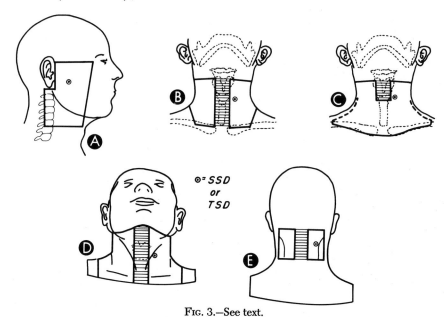

FIG. 3.—See text.

to supplement the dose, which is calculated at the sagittal midplane. In cases with persistent nodes at the completion of this therapy, an additional boost of 1,000 rads is given to the residual mass through small ports with an electron beam (9 to 15 Mev). If there are no nodes anterior to the subdigastric area, the submaxillary gland is excluded to prevent excessive dryness of the mouth. The lower neck is irradiated by an anterior field, with a midline block to protect the larynx. If there are no palpable lymph nodes, the given dose is 5,000 rads. When lymph nodes are present, 6,000 rads are delivered.

The involved neck only was treated in seven cases to doses of 6,000 rads; two additional patients were treated with other irradiation techniques.

Four of the 52 patients had secondary treatment for recurrent disease in the neck or a subsequently diagnosed primary tumor. One patient treated surgically was free of cancer three years following the treatment.

COMBINED THERAPY

A combination of radiation therapy and surgery was used, particularly on patients with large, fixed nodes.

TABLE 2.—THREE-YEAR ABSOLUTE CURE RATES
IN PATIENTS TREATED FOR CURE

	SURGERY	IRRADIATION	COMBINED RX
Nx	31/39 (79%)	8/9 (89%)	3/3 (——)
N1	4/6 (67%)	1/3 (——)	1/3 (——)
N2	10/22 (45%)	3/4 (75%)	5/9 (55%)
N3	14/37 (38%)	13/36 (36%)	4/13 (31%)

Preoperative irradiation to doses in the range of 2,000 rads in one week (5 fractions) to the involved side of the neck was used in six patients. Preoperative doses between 4,000 and 5,000 rads were given in 11 patients.

In 11 additional patients, postoperative irradiation was delivered to doses of 5,000 to 6,000 rads, usually to both sides of the neck and the nasopharynx.

Secondary treatment was administered to five patients who had recurrence in the treated side of the neck or for the appearance of a primary tumor. One patient treated surgically survived three years after the second treatment.

RESULTS AND FACTORS AFFECTING PROGNOSIS

The clinical stage was the most reliable prognostic indicator. Patients with Nx lesions have three-year cure rates of about 80 per cent, as opposed to 50 to 60 per cent for N1 to N2 and about 36 per cent for stage N3 nodes (Table 2). The cure rates five years after treatment are essentially the same (Table 3).

The location of the largest node, whether this was in the upper or middle neck, did not significantly affect the prognosis. The survival according to clinical staging in the various treatment methods is approximately the same in any of these locations. However, there were no survivors in a group of eight patients with large fixed lower cervical nodes.

The histology of the tumor did not significantly influence the prognosis.

TABLE 3.—FIVE-YEAR ABSOLUTE CURE RATES
IN PATIENTS TREATED FOR CURE

	SURGERY	IRRADIATION	COMBINED RX
Nx	21/34 (62%)	6/8 (75%)	3/3 (——)
N1	1/5 (20%)	0/2 (——)	1/2 (——)
N2	8/20 (40%)	2/2 (——)	4/9 (44%)
N3	10/34 (29%)	8/26 (30%)	1/6 (16%)

Stage by stage, the survival was approximately the same for squamous cell carcinoma, undifferentiated or unclassified carcinoma, or adenocarcinoma.

SITES OF FAILURE

Approximately 80 per cent of the patients who developed a recurrence did so within 24 months after the completion of therapy. The cumulative rates of failure were approximately the same, regardless of the method of treatment.

A detailed analysis of the sites of failure (Table 4) shows that in early lesions (Nx, N1), the proportion of treated neck recurrences was approximately the same (10 per cent) in all groups. In the surgical patients, there were five contralateral failures (12.5 per cent) as opposed to none in those treated with irradiation alone or in the combined therapy groups.

In patients with N2 lymph nodes treated surgically, both ipsilateral (6 of 22) and contralateral failures (7 of 22) were more frequent.

In the patients with N3 nodes, nine of 30 surgical cases (30 per cent) showed a failure in the treated neck as opposed to five of 23 (21 per cent) in the group receiving radiation therapy alone, and two of 13 (15 per cent) in the combined therapy groups.

Of 97 patients with unilateral neck dissections treated surgically, 16 (16.5 per cent) developed contralateral lymph nodes in contrast to none in the group receiving radiation therapy alone or in the combined therapy patients.

In the patients with bilateral nodes, the failure rate in the neck was slightly higher in the surgical group (4 of 7) as opposed to the radiation therapy groups (4 of 13). The incidence of distant metastasis was approximately the same in all groups.

TABLE 4.—CERVICAL LYMPH NODES, UNKNOWN PRIMARY:
INCIDENCE OF FAILURE IN THE NECK

TREATED NECK	SURGERY	IRRADIATION	COMBINED RX
Nx	4/39 (10%)	1/9 (11%)	0/3
N1	2/6	1/3	0/3
N2	6/22 (27%)	0/4	2/9 (22%)
N3A	9/30 (30%)	5/23 (21%)	2/13 (15%)
N3B	4/7 (57%)	4/13 (31%)	——
Contralateral Neck	16/97 (16.5%)	0/39	0/28

TABLE 5.—METASTATIC CARCINOMA IN CERVICAL LYMPH NODES,
UNKNOWN PRIMARY SITE: INCIDENCE OF PRIMARY
TUMOR FOUND AFTER Rx TO NODES

SITE OF PRIMARY	SURGERY° (104 CASES)	IRRADIATION° (52 CASES)	COMBINED Rx. (28 CASES)
Head and Neck	21 (20%)	3 (5.7%)	4 (14.3%)
Thorax, Abdomen, Other Sites	5 (4.8%)	3 (5.7%)	1 (3.6%)

°Difference in surgical and irradiation groups significant at $P < .05$ (Chi square test).

APPEARANCE OF A PRIMARY TUMOR AFTER DEFINITIVE TREATMENT

A primary tumor was diagnosed in 36 of the 184 patients with cervical lymph nodes. Table 5 shows the proportion of patients developing head and neck primary tumors. The largest percentage (20 per cent) is in the surgical group followed by the combined therapy group (14 per cent) in contrast to only three patients in the irradiation alone group (5.7 per cent). The proportion of patients with evidence of primary tumors below the clavicle, either in the thorax or the abdomen, is approximately the same in the three different treatment method groups (4 to 5 per cent). Over 90 per cent of the primary tumors appeared within three years after the initial treatment of the neck lymph nodes.

The three-year absolute cure rate is significantly better in the group of patients in which a primary tumor was not found—86 of 148 patients surviving without evidence of disease (58 per cent) in comparison with only 11 of 36 patients (31 per cent) in whom a primary tumor occurred.

LOCATION OF PRIMARY TUMOR CORRELATED WITH LEVEL OF LYMPH NODE INVOLVEMENT

The sites of primary tumors found in the patients treated by the different therapeutic modalities are listed in Table 6. A large proportion of the patients in the surgical group with upper cervical nodes later presented lesions within the oropharynx or hypopharynx. Patients with upper or middle cervical nodes have a fairly high incidence of pyriform sinus tumors.

Only three patients in the irradiation alone group developed a primary tumor, one in the uvula, another in the pyriform sinus, and the third in the

TABLE 6.—METASTATIC CARCINOMA IN CERVICAL LYMPH NODES,
UNKNOWN PRIMARY SITE: LOCATION OF PRIMARY
TUMORS IN THE HEAD AND NECK

	SURGERY	IRRADIATION	COMBINED RX.
Hypopharynx	6	1	1
Tonsil or Faucial Arch	4	–	1
Base of Tongue, Valleculum	4	–	–
Oral Cavity, Salivary Glands	2	2	–
Nasopharynx	2	–	–
Maxillary Antrum	–	–	1
A-E Fold, Epiglottis	1	–	1
Cervical Esophagus	1	–	–
Thyroid	1	–	–

floor of the mouth. These three patients were initially treated with ports that encompassed the nasopharynx and oropharynx but, except for the uvula, the location of these primary tumors was not included in the originally irradiated volume. The largest number of primary tumors found below the clavicles was in the lungs (8 patients).

COMPLICATIONS

Fatal complications were rare, regardless of the method of treatment (Table 7). Nonfatal complications were also comparably low in the various groups treated by operation, radiation alone, or a combination of both (Table 8). The most frequent complication in the surgical group was severe shoulder pain; in the radiation therapy patients, it was laryngeal edema and subcutaneous fibrosis.

TABLE 7.—METASTATIC CARCINOMA IN CERVICAL LYMPH NODES,
UNKNOWN PRIMARY SITE: FATAL COMPLICATIONS

		SURGERY	IRRADIATION	COMBINED RX.
Post-Op	Pulmonary Infarct	1		
	Myocardial Infarct	1		
	Perforated Peptic Ulcer			1
	Unknown Cause			1
Radiation Myelopathy			1	
Carotid Perforation				1
Pharyngeal Necrosis			1*	

*After irradiation of primary tumor.

TABLE 8.—METASTATIC SUPRACLAVICULAR NODES,
UNKNOWN PRIMARY SITE: SURVIVAL,
NO EVIDENCE OF DISEASE

	IRRADIATION		SURGERY	
	3 Yrs.	5 Yrs.	3 Yrs.	5 Yrs.
Nx	1/3	1/2	0/4	0/3
N1	—	—	1/1	1/1
N2	—	—	1/2	1/2
N3	0/13	0/12	0/3	0/3
	1/16	1/14	2/10	2/9

SUPRACLAVICULAR NODES, UNKNOWN PRIMARY SITE

Twenty-six patients presented with metastatic lymph nodes in the supraclavicular region, without an apparent primary tumor. Table 8 shows the clinical stage and the method of treatment distribution as well as the three- and five-year results. Most of the patients in the radiation therapy group presented with large N3 lesions, and only one patient was cured. Of the patients treated by a surgical procedure, either palliative wide local excision or a radical neck dissection, only two survived for more than three years. Six of the 26 patients developed a primary tumor after treatment of the lymph nodes (23 per cent), three of them in the lung and the other three in the abdominal viscera.

Discussion

A significant proportion of patients with diagnosed malignant disease of the head and neck show a "lump" in the neck as the first manifestation of the disease (Comess, Beahrs, and Dockerty, 1957; Martin and Morfit, 1944). The usual location of metastatic cervical lymph nodes in relation to the primary tumors is discussed by Lindberg (1972). However, in about 10 per cent of the patients, a primary lesion cannot be found, despite thorough initial examination and careful follow-up (Acquarelli, Matsunaga, and Cruze, 1961; Barrie, Knapper, and Strong, 1970; Comess, Beahrs, and Dockerty, 1957; Marchetta, Murphy, and Kovaric, 1963; Pico, Frias, and Bosch, 1971; Ridenhour, Yeun, and Spratt, 1967).

Survival rates in the range of 15 to 40 per cent at three years have been reported after surgical treatment (Barrie, Knapper, and Strong, 1970; Jesse and Neff, 1966; Marchetta, Murphy, and Kovaric, 1963; Pico, Frias, and Bosch, 1971; Ridenhour, Yeun, and Spratt, 1967), and comparable results have been obtained following radical irradiation (Jesse, Perez, and

Fletcher, 1973; Marchetta, Murphy, and Kovaric, 1963). In the present series, the three-year survival rate free of cancer was 48 per cent. If the patients with supraclavicular nodes are excluded, the three-year survival rate without tumor is 53 per cent. The therapeutic results obtained with the various treatment modalities are comparable.

The development of contralateral neck nodes was appreciably higher in the surgical group (16.5 per cent), in contrast to that in the patients treated by irradiation alone or by irradiation combined with a neck dissection, neither of which failed in the contralateral neck. Likewise, the patients treated with irradiation showed a significantly lower incidence of subsequent primary tumors (5.6 per cent) while 20 per cent of the patients initially treated surgically subsequently developed a primary lesion.

So, the question is not only what is the most effective method of therapy, but also which one is indicated in the individual patient that will yield the highest tumor control with a low morbidity.

Depending on the location of the node, the stage of disease, and the histology, different treatment methods may be selected. Partial or radical neck dissection is an adequate procedure to control single mobile lymph nodes in the submaxillary triangle and in the subdigastric region. Radiation therapy produces equal results with a lesser incidence of subsequent contralateral lymph nodes. However, if these patients are irradiated, a significant portion of the mucosa of the oral cavity and pharynx must be included in the irradiation portals, which may result in severe dryness of these areas. Because of this, a surgical procedure is preferred, since it can easily manage the lymph nodes as well as contralateral neck metastasis. Likewise, a radical neck dissection is preferred for single mobile nodes in the low subdigastric or midjugular region, since the irradiation fields will include the larynx and hypopharynx.

Patients with mobile, multiple ipsilateral, or bilateral lymph nodes may be treated by radiation alone to doses of 6,000 rads in the involved areas.

Patients with small high jugular nodes or posterior cervical nodes are effectively treated by radical irradiation with fields that include the nasopharynx, tonsillar fossa, and base of the tongue, as well as the entire lymph node-bearing tissues of both sides of the neck. The larynx is usually shielded with a small block.

Large or fixed nodes may be treated by irradiation alone to the entire neck (6,000 rads) with an alternative plan which may include a radical or partial neck dissection if there is no complete regression of the enlarged node four to six weeks after completion of the irradiation. Low dose preoperative irradiation (Henschke et al., 1964) failed to show any significant benefit.

Postoperative irradiation is indicated in those patients primarily treated by operation in whom pathological examination of the specimen shows more extensive involvement of the neck tissues than was anticipated pre-operatively.

The high proportion of patients treated initially by operation who develop primary tumors in the oropharynx or hypopharynx emphasizes the need for random biopsies of these areas. This procedure should be performed routinely, before initiation of therapy.

Even if a primary tumor develops sometime after the treatment to the cervical lymph nodes, an aggressive surgical or radiotherapeutic management will yield satisfactory results, with approximately 40 per cent of the patients being cured. The complications of these patients, whether treated surgically or by radiation therapy, are of the same nature and incidence as those observed in the treatment for other head and neck neoplasias.

Summary

A retrospective study was made of 210 patients receiving definitive therapy for a metastatic cervical lymph node with an unknown primary. The three-year survival rate without evidence of tumor was about 80 per cent in the patients with early lesions and 35 per cent in those with large fixed nodes.

A surgical procedure or radiation therapy was equally effective in controlling the disease in the more favorable clinical stages (Nx–N1). Radiation therapy was highly effective in preventing the development of subsequent contralateral metastatic nodes or a primary cancer in the nasopharynx, oropharynx, or hypopharynx. However, because of the potential morbidity of irradiation, a radical neck dissection is preferred in these patients unless the lymph nodes are located in the upper jugular or posterior cervical chains.

More advanced lymph nodes are best treated by preoperative irradiation to the entire neck, including the pharynx, to doses of 5,000 to 6,000 rads, followed by partial or radical neck dissection.

The necessity of a thorough initial work-up and aggressive management is emphasized, since many of these patients can be cured.

REFERENCES

Acquarelli, M. J., Matsunaga, R. S., and Cruze, K.: Metastatic carcinoma of the neck of unknown primary origin. *Laryngoscope*, 71:962-974, 1961.

Barrie, J. R., Knapper, W. H., and Strong, E. W.: Cervical nodal metastases of unknown origin. *American Journal of Surgery*, 120:466-470, 1970.

Comess, M. S., Beahrs, O. H., and Dockerty, M. B.: Cervical metastasis from occult carcinoma. *Surgery, Gynecology and Obstetrics,* 104:607-617, 1957.

Fletcher, G. H.: *Textbook of Radiotherapy.* Philadelphia, Pennsylvania, Lea & Febiger, 1966, 580 pp.

Henschke, U. K., Frazell, E. L., Hilaris, B. S., Nickson, J. J., Tollefsen, H. R., and Strong, E. W.: Local recurrences after radical neck dissection with and without preoperative x-ray therapy. *Radiology,* 82:331-332, 1964.

Jesse, R. H., and Neff, L. E.: Metastatic carcinoma in cervical nodes with an unknown primary lesion. *American Journal of Surgery,* 112:547-553, 1966.

Jesse, R. H., Perez, C. A., and Fletcher, G. H.: Cervical lymph node metastasis: Unknown primary cancer. *Cancer,* 31:854-859, 1973.

Lindberg, R.: Distribution of cervical lymph node metastases from squamous cell carcinoma of the upper respiratory and digestive tracts. *Cancer,* 29:1446-1449, June 1972.

Marchetta, F. C., Murphy, W. T., and Kovaric, J. J.: Carcinoma of the neck. *American Journal of Surgery,* 106:974-979, 1963.

Martin, H., and Morfit, H. M.: Cervical lymph node metastasis as the first symptom of cancer. *Surgery, Gynecology and Obstetrics,* 78:133-159, 1944.

Pico, J., Frias, Z., and Bosch, A.: Cervical lymph node metastases from carcinoma of undetermined origin. *The American Journal of Roentgenology, Radium Therapy and Nuclear Medicine,* 111:95-102, January 1971.

Ridenhour, C. E., Yeun, P. F., and Spratt, J. S., Jr.: Metastatic carcinoma in cervical lymph nodes from occult primary sites. A review. *Missouri Medicine,* 64:988-993, 1967.

Nursing Care of the Patient with Head and Neck Cancer

RENILDA HILKEMEYER, R.N., B.S.

Department of Nursing, The University of Texas System Cancer Center, M. D. Anderson Hospital and Tumor Institute, Houston, Texas

THE PATIENT WITH CANCER of the head and neck requires comprehensive, individualized nursing care including skilled physical nursing care, emotional support, teaching of self care, and an understanding of the psychological, social, and economic implications during the diagnostic, therapeutic, and rehabilitative period.

To be an effective team member in caring for the patient with head and neck cancer, the professional nurse needs to work collaboratively with the physician to understand and aid in carrying out the medical plan of treatment, and with other disciplines such as medical social service. She needs to have a positive, hopeful attitude and to be secure in her nursing skills, so that she can by verbal and nonverbal communication transmit support to the patient. Many nurses have had minimal experience with head and neck patients; orientation and continuing education are essential. I would like to pay tribute to our nursing staff, and particularly the head nurses, who care for these patients, and teach our staff.

The nurse needs to accept the patient as he is. By her physical presence she can communicate to the patient and his family that he is accepted as a human being even though his appearance may be significantly altered.

While each patient's care must be individualized, I would like to discuss some nursing care aspects common to many patients with head and neck cancer. Some are immediate needs during the diagnostic, pre-, and postoperative phases, which may be short-term goals; others are long-term goals for future rehabilitation of the patient. Working with the patient and

303

his family in a total team concept is essential to accomplishment of these goals.

The nurse's initial contact with the patient is very important in establishing the rapport and communication which are so essential. We believe that it is important for the professional nurse to be available during the physical examination and discussion of the diagnosis and treatment plan so that the nurse knows what the physician has told the patient. It is much easier for the nursing staff here, since our physicians openly discuss the diagnosis and treatment with the patient. The patient's initial shock at the diagnosis of cancer may be such that he may not hear all, or forget some, of what the physician has said. Or he may forget to ask further questions for clarification. The nurse can assist and help to allay his fears by reinterpretation of the diagnostic tests and procedures and reinforcement of the treatment plan.

When the patient is admitted for surgery, pre- and postoperative teaching is necessary. For example, if the patient is scheduled for total laryngectomy, the nurse can explain to the patient that he will not be able to communicate postsurgery, but that he will use the magic slate (Fig. 1). For patients who cannot write, flash cards can be used, or pictures for those who can neither read nor write. The nurse also can explain that he will have a tube in his throat through which he will breathe, that we will have to keep the tube free from drainage, and that we will be using suction which will make the patient cough, sometimes violently. The patient is also shown the film "To Speak Again." Another laryngectomy patient

Fig. 1.—Explaining use of a magic slate preoperatively to a laryngectomy patient.

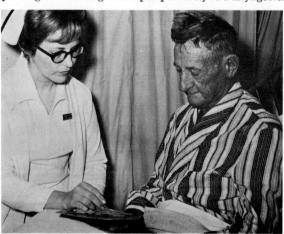

who can speak again, as well as the speech therapist, will probably also visit preoperatively. The patient is taught the importance of coughing and deep breathing.

This preoperative teaching on the nursing unit is reinforced by the preoperative visits of the registered nurse from the recovery postoperative care unit. She will explain to the patient about the postoperative care unit and what to expect there, and will reassure him regarding his care. The head nurse in the postoperative care unit tells me that in their preoperative visits to these patients, the patient has felt reassured by knowing how he would communicate. Patients often felt they were choking or smothering because of the massive pressure dressings.

The period of time that the patient's family has to wait can be very stressful since cancer operations are long. We have a waiting room in conjunction with our recovery postoperative care unit where the family can wait and receive periodic information about the patient. Volunteers or a ward clerk work in this area. When the patient returns from the operating room, an adjacent conference room is used by the physician to talk with the family.

Some important aspects of postoperative nursing care are: (1) providing an open airway, (2) care of the laryngectomy or tracheostomy tube, (3) positioning, (4) checking vital signs, (5) maintenance of nutrition, (6) patient teaching, and (7) rehabilitation and continuity of care.

On admission to the recovery room, the patient who has undergone major head and neck surgery is placed in an upright sitting position to facilitate breathing and to alleviate venous congestion (Fig. 2). To prevent the patient's slipping down in bed, the bed is elevated and the patella supported by breaking the bed slightly. Minimal hyperextension of the neck prevents pull on the sutures. The patient can be turned by supporting the head when moving him to prevent strain on sutures. Early ambulation is expected, and this same patient is out of bed on the first postoperative day—sitting and walking three to four times.

A patent airway must be maintained at all times whether the patient has a permanent or temporary tracheostomy. Laryngectomy and also tracheostomy tubes with extensions facilitate care. In the immediate postoperative period, the patient will need frequent suctioning.

The inner cannula should be removed frequently for cleaning. The dressing and the tape on the patient shown in Figure 3 have been placed in a manner so as not to obstruct the airway or prevent access to the laryngectomy tube. With the heavy pressure dressings, the flange for the tube may be difficult to open and the use of a forcep may be necessary. The inner cannula should be cleaned under cool running water to prevent con-

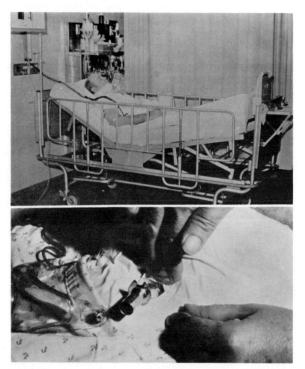

Fig. 2 (*top*).—Positioning of patient to facilitate breathing and alleviate venous congestion.

Fig. 3 (*bottom*).—Dressings and tapes are positioned so as not to obstruct airway or prevent access to laryngectomy tube.

gealment of secretions. We use a nylon bristle brush rather than cotton or gauze which may adhere and be aspirated. The patient is taught to remove, clean, and replace his tube as soon as feasible.

To prevent the formation of crusts, to provide humidity, and to thin secretions, humidifiers or mist collars are used (Fig. 4). These are used with compressed air rather than oxygen. Moisture will collect in the end of the tubing, and care needs to be taken when disconnecting and emptying so as not to get moisture in the stoma. When the humidifier is discontinued, a moist 4 × 4 gauze dressing can be used as a curtain for humidity and to act as a filter. At home, the patient can use a vaporizer or steam kettle, or can run hot water in the sink and hold the stoma area over it to prevent dryness. The use of a tonsil tip to aspirate oral secretions can prevent trauma to the suture line.

Proper suctioning is important to maintain a patent airway and to pre-

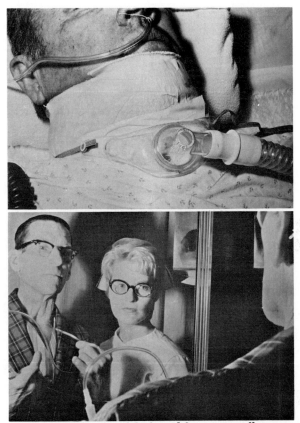

Fig. 4 (*top*).—Use of the humidifier or mist collar.
Fig. 5 (*bottom*).—Training the patient to suction the laryngectomy tube.

vent crusts and damage to the tissues. Patients are taught to do their own suctioning as soon as possible (Fig. 5). We use plastic disposable catheters with a "Y" connection. The catheter is inserted with suction off; placing a finger on the "Y" permits suction. The catheter is removed with a swirling rotating movement with suction off. It is important not to hold the catheter in for long periods as tissue damage can result. We use clean rather than sterile technique. Catheter plug drainage protectors cover the tip of the catheter between uses. The irritation from the suctioning will make the patient cough and aid in getting up secretions. If you do not get a vigorous coughing reflex, the catheter may not have been down far enough.

Patients with a neck dissection will have wound catheters connected to regulated suction, usually 80–120 mg. mercury. The nurse needs to observe that it is working properly by noting the movement of fluid in the tube. She also needs to note the color and the amount of drainage. The catheters are usually removed in six to eight days. Warm, moist packs to the suture line are used to aid in promoting healing and preventing edema. The patient can use a bath towel and warm water over the lavatory.

The nurse needs to be alert to any possible respiratory difficulty and must be able to distinguish between true respiratory difficulty versus venous stasis. The patient may be in respiratory difficulty without being cyanotic. Place the hand on the tracheostomy tube to check the breathing. Check the nail beds. Restlessness and disorientation may also indicate respiratory difficulty, even though the patient may not be cyanotic. Check dressings for possible constriction.

Patients return to the recovery room with a nasogastric tube sutured in place to prevent displacement. The tube may be connected to gravity drainage or intermittent suction, or may be clamped off. When the patient is discharged to the nursing unit, unless ordered otherwise, the nurse removes the stitch and the tube is fastened to the forehead with paper tape which is less irritating.

The same nasogastric tube is used for feeding the patient. Before beginning to feed the patient, be sure the tube is in the stomach. It can be checked by placing air by syringe into the nasogastric tube and listening with stethoscope over the abdomen. Patients are taught to do their own tube feedings (Fig. 6). Initially, patients start with clear liquids and progress to full tube feedings. Our formula provides for 2,700 calories per

Fig. 6.—Tube feeding. *A*, instructing the patient in tube feeding. *B*, self care.

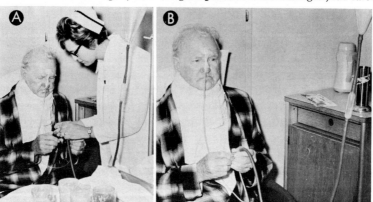

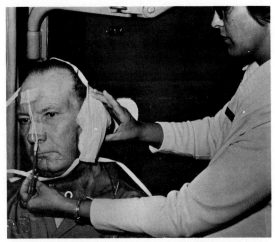

Fig. 7.—Holding dressings in place.

day. Feedings are usually given at mealtime three times per day with in-between supplement if needed. The amount, type, and quantity can be adjusted for individual patients, based on tolerance or special problems, such as diarrhea. Patients progress to mechanical soft diets.

We have not found a satisfactory disposable tube feeding set for patient use; therefore, we still purchase the Pyrex type locally. Patients going home on tube feedings usually prefer the bulb syringe. Mouth care is essential to keep the area clean, and to prevent infection and odors. A power spray, usually with 1 per cent neomycin, is used. Patients are also taught to do mouth irrigations, using one tablespoon of soda and one tablespoon of salt in a quart of warm water. We use a regular quart irrigating can with rubber tubing and a blunt medicine dropper attached for easy access to areas in the mouth.

Keeping dressings on without tape often takes ingenuity. Volunteers make a variety of cotton washable masks which we use and send home with patients (Fig. 7). Disposable surgical masks can also be used.

Patients receiving radiotherapy, such as the postsurgical laryngectomy patient, also have need for good mouth care. Depending on their nutritional status, they may need to be placed on tube feedings. They are instructed not to disturb or wash off the treatment area markings, to keep the skin exposed during the treatment, and to place nothing on it (Fig. 8). They may start to bathe the area with mild soap two weeks after therapy

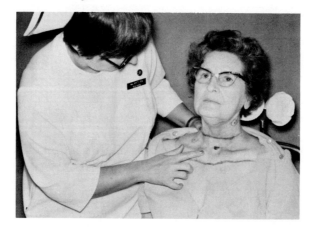

Fig. 8.—Radiotherapy patients are instructed in care of treatment area.

and to pat it dry. Aquaphor ointment is used after treatment. Protection from sunlight is necessary. Radiotherapy staff and clinic nurses work closely together with these patients.

Patients who have had a laryngectomy can learn esophageal speech. Special precautions are necessary, however, such as no showers, no swimming. They learn to cover their stomas with bibs and fancy or plain jewelry; men can wear their shirts buttoned up. Our volunteers make the bibs for us so we can send them home with the patient.

Patients with laryngectomies may wish to join a local unit of the International Association of Laryngectomees. We give these patients a card to carry so that in an emergency persons will know they have a laryngectomy. Literature from the American Cancer Society and our local Speech and Hearing Center is also given to them.

In summary, the professional nurse can contribute to the care of the patient with head and neck cancer by providing skilled nursing care, lending emotional support, and aiding in his rehabilitation.

REFERENCES

Alt, Joyce: Personal communication.
Hilkemeyer, R. N.: *Meeting the Nursing Needs of the Patient with Total Laryngectomy.* Technical Innovations in Health Care: Nursing Implications, Monograph No. 4. New York, New York, The American Nurses' Association, 1962.
Weenig, Ernestine: Personal communication.
White, Georganne: Personal communication.

Palliation for Head and Neck Cancer Patients: Hospitalized or Home Confined

ROBERT C. HICKEY, M.D.

Director and Professor of Surgery, Department of Surgery, The University of Texas System Cancer Center, M. D. Anderson Hospital and Tumor Institute, Houston, Texas

THE ANATOMICAL AREA of the head and neck is singular by reason of its compactness, diversity of tissue types, and the fact that it is transversed by significant nerves, blood vessels, and food and air passageways. It is subject to a multiplicity of tumor types, and consequently the problems encountered in palliation are unique.

While the major effort in the management of head and neck cancers is always to eradicate the cancer, a proportion of these extracranial neoplasms cannot be cured. Therefore, efforts must be made to help these patients through their final days. Many disciplines and skills are required in the over-all palliative effort.

Palliation may be accurately defined as those events, procedures, and training whereby life is prolonged and made useful, socially acceptable, and comfortable. This includes dealing with the complications of therapy, is intertwined with rehabilitation, and ultimately concerns itself with the terminal care of the patient. The setting may be hospital based, home based, or in an intermediary care facility.

In preparing this essay, consultations were held with persons knowledgeable about head and neck cancer—physicians, clinic and floor nurses, social workers, pharmacists, and patients and their families. Repeatedly during these consultations, the need for control of local disease, proper nutrition, management of pain, common hygiene procedures, and support for the patient through the family and community agencies was stressed.

311

Control of Local Disease

CASE 1.—F.L. (combined therapy). This patient had a squamous carcinoma arising in the submaxillary region, with massive invasion of the mandible (Fig. 1A). He was treated with a combination of modalities. Initially he underwent irradiation therapy with approximately 5,000 rads depth dose (Fig. 1B). A radical neck-jaw resection with mobilization of skin flaps was done six weeks (Fig. 1C) after irradiation. The patient was doing well one year later with local control (Fig. 1D), but ultimately died of systemic disease.

CASE 2.—T. McA. (palliation, including complication). This 88-year-old man had multiple skin cancers of 44 years' duration. His systemic illnesses have included a fractured hip, and coronary and cerebral arterial occlusive disease; he also had a severe auto accident.

He had a recurring right temporal cancer. Corneal ulceration occurred with ocular globe penetration and rupture. Evisceration of the globe was an essential step in his further palliation.

In Palliation, Not All Illnesses Are Cancer

In Case 2 cited above, the patient has a multitude of other systemic illnesses which are often overlooked in the cancer patient.

Other illustrative examples may be cited: A patient with a successfully resected carcinoma of the colon had a return urgent admission to a cancer institution because of gastrointestinal bleeding, and en route he exsanguinated. At necropsy there was no evidence of cancer; the bleeding was from an artery eroded by a benign peptic ulcer. Another patient was being treated by irradiation for carcinoma of the parotid and developed an intra-abdominal mass. The diagnosis of the latter was proved to be a walled-off appendiceal abscess.

In a study directed toward involvement of cancer patients in broadly oriented undergraduate medical educational purposes (Hickey, 1972), the data upon patients with carcinoma of other anatomical sites (breast and rectum), but within the same age group, showed that the vast majority had other systemic illness, i.e., 70.8 per cent of males and 67.8 per cent of females with rectal cancer, and 72.7 per cent of males and 49.5 per cent of females with breast cancer.

Nutritional Support

Head and neck cancer patients are prone to nutritional deficits, particularly from past social-dietary indiscretions and alcoholism. Nutritional re-

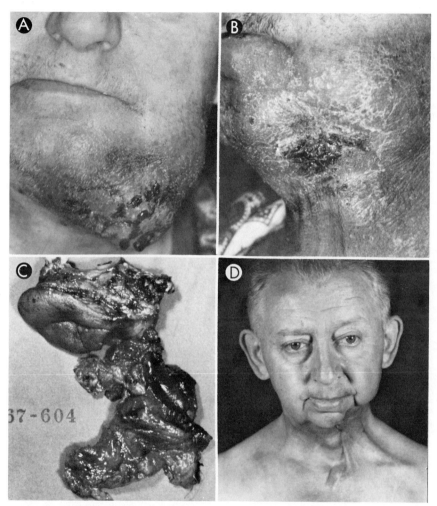

FIG. 1.—*A*, a 60-year-old man with squamous cell carcinoma destroying the left hemimandible. *B*, radiation therapy was delivered with 5,000 rads to the tumor and 3,000 rads to the neck area by a ⁶⁰Co radiator. *C*, after six weeks, a hemimandibulectomy, left radical neck dissection, and tracheostomy were performed with mobilization of skin flaps to cover the defect. *D*, patient at one year. The patient died of disseminated disease one year later, but had an excellent interim period.

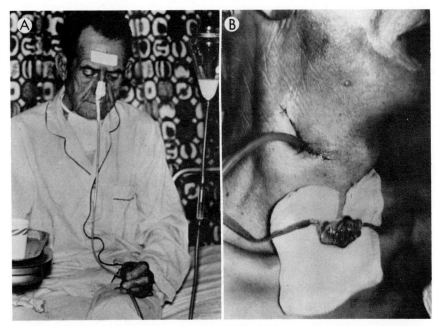

FIG. 2.—Nutritional support. *A*, patient being fed through a nasogastric tube after a laryngectomy. *B*, patient being fed through a lateral cervical esophagostomy.

quirements must not be overlooked in cancer palliation (Hickey and Tidrick, 1967). In brief, if the patient retains reasonable gastrointestinal digestive capability, he may be capable of being made ambulatory, is happier, and is less of a nursing problem. The gastrointestinal tract is preferred to other feeding routes, *i.e.*, through a large-caliber vein. If the patient can swallow (although many cannot), the importance of nutrition can be explained to him. Many patients are fed adequately via a plastic transnasal polyvinyl catheter with a variety of individualized formulas (Fig. 2A). These catheters may be introduced through a lateral pharyngeal stoma as fashioned by an elective cervical esophagostomy (Fig. 2B) using a surgical approach very similar to that used in the repair of a Zenker's diverticulum. If these techniques are impractical or impossible, the following intradiaphragmatic surgical fistulae may be fashioned (Hickey, 1967): (1) Stamm gastrostomy, (2) Witzel gastrostomy, (3) Janeway gastrostomy, (4) Mäydl jejunostomy, and (5) Witzel jejunostomy.

The Witzel jejunostomy (Fig. 3A) is the most frequently used technique

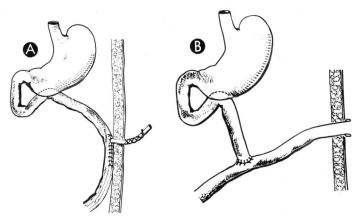

FIG. 3.—*A*, Witzel jejunostomy. *B*, Mäydl jejunostomy. (Courtesy of Brintnall, Dahm, and Womack, 1952.)

for constructing a feeding stoma. The Janeway gastrostomy and the Mäydl jejunostomy (Fig. 3B) are conduits constructed from the patient's alimentary tract tissues. These are employed less frequently than tube feedings, are permanent, and demand a larger surgical operation. They may cause skin excoriation from leakage.

It is important that all patients be adequately instructed in the use and care of a Levin tube and asepto syringe. Food idiosyncrasies, such as allergies to milk, and digestive tract responses to food must not be overlooked.

Wound Care, Hygiene, and General Measures

A patient who has had the full measure of treatment for cancer control can have few definitive additional procedures. Certain guidelines for specific management may be helpful.

Ulcerated wounds in particular are burdensome. They may be odoriferous, cause protein loss, and are of emotional concern to the patient, his family, and his friends. They can even be life-threatening, leading to hemorrhage from the great vessels and the consequent hazard of paraplegia. Topical care of these wounds is important. Cleansing by dilute solutions of hydrogen peroxide, Clorox, an antibacterial preparation such as 1 per cent neomycin, or soda and saltwater power sprays may be helpful (White, personal communication).

The tissue putrefaction may be extremely disquieting. Elements of good

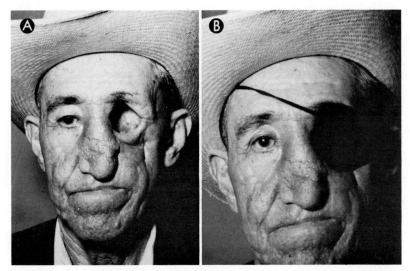

Fɪɢ. 4.—*A*, this man had an exenteration of the left orbit for squamous cell carcinoma. *B*, the simple eye patch used to achieve cosmetic palliation.

nursing care should include open dishes of vinegar, room deodorants, and aerosol spray deodorants. When possible, judicious dressing of the wound and control of infection may aid.

A patient undergoing palliative irradiation therapy should be advised to anticipate an erythema, and that the discomfort may be ameliorated by Aquaphor ointment. Additionally, he should be advised to avoid sunlight and that moisture next to the irradiated surface may augment the general tissue reaction. In irradiation of the oral cavity or of fields which include the salivary glands, oral dryness caused by the lack of saliva may be a problem. The patient may combat this by carrying a liquid-filled container for use in keeping his oral cavity moistened. Further, the sense of taste may be lessened or altered, thus handicapping his natural desire for food.

In palliation of head and neck regions, good oral hygiene is essential, and instructions must be given to continue this care at home. The patient's teeth and oral cavity should be checked by a dentist or oral hygienist at periodic intervals (Daly and Drane, 1974; see pages 225 to 231, this volume).

Laryngectomized patients are a special group and consideration must be given to the task of speech relearning or substitution. Communication is an important human function. A magic slate, a pad, or other writing materials may be a real comfort to the laryngectomized patient. Tracheal

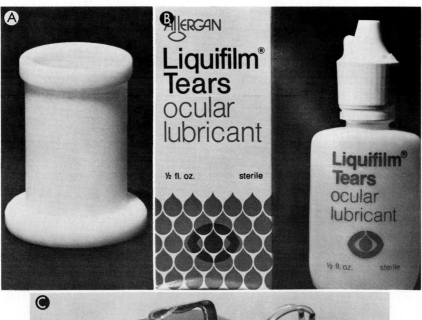

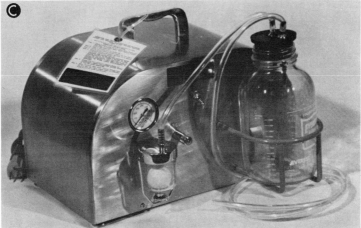

Fig. 5.—Home comfort items. *A*, tracheostomy button. *B*, ocular lubricant. *C*, home suction apparatus.

mucosa deterioration must be guarded against by room humidifiers, breathing through moistened gauze (which also protects against foreign bodies), or by inserting intratracheally a few drops of saline with a simple medicine dropper several times daily.

Figure 4 directs attention to the use of cosmetic resources in palliation.

This man had a complete exenteration of the left orbit for squamous cell carcinoma. A simple eye patch was worn over his eye for cosmetic palliation which satisfied both the patient and his family. Figure 5 illustrates three of the many items used in "comfort" palliation.

Pain Control

Pain is often a dehumanizing, agonizing experience which is not compatible with current concepts of palliation. After analysis of the pain, drug therapy may be introduced beginning with the milder analgesic agents and then resorting to the narcotics in rotation or in various combinations (Roberts, 1967).

In the upper areas of the face, such as the forehead, orbit, and frontal sinuses, pain is transmitted over the branches of the trigeminal nerve and can be relieved by a rhizotomy behind the gasserian ganglion. Neoplasms which involve the pharynx, pterygoid region, eustachian tube, or ear necessitate, for relief, a rhizotomy of multiple cranial nerves including the fifth, the nervus intermedius, the ninth, and the upper fibers of the tenth nerves. It may be necessary to extend the rhizotomy to C-2 through 4, for cervical pain. If the brachial plexus distribution is involved, a complete sensory denervation of the extremity may be necessary by rhizotomy (Leavens, 1972).

Agency Resources to Aid the Cancer Patient

The cost of care cannot help but be a factor in either primary or secondary therapy. If the advanced cancer patient can be cared for in his home, this should be done. Of interest, in Sheffield, England, 3,500 deaths from malignant disease were recorded in 1963 and 55 per cent of these deaths took place at home (Wilkes, 1965). Levels of care are essential in palliation because at the present the per diem cost of hospitalization at M. D. Anderson Hospital is $112.50 per day.

The ability to seek out and therefore to fully utilize the community resources may require expert consultation, since regulations are ever changing. Further, state and regional variations exist so that an analysis of one area is not appropriate elsewhere. Anderson Hospital is fortunate to have an excellent social service department.

The need for aid may be very real. The Texas Office of Economic Opportunity reported recently (Editorial, *Houston Post*, 1972) that one of every five Texans lives in poverty under the OEO formula. An urban resident with less than $1,900 annual income, a rural resident with less than $1,600, an urban family of four with less than $3,800 annual income, and a farm family with less than $3,200 are considered to be in poverty. The burden of poverty falls most heavily on the young and the old, and by OEO criteria, one fourth of Texas children and 40 per cent of its elderly are in poverty. Inasmuch as cancer often strikes these ages, the data are particularly pertinent to the discussion of aids from the community.

Among weaknesses in our essentially strong health care system (regardless of criticisms) is the maldistribution of the health professionals; consequently, this results in a shortage of those available to engage in palliative care. Another weakness is inadequate insurance coverage in Texas, and nation-wide, for catastrophic illness. A third weakness is the tendency for a major concentration of care to be in beds within medical centers. A fourth major deficit is the day-to-day ever-increasing cost of hospitalization. There may well be abuses or alleged abuses as serialized or editorialized in the popular press (Editorial, *Washington Post,* 1972), but, over-all intentional neglect, conflict of interests, excessive profits, and other administrative abuses are not related to the usual behavioral pattern of the health science servants. Other writings in the public press (Zehr, 1972), and there is no dearth of such, dealing with health care delivery point out that nationalized programs in Canada and Great Britain have not proved a panacea. Our system must be designed and developed for the future so as to lessen costly hospitalization, emphasize less expensive outpatient care, foster preventive measures, and encourage transportation to the most expeditious site for the patient-physician exchange. These facets are especially important in the palliation of cancer.

Senator Edward Kennedy (1972) has involved himself in the development of a comprehensive National Health Insurance Legislative Program, but the financing methods to be employed have been unclear. He has proposed that this program be financed variously—by the general revenues of the Treasury, out of tax credits, from Social Security trust funds, or from other independent trust funds created for this purpose. He proposes to avoid the vagaries of the appropriations process which have been a past problem. Social Security financing, a mechanism used for nearly three and one-half decades, has an established confidence. In the 1960's, it demonstrated efficiency in implementation of the Medicare Program, and therefore it could be a vehicle to soothe doubts and suspicions. This insurance approach, regardless of its directional source, is a projection for the foreseeable future, and it, along with other current programs under Social Security amendments (HR-1, 1972), will have a further immediate effect on medical practice, health care, and palliation for cancer. This legislation, signed by President Richard M. Nixon on October 30, 1972, is extensive. It increases both the tax rate and salary levels subject to tax, and anticipates an increase in the taxable wage base to $12,000 in 1974. Further, the tax rate now raised to 5.85 per cent will increase to 6 per cent in 1978. There are 100 changes related to Medicare, Medicaid, and Maternal and Child Health in Title II of the Bill. Several of these are applicable to patients with cancer and to the palliative effort.

Major Tax-Supported Agencies

SOCIAL SECURITY

It is estimated that nine of every 10 working persons in the United States contribute to Social Security and are therefore properly entitled to some benefit in the event of retirement, disability, or death (Table 1). The laws are complicated, and numerous booklets are available as are trained counselors from the Social Security offices. The patient or his family is well advised to look into these benefits. The local post offices will usually have the appropriate address of the Social Security office nearest the patient's home. When the patient is unable to go to the Social Security office, the Social Security counselor will respond to a telephone inquiry or will visit the patient.

In the decade of the 60's, there occurred a sixfold increase in Federal expenditures for health, with 10 per cent of the total Federal Budget going for health; the major share of this was for Medicare and Medicaid under Social Security. This support is very significant.

VETERANS ADMINISTRATION

In general, the Veterans Administration compensates veterans with service-connected disabilities. Nonservice-connected disability or illness benefits can be obtained, under certain conditions, for patients with can-

---

TABLE 1.—GOVERNMENTAL AGENCIES, FEDERAL

Social Security Administration	*Veterans Administration*
Medicare—Medicaid	Veterans' benefits
Retirement benefits	Widow, other dependents'
Disability benefits	benefits
Death benefits	Death benefits

cer. In fact, a variety of benefits are available for the veteran, his widow, or his immediate dependents (Table 1). These benefits extend beyond those medically available to the veteran that are directly related to his needs for definitive care. For example, a veteran who needs nursing home care may obtain this assistance at either a Veterans Administration facility or in a private nursing home at government expense. Applications for assistance may be made through the nearest regional Veterans Administration Office where clarification of benefits can be obtained. The local Red Cross or the American Legion can refer the patient to the appropriate Veterans Administration Office.

STATE DEPARTMENT OF PUBLIC WELFARE

This department is a valuable resource in Texas and elsewhere for those with limited income (Table 2). Since there are many variables in each instance, the State Department of Public Welfare has workers for individualized consultation. In rural communities, the State Department of Public Welfare worker is usually located in the county courthouse. Cities generally have several workers who may be found by consulting the telephone directory. These workers may be helpful, particularly in making nursing home plans for patients who need this assistance. There are three levels of care paid for by the Texas State Department of Public Welfare: (1) custodial care—ambulatory patients who need general supervision, meal preparation, medicinals, etc., (2) intermediate care—that which may be given by an L.V.N., such as irrigation of a catheter, injections, or close supervision of medicines, etc., and (3) skilled nursing home care—applies to many cancer patients and requires the supervision of a registered nurse.

TABLE 2.—GOVERNMENTAL AGENCIES, STATE AND COUNTY

State Department of Public Welfare	*City-County Medical District*
Old age assistance (over age 65)	*County Judge*
Aid to the needy blind	City-County Welfare Departments
Aid to totally and permanently disabled	County Nurses
Aid to families of dependent children	*State Department of Health*
State Rehabilitation Commission	Crippled Children's Program
Division of Vocational Rehabilitation	County Health Departments
Social Security Disability Determination	County Health Nurses

---

State Department of Health

The Crippled Children's Division of the Texas State Department of Health is an important source for aid to needy children in medical costs, transportation, and appliances. This department may be contacted directly, via the local county judge's office, or through a county health unit.

Rehabilitation Commission

This is an independent State agency funded through Federal and State monies. Its purpose is to rehabilitate patients and return them to a productive life. The counselors are very helpful and may provide speech lessons, prostheses, and job counseling. In certain instances, the cost of therapeutic undertakings which return the patient to a productive life may be defrayed by the Commission. The Vocational Rehabilitation service is active in bringing handicapped individuals to a productive life.

County Welfare Department and Office of the County Judge

In Texas, the County Welfare Department may work out of the County Judge's Office. The County Judge may also have attached to his office a county social worker and/or a county nurse. It is possible for them to perform a variety of services, particularly in the tendering of emergency aid. Often, the sheriff's office will assist with transportation.

A public health nurse or a public health physician may be attached to the County Public Health Department, and some assistance may be offered through this means. In the larger towns and cities, Family Service Agencies can often provide temporary homemaking service for cancer patients, especially if care of children is involved. The Visiting Nurse Association is another valuable resource.

Voluntary Health Agencies

American Cancer Society, Incorporated

The American Cancer Society, Inc., with its numerous divisions was established in 1913 and is volunteer-oriented in aid to the cancer patient. Transportation of cancer patients may be offered by volunteers, as well as the preparation of dressings and the management of loan closets of home-care essentials which include certain "comfort" items such as gowns, nonsterile dressings, bedpans, etc. In addition, the rehabilitation programs such as "Reach to Recovery" (breast cancer), the "Lost Chord Club" (laryngectomy), and the "Ostomy" clubs are designed and projected to assist the cancer patient through participation by oriented volunteers.

LEUKEMIA SOCIETY OF AMERICA, INCORPORATED

This Society, with its many chapters, is noted especially for its work with the leukemia and lymphoma groups of neoplasms. Its blood and blood fractionation program contributes an inestimable aid in palliation. Further, the Society assists in knowledgeable referrals for patients suffering from these diseases, pointing out where further assistance might be obtained. Fiscal relief from some outpatient charges also is offered, within the limits of the Society's resources, and includes such things as travel, drugs, laboratory fees, and dressings.

SERVICE ORGANIZATIONS

The local Chamber of Commerce, Kiwanis Club, or Lions Club will guide inquiries to other organizations which may assist in the care of the advanced or troubled cancer patient. Other service organizations which may be of aid indirectly or directly include: Knights of Columbus, Eastern Star, Salvation Army, Volunteers of America, American Legion, Rotary Club, Optimist Club, and a variety of church groups. The United Fund and Community Chest may be involved indirectly by supplying resources to others who are actively involved (Table 3).

Summary

Palliation extends unto death for the patient with head and neck cancer, or any other cancer. The care of the dying patient is a skill and an art that extends beyond science.

TABLE 3.—VOLUNTARY AGENCIES

American Cancer Society, Inc.	Leukemia Society, Inc.
American Legion	Lions Club
American Red Cross	Optimist Club
Chamber of Commerce	Rotary Club
Church Groups	Salvation Army
Eastern Star	United Fund
Kiwanis Club	Volunteers of America

After therapy fails, the patient's own emotional and physical strengths and those of his family must be marshalled in palliation.

Cancer care is costly care and all resources, medical and sociological, must be woven into the scheme to aid the stricken victim.

REFERENCES

Brintnall, E. S., Dahm, K., and Womack, N. A.: Maydl jejunostomy. Technical and metabolic considerations. *Archives of Surgery*, 65:367-372, 1952.

Daly, T. E., and Drane, J. B.: Dental care for irradiated patients. *In Neoplasia of Head and Neck*, A Collection of Papers Presented at the Seventeenth Annual Clinical Conference on Cancer, 1972, at The University of Texas M. D. Anderson Hospital and Tumor Institute at Houston, Houston, Texas. Chicago, Illinois, Year Book Medical Publishers, Inc., 1974, pp. 225-231.

Editorial: *The Houston Post*, August 29, 1972.

Editorial: *The Washington Post*, November 6, 1972.

Hickey, R. C.: I. Education and training. Cancer center participation in biomedical education—opportunity or hazard? *Cancer*, 29:826-829, April 1972.

————: Terminal care. In MacComb, W., and Fletcher, G.: *Cancer of the Head and Neck*. Baltimore, Maryland, The Williams and Wilkins Company, 1967, pp. 575-584.

Hickey, R. C., and Tidrick, R. T.: Nutritional support in cancer palliation: General concepts and palliative surigcal aids. In Hickey, R. C., Ed.: *Palliative Care of the Cancer Patient*. Boston, Massachusetts, Little, Brown, and Company, 1967, pp. 511-536.

House Resolution—1. Social Security Amendments. October 30, 1972. United States Congress.

Kennedy, E.: A health policy of the 70's. In Lowell Institute Lecture Series: *Doctors and People Talking*. Boston, Massachusetts, Boston University Medical Center, 1972, pp. 22-36.

Leavens, M. E.: The neurosurgeon's role in rehabilitation of the cancer patient. In *Rehabilitation of the Cancer Patient*, A Collection of Papers Presented at the 15th Annual Clinical Conference on Cancer, 1970, at The University of Texas M. D. Anderson Hospital and Tumor Institute at Houston, Houston, Texas. Chicago, Illinois, Year Book Medical Publishers, Inc., 1972, pp. 139-156.

McNerney, W.: Why does medical care cost so much? In Lowell Institute Lecture Series: *Doctors and People Talking*. Boston, Massachusetts, Boston University Medical Center, 1972, pp. 117-131.

Medical News: High cancer "cure" rates create human problem—rehabilitation. *Journal of the American Medical Association*, 222:418-421, October 23, 1972.

Roberts, L. M.: Drugs in the palliative care of the cancer patient and emotional aspects of the cancer illness. In Hickey, R. C., ed.: *Palliative Care of the Cancer Patient*. Boston, Massachusetts, Little, Brown and Company, 1967, pp. 559-596.

White, G.: Personal communication.

Wilkes, E.: Terminal care at home. *Lancet*, 1:799-801, April 10, 1965.

Zehr, L.: The hypochondriac's Valhalla. *The Wall Street Journal*. November 6, 1972.

Nutritional Concepts in Head and Neck Cancer

STANLEY J. DUDRICK, M.D., AND
EDWARD M. COPELAND, M.D.

Departments of Surgery, The University of Texas Medical School at Houston, and The University of Texas System Cancer Center, M. D. Anderson Hospital and Tumor Institute, Houston, Texas

OUR SURGICAL TEAM has been interested in nutrition and metabolism for many years, primarily because many patients who undergo major operations experience prolonged impairment of gastrointestinal tract function. It was thought that these patients had not fared as well as they might have if their preoperative and postoperative nutrition had been adequate. Based on this premise, a feeding regimen designed to provide adequate calories and other nutrients entirely by peripehral vein was instituted and tested at the Hospital of the University of Pennsylvania in 1961. The program involved infusing 5 to 7 liters of a slightly hypertonic nutrient solution and stimulating the patients with intravenous diuretics to excrete the excess water load via the urine (Rhoads *et al.*, 1965). This technique was successful in approximately 40 patients, but often fell short of achieving positive nitrogen balance and required close physician supervision. With the advent of percutaneous subclavian venous catheterization, hypertonic solutions could be delivered safely with fewer complications, particularly thrombophlebitis, than were encountered peripherally (Wilmore and Dudrick, 1969). Using an animal model, normal growth and development were accomplished by supplying all nutrients by the intravenous route (Dudrick, Rhoads, and Vars, 1967). Based upon this experimental evidence, neonates with severe congenital anomalies of the gastrointestinal tract were fed hypertonic nutrients intravenously, and normal growth and development were achieved. We have now used hyperalimentation in almost 2,000 patients, with minimal septic and metabolic complications secondary to long-term nutritional support and percutaneous subclavian catheterization. The technique of hyperalimentation was not used initially on cancer patients because of the possibility of complicating an already poorly understood process, as well as possibly postponing unnecessarily an inevitable death. Our colleagues, however, pointed out that many of the oncologic patients were being treated desperately by their physicians and certainly deserved nutritional and metabolic support to the maximum extent possible. Our nutritional resuscitative efforts in oncologic patients were limited initially to that period of time when their metabolic requirements were the highest, *i.e.*, during or following radiation therapy, chemotherapy, or operative trauma. In reviewing the results, it became apparent that these patients did not die from complications related to their primary modality of therapy, but died eventually because of progression of the primary disease process.

Data on the effects of nutritional support of oncologic patients are sparse. Schwartz and co-workers (1971) recently reported the effect of hyperalimentation on oncologic patients undergoing chemotherapy for a variety of metastatic malignant diseases. These patients did not appear to have increased longevity; however, their tolerance for chemotherapy was much improved in that nausea and vomiting decreased and their general feeling of well-being was much improved. The hyperalimentation program has now been underway at M. D. Anderson Hospital and Tumor Institute for a period of eight months. Approximately 90 patients have undergone nutritional support during radiotherapy, chemotherapy, or the parasurgical period. Various protocols are in effect, and it is much too early to give results of comparative groups of patients. In this larger series of patients, however, our data definitely support those of Schwartz's group. The patients undergoing chemotherapy appear to tolerate their drugs much better. They often gain weight during treatment even though nutritional intake by mouth is poor. Preliminary evidence also suggests that, in some patients, an increase in the maximally tolerated dose of chemotherapy may be possible. In those patients manifesting bone marrow depression, leukocyte counts drop, but the length of time that the bone marrow remains depressed appears to be shortened. There have been minimal infectious complications secondary to the subclavian catheter remaining in the vascular system during periods of time when the white blood cell count remained below 1,000 cells per cubic millimeter for several days. M. D. Anderson Hospital and Tumor Institute has the staff expertise and the volume of patients which should allow us to determine once and for all to what extent nutrition might benefit cancer patients during therapy.

Most pathologic processes increase the energy requirement significantly (Table 1). The absolute basal caloric requirement in a patient who is virtually comatose is between 600 and 800 calories per day. At the functional basal state of minimal activity but normal mentation, 1,500 to 1,800 calories are expended per day. The busy doctor or nurse engaged in ward activities would utilize between 2,000 and 3,000 calories per day. Postoperatively, after an operation of the magnitude of a radical neck dissection, the patient will expend a minimum of 3,000 to 3,500 calories daily. This caloric expenditure would last for seven to 10 days if no infection or other stress related to the procedure occurred. Inflammatory diseases, such as wound infections, pneumonia, or bladder infection, raise the daily energy expenditure to as high as 5,000 calories. In hypermetabolic states such as hyperthyroidism and major third-degree burns, the caloric expenditure may rise to 10,000 calories per day.

The mythical 70-kilogram man is composed of 49 kilograms of noncalorigenic water and minerals. He has only 300 to 400 grams of carbohydrate available for immediate use. Two thirds of this carbohydrate is stored as glycogen in the skeletal muscle and the remaining one-third is in the liver. This glycogen is utilized during simple starvation to yield 4 calories per gram within the first 18 hours of the starved period.

There are 6 kilograms of protein in the carcass of the 70-kilogram man which theoretically could be used for energy by the process of gluconeogenesis. Since every molecule of protein has a specific function within the viable organism, the utilization of protein for energy through gluconeogenesis is done at the expense of functional body tissue. There is no storehouse of protein readily available for such purposes. Each of us is familiar with the low serum albumin in patients in negative nitrogen balance. Recent evidence would also indicate that the nutritionally depleted patient has reduced immunological tolerance. From the surgical standpoint,

TABLE 1.—DAILY ENERGY REQUIREMENTS

METABOLIC STATUS	CALORIES
Absolute Basal	600 to 800
Functional Basal	1,400 to 1,800
Moderate Activity	2,000 to 3,000
Postoperative State	2,500 to 3,500
Inflammatory Disease	3,000 to 5,000
Hypermetabolic States	5,000 to 13,000

the catabolism of endogenous protein for energy reduces the muscle mass of the shoulder girdle, intercostal muscles, diaphragm, and abdominal wall. As these muscle masses diminish, the efficiency and effectiveness of respiration and ventilation are reduced. These patients do not take deep breaths, do not cough, and eventually develop patchy atelectasis which lays the groundwork for pneumonia. A quick personal reflection will reveal that many patients who are nutritionally depleted die of pneumonic complications. It is quite possible that some 90 per cent of all patients dying with terminal pneumonia on the surgical services should be signed out as death secondary to malnutrition, for extreme negative nitrogen balance is often the common denominator causing the death of patients with multiple associated problems.

There are apparently at least two distinct metabolic mechanisms for the utilization of fat. Fat can provide 9 calories per gram; unfortunately, however, fat is stored much easier than it is utilized. In simple starvation, without stress or sepsis, one can utilize fat calories very readily. However, with superimposed surgical and anesthetic stresses or the stress of neoplastic growth, something appears to go awry in the metabolic pathways and fat is not as readily utilizable as an energy source as it is with simple starvation. Many patients die of malnutrition with a relatively thick layer of fat remaining in the subcutaneous tissue. In these instances of stressful malnutrition, fat and protein are burned simultaneously. As mentioned, protein malnutrition leads to the malfunction of enzyme systems, respiratory musculature, immunological mechanisms, etc., which eventually results in the demise of the patient. Interestingly enough, in stressful starvation, protein utilization can be significantly reduced by the provision of 500 to 600 carbohydrate calories (Cuthbertson, 1935). The administration of 2½ to 3 liters per day of 5 per cent dextrose solution will provide this caloric equivalent. What is not supplied, however, is the energy and protein substrates necessary for repair of injured tissues, repletion of serum albumin, normal function of the body muscle mass, and adequate function of the immunological mechanisms necessary to combat infection. The utilization of 10 per cent dextrose solutions by peripheral vein will supply as much as 1,200 calories per day, but this is still much below the functional basal requirement of 1,500 to 1,800 calories.

Intravenous hyperalimentation solutions deliver approximately 1 calorie per milliliter. The majority of patients can tolerate 3,000 to 4,000 calories per day. Within the hyperalimentation solution are the amino acid substrates, the minerals, and the vitamins necessary for the repletion of the body protein stores (Table 2). Interestingly and for unexplained reasons, utilization of the caloric substrates provided by hyperalimentation appears

TABLE 2.—EXAMPLE OF HYPERALIMENTATION UNIT SOLUTION

AMINO ACID SUBSTRATE SOLUTION	PROTEIN HYDROLYSATE SUBSTRATE SOLUTION
500 cc. 50% Dextrose plus	350 cc. 50% Dextrose plus
500 cc. 8.5% Amino Acid Solution	750 ml. 5% Dextrose in 5% Protein Hydrolysate
Additives:	Additives:
40–50 mEq. Sodium Acetate	40–50 mEq. Sodium Chloride
20 mEq. Potassium Acetate	20 mEq. Potassium Chloride
15 mEq. Potassium Acid Phosphate	15 mEq. Potassium Acid Phosphate
15 mEq. Magnesium Sulfate	15 mEq. Magnesium Sulfate
5 ml. Multivitamins (MVI)*	5 ml. Multivitamins (MVI)*
1 gm. Calcium Gluconate*	1 gm. Calcium Gluconate*

*Added to only one unit of solution daily.

greater in patients undergoing surgical procedures of the head and neck than in those patients with major abdominal or thoracic operative procedures.

Frequently, patients with major malignant disease of the head and neck are elderly, malnourished, cirrhotic, emphysematous, and have poor oral hygiene. Most will agree that this type of patient will tolerate radiotherapy, chemotherapy, or surgical therapy much better if his nutritional status is improved before institution of treatment. Methods of alimenting such a patient are through a nasogastric feeding tube, gastrostomy, esophagostomy, feeding jejunostomy, and intravenous tube. A normal diet introduced into a normal gastrointestinal tract with the appropriate brush border enzymatic systems for absorption is the ideal method of alimenting any patient. Assimilation of food across the gastrointestinal tract is depressed in chronically malnourished patients, particularly those with cancer, and much of the administered caloric load is lost in the stool. Many aging patients have discovered this mechanism and do not challenge their gastrointestinal tracts with large volumes of food, but maintain themselves on simple diets such as tea and toast.

The chemically defined diets are designed to supply the basic nutrients in the most readily utilizable form for absorption across the proximal small bowel. These diets are usually provided as a powder which must dissolve before administration. The standard solution provides 1 calorie per milliliter. Thus, to administer 3,000 calories to a patient, the gastrointestinal tract must be challenged with a volume of 3,000 milliliters. The powdered diet must be dissolved in the recommended volume to control the osmolarity of the solution. Hyperosmolar solutions produce diarrhea and hypovolemia and symptoms usually associated with the postgastrectomy dumping syndrome. Another drawback of the chemically defined diets is the unattractive taste caused by the high amino acid content. Though these diets are administered via a gastrostomy or nasogastric feeding tube, regurgitation of small amounts into the oropharynx invariably leaves the patient with an unpleasant aftertaste. In our experience, only one in six patients fed with the chemically defined diets has tolerated them for longer than a week. Often the diet must be diluted with twice the recommended volume in order to prevent diarrhea when introduced into the gastrointestinal tract. Several days are usually necessary for the bowel to adapt to assimilating the diets in the concentration of 1 calorie per milliliter. Frequently, only 1,800 to 2,000 calories can be delivered daily without producing untoward effects. We have administered 4,000 to 5,000 calories per day using chemically defined diets, but two to three months were necessary for the gastrointestinal tract to adapt to this caloric load.

To deliver a large volume to the stomach, a constant drip infusion mechanism must be utilized. The stomach empties only sporadically in the normal patient and much less so in the debilitated patient. Gastric distention and aspiration of gastric contents are constant threats when gastric infusion of nutrients is utilized. Aspiration during sleep is particularly troublesome, and it is no longer recommended that patients receive intragastric infusions during the night. Even with intermittent infusion of 300 to 400 milliliters of a nutrient solution, the stomach should be periodically aspirated to prevent inadvertent gastric distention.

Realizing the mechanism of gastric emptying in those patients with normal gastrointestinal assimilative mechanisms, we recommend the use of blenderized diets of regular table foods given intermittently via a nasogastric feeding tube or esophagostomy. Calorie counts on the actual delivered nutrients should be tabulated. Diarrhea and the physical characteristics of the stool produced should be noted to detect the possibility of malabsorption. Frequently, the tolerated caloric load given via nasogastric tube is below 1,800 calories per day and thus below the functional basal caloric requirement. One would not expect repletion of body protein stores and weight gain at this caloric level. In this setting, intravenous hyperalimentation can deliver an additional 2,000 to 3,000 calories by bypassing gastrointestinal digestive and absorptive processes. With improved nutrition, gastrointestinal assimilation improves, and the patients will tolerate a larger caloric load via the gastrointestinal tract. Experimental evidence for repletion of brush border enzymes following return to positive nitrogen balance is sketchy; however, a nutritionally depleted patient's capacity of assimilating foodstuffs from the gastrointestinal tract increases linearly with the increase in the over-all nutritional status of the patient.

Parenteral hyperalimentation is indicated for use in those patients who cannot eat, will not eat, or should not eat. A patient with a large oropharyngeal lesion is often incapable of glutition, and the introduction of a nasogastric feeding tube may be difficult. Those patients on either pre- or postoperative radiation therapy often reach a stage where chewing and swallowing become impossible. Erosions from long-term intubation with a nasogastric feeding tube can be eliminated with the use of intravenous hyperalimentation. A long-term, indwelling, intragastric plastic tube can cause superficial gastric erosions. These erosions are more frequent in the debilitated, malnourished patient. Hyperalimentation eliminates the necessity for a nasogastric tube, improves the nutrition, and reduces the chances of an upper gastrointestinal bleeding episode. Patients who should not eat are represented by individuals with laryngeal and/or esophageal incompetence, who are prime candidates for aspiration pneumonia. Those patients who will not eat enough are most often in the geriatric age group, and supplemental caloric intake via the intravenous route may be lifesaving.

Selected Case Reports

CASE 1.—B.N. is a 69-year-old white man admitted to M. D. Anderson Hospital on September 15, 1972. The patient's primary complaints were pain in his left ear and an increasingly severe sore throat. He had experienced a 15- to 20-pound weight loss, secondary to anorexia and inability to swallow food during the previous three to four months. The patient had a previous aortoiliac graft inserted in 1969. His alcohol intake had remained at a quart of wine per day for several years, and he smoked one to two packs of cigarettes per day. On physical examination he was a well-developed but chronically malnourished male who weighed 108 pounds. Examination of his oral cavity and oropharynx were within normal limits. Mirror laryngoscopy revealed a large lesion which appeared to arise from the area of the left aryepiglottic fold, filled the left pyriform sinus, and involved the left lateral pharyngeal wall, making examination of the larynx impossible. A 1-cm., soft palpable node was present in the left midjugular chain. The remainder of the physical examination was within normal limits. A chest X-ray film was within normal limits also. Laryngogram confirmed the anatomical location of the lesion. Preoperative studies included a normal coagulation profile, complete blood count, urinalysis, electrocardiogram, and liver function profile. His serum albumin was 2.3 gm%. The patient was taken to the operating room on September 28, 1972, and under general anesthesia, a left radical neck dissection was performed in combination with a total laryngectomy and left lateral pharyngectomy. Closure was accomplished with skin flaps, leaving a large pharyngocutaneous stoma.

Because of the magnitude of the operative procedure, the patient was begun on intravenous hyperalimentation on the first postoperative day; he was receiving 3,000 intravenous calories by the fourth postoperative day. Supplementation with about 1,000 calories per day was achieved via a nasogastric tube. On October 2, 1972, the flaps covering the left lateral neck dissection, particularly the area around the tracheostomy stoma, were blue in color. By the following day, total necrosis of all the skin flaps on the left side of the neck had occurred.The patient was returned to the operating room where debridement of these flaps was done. The tracheostomy stoma had retracted dangerously below the sternal notch. Hyperalimentation was continued. On October 12, 1972, healthy granulation tissue appeared throughout the left neck wound. The patient was returned to the operating room and sliding grafts were placed to fill the gap between the trachea and the viable skin. These flaps healed perfectly. At this time, the patient's weight was 118 pounds, 10 pounds above his weight upon admission to the hospital. On November 5, 1972, pedicle flaps were raised in order to reconstruct the lateral pharyngeal wall and to close the pharyngocutaneous stoma. On November 29, 1972, the patient spiked a temperature to 102.3° F. No source of infection could be identified and the subclavian catheter was removed and the tip cultured. The catheter tip and a simultaneous blood culture grew *Candida albicans.* The elevated temperature abated within 48 hours. A subclavian catheter was again inserted into the right subclavian vein and hyperalimentation was reinstituted. The patient received 2,000 calories by vein, supplemented by 1,000 calories via nasogastric tube for the next three months as the various plastic procedures were successfully performed to reconstruct the left lateral pharyngeal wall and to close the pharyngocutaneous stoma. An attempt to increase the nasogastric feedings produced diarrhea, regurgitation, and abdominal discomfort. During this period of time, the patient's weight rose to 122 pounds and remained stable throughout his entire healing process.

CASE 2.—W.R., a 70-year-old Negro was admitted to M. D. Anderson Hospital on August 10, 1972. His chief complaint was difficulty swallowing since December 1, 1971. The dysphagia had progressed to inability to swallow his own saliva by the time of admission. In the 12 months prior to admission, the patient had lost 57 pounds—from 125 pounds to his admission weight of 68 pounds. Past medical history was noncontributory. He drank only socially and smoked minimally. On physical examination, he was a cachetic elderly gentleman who continually expectorated saliva into a coffee can that he kept constantly available. His oral cavity and oropharynx were within normal limits. Examination of the hypopharynx revealed a large, ulcerating, exophytic lesion in the posterior pharynx; the lesion was horseshoe-shaped, and extended into the larynx, particularly onto the area of the right aryepiglottic fold. Palpation of the neck revealed bilateral cervical adenopathy. The remainder of the physical examination was within normal limits. His chest X-ray films, electrocardiogram, complete blood count, urinalysis, and coagulation profile were within normal limits. Larynx tumor survey and barium swallow revealed a tumor mass arising from the posterior wall of the hypopharynx with paralysis of the right vocal cord and inability to swallow the contrast material. His liver profile was within normal limits with the exception of a serum albumin count which was 1.6 gm.%. The patient was thought to be a candidate for preoperative hyperalimentation rather than gastrostomy or jejunostomy for feeding purposes. A catheter was placed in the right subclavian vein, and the patient was maintained on 3,000 calories per day. On September 1, 1972, after the patient had gained 22 pounds (weight, 90 pounds), he underwent a laryngopharyngectomy, total thyroidectomy, and tracheostomy. An esophagostomy and pharyngostomy stoma were fashioned. The patient's nutrition was maintained in the postoperative period with blenderized regular diet instilled through a feeding tube inserted into the stomach through the esophagostomy stoma. The patient was able to tolerate between 2,000 and 3,000 calories via this route with normal assimilation and normal bowel movements. He was discharged on the same nutritional regimen. He was readmitted on January 5, 1973, and underwent closure of the pharyngostomy stoma. The postoperative course was uncomplicated. The patient was last examined on March 21, 1973, following a course of radiotherapy to an area of recurrence lateral to the trachea. At this time, the patient weighed 101 pounds and was tolerating feedings through the esophagostomy stoma quite well.

These two case histories represent examples of patients operated upon following extreme inanition from lack of adequate oral food intake. The first patient underwent operation without prior intensive nutritional resuscitation. Although hyperalimentation was begun in the immediate postoperative period, he still suffered wound complications. During the next three and one-half months, the patient both gained weight and healed the wounds of multiple reconstructive procedures. Attempted oral alimentation throughout this period met with constant failure. One cannot adequately postulate the healing capacity of this patient's wound if hyperalimentation had been initiated several days before operative intervention. It is quite doubtful, however, that adequate wound healing and closure of the pharyngocutaneous fistula could have been accomplished without the aid of intravenous nutritional support.

The second patient had an equally large lesion with much more severe inanition. Hyperalimentation was begun two weeks preoperatively, and the patient was operated upon in positive nitrogen balance after having gained 22 pounds. A laryngopharyngectomy was carried out with primary wound healing. Adequate postoperative nutritional support was delivered via a feeding tube passed into the stomach through the cervical esophagostomy. The patient assimilated 2,500 to 3,000 calories, delivered as a blenderized regular house diet. He had no problems with malabsorption or diarrhea. Though his gastrointestinal tract was not challenged with food preoperatively, experience with many other malnourished geriatric patients allows us to predict that assimilation of foodstuffs across his gastrointestinal mucosa would have been grossly impaired. Following nutritional repletion and positive nitrogen balance, this patient was totally maintained in the postoperative period with oral feedings without any untoward effects.

Hyperalimentation is recommended as an adjunct to therapy in patients who are nutritionally depleted, particularly elderly patients and patients with large borderline operable lesions. For detailed descriptions of catheter insertion technique, catheter and hyperalimentation delivery system maintenance, mixing of solutions, and the diagnosis, treatment, and prevention of complications associated with the use of hyperalimentation, the reader is referred to the literature (Wilmore and Dudrick, 1969; Dudrick, Wilmore, Vars, and Rhoads, 1968, 1969; Dudrick and Ruberg, 1971; Dudrick, Wilmore, and Vars, 1969; Dudrick et al., 1972; Ruberg et al., 1971). Briefly, the solution is made by mixing together 50 per cent dextrose and concentrated amino acids or protein hydrolysates (Table 2). The caloric equivalent of the solution is 1 calorie per milliliter. Forty to 50 milliequivalents of sodium and 30 to 40 milliequivalents of potassium as the chloride, bicarbonate, acetate, or acid phosphate salts are added to each 1,000 milliliters of solution. When amino acids are used as the protein substrate, the sodium and potassium should not be added as chloride salts. The amino acids are already in solution as the hydrochloride and chloride salts, and the addition of extra chloride will produce an extremely hyperchloremic solution leading to hyperchloremic acidosis with prolonged use of large volumes of solution. Both the fat-soluble and water-soluble vitamins should be given daily. Folic acid, vitamin K, and vitamin B_{12} are given parenterally as needed. Magnesium, calcium, and phosphate must be added to the solutions daily. As calories are provided to the depleted patient, high-energy phosphate bonds are replenished. Without additional phosphate, the patient may become severely hypophosphatemic. Similarly, with the repletion of the enzyme systems, magnesium is utilized, requiring the daily exogenous supplementation of magnesium. Moreover, there will be a reciprocal fall in serum calcium level if phosphate is provided without providing adequate exogenous calcium daily.

Percutaneous catheterization of the subclavian vein is done preferentially via the infraclavicular route. Strict aceptic technique is employed for insertion of the catheter. Following catheter insertion, a chest X-ray film must be taken to determine the correct position of the catheter in the middle of the superior vena cava. In dealing with head and neck cancer patients, the catheter should be inserted contralateral to the side of the operative procedure. A member of the hyperalimentation team, usually a nurse, changes the dressing and the intravenous tubing at least three times a week. She recleanses the skin, applies antibiotic ointment to the skin entrance site of the catheter, and reapplies a sterile, waterproof dressing. The use of water-repellent tape to secure the dressing is particularly important in head and neck cancer patients (Fig. 1). Frequently, there will be a pharyngostomy stoma or esophagocutaneous fistula, and saliva will constantly bathe the dressing. If the dressing has been applied to skin treated generously with tincture of benzoin and has been completely covered with water-repellent tape, the dressing should remain dry for 24 to 48 hours. If secretions gain access to the dressing, we also recommend covering the entire dressing and subclavian area with a plastic sheet. Electrolytes, blood sugar, magnesium, phosphate, blood urea nitrogen, and creatinine should be monitored frequently, and the appropriate manipulation of the electrolyte content and rate of delivery of the hyperalimentation solution carried out to maintain normal electrolyte and fluid balance.

The first patient had a *Candida albicans* sepsis. The organism was grown from both the blood and the catheter tip. The sepsis cleared spontaneously when the catheter was removed. Each patient undergoing hyperalimentation at M. D. Anderson Hospital has the catheter tip cultured at the termination of hyperalimentation. Eighty-eight patients are currently in the series, and the over-all catheter contamination rate is 4.2 per cent. Of the five positive cultures obtained, three were grown from the catheter tips of patients being discharged from the hospital fully recovered from their therapeutic procedure. The other two positive cultures (one

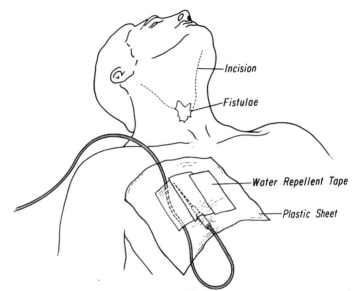

Fig. 1.—In those patients with a wound infection or pharyngocutaneous fistula, the catheter exit site should be covered with water-repellent tape and the entire subclavian area covered with a well-secured plastic sheet.

from the first patient) were from patients with a concurrent *Candida albicans* septicemia. Both of these patients were undergoing hyperalimentation for periods longer than three months, had multiple associated problems, and had a separate source of bloodstream contamination. We associate our relatively low rate of catheter contamination to strict adherence to time-honored principles of aseptic technique, and to the concept that a small number of trained personnel must be responsible for the intravenous hyperalimentation program.

Hyperalimentation is a safe and efficacious technique when properly employed. Positive nitrogen balance can be obtained in the most severely cachetic patients. Infectious complications are minimal if the care of the hyperalimentation catheter and delivery system remains in the hands of a few well-trained personnel. It is lifesaving in the patient who is unable to take and assimilate nutrients via the gastrointestinal tract. No longer should patients of this type be denied possible curative surgical procedures or combinations of surgical therapy and radiotherapy because of the fear of complications secondary to malnutrition.

REFERENCES

Cuthbertson, D. P.: Further observations on the disturbance of metabolism caused by injury, with particular reference to dietary requirements of fracture cases. *British Journal of Surgery*, 23:505-520, January 1935.

Dudrick, S. J., MacFadyen, B. V., VanBuren, C. T., Ruberg, R. L., and Maynard, A. T.: Parenteral hyperalimentation, metabolic problems and solutions. *Annals of Surgery*, 176:259-264, September 1972.

Dudrick, S. J., and Rhoads, J. E.: Total intravenous feeding. *Scientific American*, 226:73-80, May 1972.

Dudrick, S. J., Rhoads, J. E., and Vars, H M.: Growth of puppies receiving all nutritional requirements by vein. In *Fortschritte der Parenteralen Ernahrung*, Symposium of the International Society of Parenteral Nutrition in 1966. Lochham bei Munchen, West Germany, Pallas Verlag, 1967.

Dudrick, S. J., and Ruberg, R. L.: Principles and practice of parenteral nutrition. *Gastroenterology*, 61:901-910, December 1971.

Dudrick, S. J., Wilmore, D. W., and Vars, H. M.: Long-term venous catheterization—an adjunct to surgical care and study. *Current Topics in Surgical Research*, 1:325-340, 1969.

Dudrick, S. J., Wilmore, D. W., Vars, H. M., and Rhoads, J. E.: Can intravenous feeding as the sole means of nutrition support growth in the child and restore weight loss in an adult? *Annals of Surgery*, 169:974-984, June 1969.

————: Long-term total parenteral nutrition with growth, development, and positive nitrogen balance. *Surgery*, 64:134-142, July 1968.

Rhoads, J. E., Rawnsley, H. M., Vars, H. M., Crichlow, R. W., Nelson, H. M., Spagna, P. M., Dudrick, S. J., and Rhoads, J. E., Jr.: The use of diuretics as an adjunct in parenteral hyperalimentation for surgical patients with prolonged disability of the gastrointestinal tract. *Bulletin de la Société Internationale de Chirurgie*, 24:59-70, January-February 1965.

Ruberg, R. L., Allen, T. R., Goodman,M. J., Long, J. M., and Dudrick, S. J.: Hypophosphatemia with hypophosphaturia in hyperalimentation. *Surgical Forum*, 22:87-88, 1971.

Schwartz, G. F., Green, H. L., Bendon, M. L., Graham, W. P., III, and Blakemore, W. S.: Combined parenteral hyperalimentation and chemotherapy in the treatment of disseminated solid tumors. *American Journal of Surgery*, 121:169-173, February 1971.

Wilmore, D. W., and Dudrick, S. J.: Safe long-term venous catheterization. *Archives of Surgery*, 98:256-258, February 1969.

Panel Discussion: Cancer of the Oral Cavity

MODERATOR: ROBERT M. BYERS, M.D.

Assistant Surgeon, Section of Head and Neck Surgery, Department of Surgery, The University of Texas System Cancer Center, M. D. Anderson Hospital and Tumor Institute, Houston, Texas

Dr. Byers: The interaction among the multiple disciplines concerned with the diagnosis, treatment, and rehabilitation of patients with oral cancer—the team approach—is one of the important aspects or concepts we practice here at M. D. Anderson Hospital and Tumor Institute. Numerous factors come into focus when we select a particular treatment to fit a particular tumor. These factors may be tumor factors, patient factors, or, often, a blending of the two. The theme of this panel will be to explore in some detail, using case illustrations, the concept of matching the treatment with the disease so that we can employ the proper blending of the various modalities to manage the tumor and yet insure adequate function and cosmesis. We have four cases which illustrate various aspects, some controversial, in the treatment of patients with cancer of the oral cavity. These are actual case histories of patients who were treated at M. D. Anderson Hospital.

CASE 1.—This is a 57-year-old man with a "blister" in the floor of the mouth of four to five months' duration. He is a heavy smoker but did not dip snuff. He developed problems with his dentures two weeks before seeking medical attention.

Dr. Byers: Dr. Pleasants, would you have any questions concerning this patient's dental problem?

Dr. John E. Pleasants, University of Texas at Houston Dental Branch, Houston, Texas: Certainly the reason he could not wear his dentures should be investigated.

Dr. Byers: Would you be looking for something that was wrong with the dentures, something wrong with his mouth, or both?

Dr. Pleasants: I would certainly start looking for an irritated area. Quite often, dentures worn over a period of time will settle because of the absorption of the ridges and the tissues and will cause denture irritation. If I believe the lesion is only denture irritation, I would take his dentures away from him and watch the area for ten days to two weeks; if it did not get any better, then I would recommend biopsy.

Dr. Byers: This man had a lesion in the anterior floor of his mouth, measuring 2 to 3 cm. It was fixed to the periosteum of the mandible and extended into the root of the tongue (Fig. 1A). The neck was classified as N_1 because of a 1.5 cm. right submaxillary node. Dr. Strong, how would you proceed?

FIG. 1.—*A*, T_3N_1 squamous cell carcinoma of anterior floor of the mouth fixed to periosteum of the mandible. *B*, artist's sketch of resection of lesion of floor of mouth with partial mandibulectomy. *C*, artist's view from above of same lesion and same type of resection.

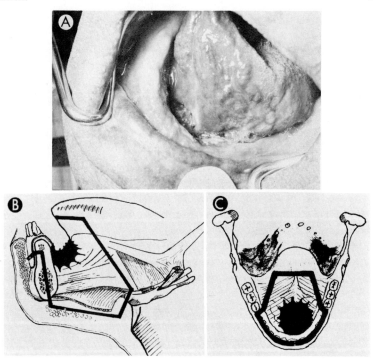

Dr. Elliot W. Strong, Memorial Hospital, New York, N.Y.: I suspect the reason the man could not wear his dentures was that his tumor had begun to interfere with their placement because of the tumor's increasing bulk. The reason that brought him to the doctors is because the tumor interfered with the comfort with which he wore his dentures. He had had this lesion for four months, at least, according to the history. I suspect for completeness' sake, I would take some X-ray films of his mandible to see if there was gross evidence of neoplastic invasion of the cortical bone, knowing full well that in the areas where we need it the most the radiographs are least likely to tell us the answer. The continuity of the mandible is so important here that we hate to resect it if we do not have to. But, certainly, if we are going to operate on him or if we are going to irradiate him, we need to know whether the cortical bone is actually invaded or whether the tumor is merely stuck to the periosteum.

Dr. Byers: The mandible and chest X-ray studies were negative. The reason that we could not get a better view of this lesion is because the mobility of the floor of the mouth was impaired by tumor infiltration. You can see the cancer creeping up over the alveolar ridge. He could not really elevate his tongue. Dr. Strong, how would you proceed now?

Dr. Strong: Well, I assume that you have already obtained a biopsy which has confirmed the clinical impression.

Dr. Byers: Yes, squamous carcinoma.

Dr. Strong: With the deeply infiltrating disease of this magnitude and with a clinically positive node in his neck, I would give him preoperative radiotherapy to include both the primary tumor and the neck. The dosage of the preoperative radiation would be about 4,000 rads in four weeks. After completion of the radiotherapy, I would then perform a combined procedure on the side of involvement. Whether I would do anything with the other side of the neck would depend on the location of the primary lesion. If it crossed the midline, I might consider doing a submaxillary dissection on the opposite side.

Dr. Byers: Would it bother you that this lesion was fixed to the periosteum initially?

Dr. Strong: It certainly would. I would be forced, obviously, to resect some bone, depending on what I found at operation. If the cortical surface of the bone appeared not to be involved, I would be content with a marginal resection of the mandible preserving the continuity of the mandibular arch.

Dr. Byers: In other words, a coronal-type resection?

Dr. Strong: Correct.

Dr. Byers: Dr. Lindberg, Dr. Strong wants to treat this patient with preoperative radiation. What are your views concerning this therapeutic approach?

Dr. Robert D. Lindberg, The University of Texas System Cancer Center, M. D. Anderson Hospital and Tumor Institute, Houston, Texas: I would prefer not to treat him preoperatively. If a combined modality of treatment were indicated, I would prefer to have the surgical procedure done first and then use postoperative radiation therapy. This is a matter of preference. I think the patients tolerate the order of treatment utilizing a surgical procedure followed by radiation better than having the radiotherapy first. If preoperative radiation therapy is going to be used, I would use a higher dose preoperatively, of at least 5,000 rads in five weeks.

Dr. Byers: I would like to ask Dr. Strong why he changed his preoperative therapy from the 2,000 rads in one week in his recently published articles to the 4,000 rads in four weeks which he is advocating today, and also whether he now includes the primary tumor area in his radiation portals instead of only including the neck.

Dr. Strong: May I answer the second part of your question first? Obviously, our initial intention in the study I reported was relative to the neck only. The same problems that occur at the primary site occur in the neck. So, I think that, as has become readily apparent, if one is going to use preoperative radiotherapy, it should be directed to both the primary site and the neck. We have satisfied ourselves that we can better locally control the cervical metastasis and, we hope, also better control the disease at the primary site with preoperative radiation. My concern about the level of dosage is not based on any statistical evaluation that I can quote, but certainly, much reference has been made in the literature and at various meetings to the fact that 2,000 rads in five days may not be adequate. The answer to that question is not yet available, but I think it is mandatory to point out that 2,000 rads in five days is not equivalent to 2,000 rads in two weeks. Biologically, it is much nearer 3,500 rads given in rather conventional fractionation, so that although 2,000 rads is an absolute figure quoted, is not the biological dose the patient receives.

Dr. Byers: Dr. Jesse, would you agree with Dr. Strong's surgical approach to the problem?

Dr. Richard H. Jesse, The University of Texas System Cancer Center, M. D. Anderson Hospital and Tumor Institute Houston, Texas: As the preoperative dose of radiation increases, the surgeon doing major procedures afterward has problems with his patients, particularly in maintaining a good nutritional level and obtaining adequate healing. However, in the radiobiologic studies, it does seem that the 5,000 rad level in five weeks kills the peripheral cancer cells, both in the neck and at primary site. It is also true that the higher dose of radiation, the more one must worry about both wound healing and subsequent bone necrosis. You might ask the question, "Well, why didn't you treat the patient with radiation alone?" I think the answer is that, in a patient with an extensive lesion and with mandibular or periosteal involvement, at the dose necessary to eradicate this lesion it will jeopardize the viability of the mandible. If radiation to full dose fails, an entire resection of the anterior arch of the mandible is necessary. Therefore, I would rather do the surgical procedure first. If the margins of the specimen were not free or were very close to the cancer and/or if more than one first level node was positive, I would give postoperative radiation therapy.

Dr. Byers: Dr. Lindberg, how would you treat him postoperatively?

Dr. Lindberg: Well, as much as I would like not to irradiate the mandible, or what's left of the mandible, I would be afraid not to. We have shown in a number of patients that whenever we irradiate only part of the surgical area, a high incidence of recurrence occurs in the area not irradiated. It is, therefore, mandatory that the entire surgical field be included.

Dr. Byers: Dr. Drane, we have stated that this man is edentulous. You have heard the surgical procedures proposed by Dr. Jesse and Dr. Strong. What would be your concern in getting this man rehabilitated?

Dr. Joe B. Drane, The University of Texas System Cancer Center, M. D. Anderson Hospital and Tumor Institute, Houston, Texas: Well, I am not sure that it is entirely decided whether he would be irradiated. This would have a crucial bearing on whether I would suggest he wear dentures posttreatment. If he did have radiation, it would depend on whether he had a radium implant or whether it was all from an external beam. If he received radium, I would certainly not recommend the wearing of dentures afterward. However, if he undergoes only a surgical procedure, I would suggest dentures because they provide support in the mouth anteriorly for the lips or the flaps used in the repair.

Dr. Byers: Thank you. Dr. Strong, we haven't talked too much about the closure of this wound after 4,000 rads in four weeks. How are you going to repair this defect?

Dr. Strong: I would close it primarily. If it became obvious that the patient was seriously incapacitated, I think an effort to release the structures involved is better undertaken at a later date, in the face of preoperative 4,000 rads, than it would be as a primary effort.

Dr. Byers: In summary, Dr. Jesse would operate and use postoperative radiation therapy, if indicated; Dr. Strong would use preoperative radiation therapy and follow with approximately the same type of surgical procedure.

Let me give you the report on the patient in Case 1. In 1966, the patient underwent a right radical neck dissection, left upper neck dissection, coronal resection of the mandible, and resection of the floor of the mouth with primary repair suturing the tongue to the anterior alveolar ridge. The surgical margins were free, according to the pathologist. Five nodes in the specimen of the right radical neck dissection contained metastatic squamous carcinoma while one node on the left contained metastatic disease. No postoperative radiation was given this patient. An artist's drawing of the surgical resection shows the anterior arch of the mandible has been preserved while the inner portion of the mandible is removed en bloc with the entire floor of the mouth and anterior tongue (Figs. 1B and 1C). Eight months later, we completed the left radical neck dissection for a single positive node which appeared in the previously undissected portion of the neck. At the same operation, we released his tongue and replaced the floor of the mouth with a skin graft. The patient is free of disease six years following this last procedure. Unfortunately, he has never been able to wear his dentures since his operation.

Dr. Lindberg: I would like to make a couple of comments. You hate to argue with success. Today, in light of what we now know, a patient having multiple nodes in the ipsilateral side of the neck and a histologically positive node in the contralateral side of the neck would probably receive postoperative radiation therapy. This would have prevented the appearance of the node in the lower neck and obviated the necessity of the second surgical procedure.

Dr. Strong: I would have completed the contralateral neck dissection soon after the pathologist told me about the histologically positive node on that side.

Question from Audience: Why could you not treat the primary with radium needles and give external irradiation to the neck?

Dr. Lindberg: This is one approach. If this patient was selected for only radiation therapy, he would receive 5,000 rads in five weeks with external beam irradiation and 3,000 rads with radium needles. The reason we chose a surgical procedure for this particular patient rather than radiation therapy as the treatment for his primary was that the surgeon thought only the inner table of the mandible needed to be removed. This is the key. If the surgeon had thought it necessary to remove a full segment of the mandible, then we would have preferred to give the patient radiation therapy. Because this tumor extended onto the superior aspect of the alveolar ridge, it would be very difficult to needle. You can needle the floor of the mouth component easily, but you have to give a high dose with external beam to sterilize the extensions over the alveolar ridge because the needles alone will not deliver a sufficient dose. With this much involvement in the periosteum, the chance of radiation necrosis of the anterior arch of the mandible is considerably more than it would be with a floor of the mouth lesion that was not attached to the inner table of the mandible. Therefore, when the surgeons can maintain the arch of the mandible by removing just the inner table, we would prefer to have the patients treated surgically.

Dr. Sam Jampolis, M. D. Anderson Hospital, Houston, Texas: Dr. Daly: In this type of patient who is edentulous and would probably be getting a 5,000 to 6,000 rad dose postoperatively, what dental complications might one expect?

Dr. Thomas E. Daly, The University of Texas System Cancer Center, M. D. Anderson Hospital and Tumor Institute, Houston, Texas: We had 32 per cent necrosis in all patients with floor of the mouth lesions. This includes those with teeth as well as those in the edentulous phase. In the patients receiving postoperative radiation, we would be most cautious. We would not consider any rehabilitation until all of the treatments were completed. Necrosis is very rare in patients who receive postoperative radiation therapy if they have good postoperative healing before radiation therapy starts.

Dr. Jesse: Is necrosis as prevalent in edentulous patients treated by radiation therapy?

Dr. Daly: We had a 10 per cent incidence of necrosis in the edentulous patients. They did better than any dental group. We have seen necrosis in many patients who have had 3,000 to 5,000 rads in three to five weeks and then received a marginal resection of the mandible. I think such a combination of treatment would not likely result in the patient eventually losing his entire mandible.

CASE 2.—This is a 60-year-old man with burning under his tongue and swelling under his left jaw. The patient was a heavy smoker and an alcoholic. The lesion involved the entire anterior floor of the mouth extending into the root of the tongue but not fixed to the periosteum of the inner mandible (Fig. 2A). There was very little loss of mobility of the tongue. Numerous areas of leukoplakia were evident in the oral cavity. The lesion was classified as a T_2N_0 anterior floor of the mouth.

Dr. Byers: Dr. Jesse, how would you analyze this problem in comparison to the previous one?

Dr. Jesse: There are two or three basic differences in the two cases. I would guess from what you tell me that this lesion may be not quite as big

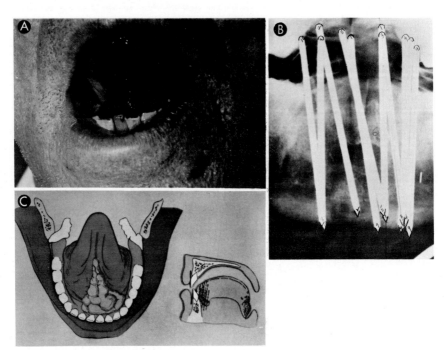

Fig. 2.—*A*, T2N0 lesion of the anterior floor of mouth which extends to root of the tongue but not to mandible. *B*, X-ray film showing modified volume implant in floor of the mouth. *C*, artist's drawing of T2 squamous cell carcinoma floor of the mouth volume radium implant.

and not quite as deep. It also does not run over the anterior arch of the mandible. He also is a heavy drinker. He also has mobility of the tongue.

Dr. Byers: Would you treat this patient surgically?

Dr. Jesse: The lesion is ideal for radiation therapy but before I made that decision, I would have to know the patient. I would hope that he would stop smoking and cut down on his drinking. If I thought he would, radiation therapy would be my choice.

Dr. Byers: Dr. Lindberg, what about these numerous areas of leukoplakia in the oral cavity? Is this going to modify your preferred choice of therapy?

Dr. Lindberg: This patient is, of course, an ideal candidate to develop other primary oral cancers. He is a heavy smoker, a heavy drinker, and already has some mucosal changes, so he falls into the high-risk group for developing other primaries in the upper respiratory tree. If we were considering radiation for the floor of the mouth lesions, we would ignore the leukoplakia. We don't treat leukoplakia with radiation therapy.

Dr. Byers: Dr. Strong, if this patient presents to you, how would you handle him at Memorial Hospital?

Dr. Strong: Much the same as I did the previous one. I feel a little bit more optimistic about him for the same reasons that Dr. Jesse does. The lesion seems to be more of a spreading type than a deep infiltrative lesion. I am concerned about "leukoplakia." I wish we would get away from that term because it is solely a descriptive term. It has no relationship, whatsoever, to the actual nature of the lesion. Leukoplakia may be lichen plantis or an infiltrating epidermoid carcinoma, and without biopsy, or without a very well-trained clinical eye, it is very difficult to be certain about these lesions. I think this is exactly the type of patient who represents a prime candidate for second, third, fourth, or fifth primary lesions. You may want to save radiotherapy for those other lesions when they occur. I would like to ask Dr. Jesse what he does to get his heavy smokers to stop. I have not been very effective.

Dr. Jesse: Nor I. I agree that this is a very, very difficult problem. What I usually try to do is to barter the booze for the cigarettes. I think you cannot ask them to give up both. I tell them, "Now, you can have the drinks that you are used to, but please dilute them with water and see if you can't quit smoking." If you barter one for the other, they will often cut down on smoking. Often, however, they will stop smoking for a while and start again after treatment.

Dr. Byers: Dr. Lindberg, you are outnumbered by the surgeons here. Let's put you in an environment where you do not have experienced head and neck surgeons and hear your views on how you would treat this lesion primarily by radiation therapy.

Dr. Lindberg: Well, I think the patient could be handled very well by radiation therapy. This lesion is, in comparison to the last lesion, a much more favorable lesion. The probability of late and serious sequelae of the radiation is much less. On a patient like this, we would use a combination of external beam radiation therapy and radium needles. We would include the first relay of nodes if the neck is negative, or if clinically positive, treat the entire neck and then follow it with a radical neck dissection.

Dr. Byers: How much of the radiation dosage would be with external beam and how much by needles?

Dr. Lindberg: As the lesion increases in size, we increase the dose delivered by the external beam. If the patient was not able to tolerate anesthesia for the radium needles, he would be considered for intraoral cone or a submental electron beam field as a boost. In general, we would prefer to boost him with the radium needles.

Dr. Byers: Dr. Daly, this patient has been selected for radiation therapy. How would you proceed from the dental standpoint?

Dr. Daly: We would do a complete dental work-up, including all necessary X-ray studies and determine whether this patient has restorable teeth or whether he is in the group of patients needing extractions. The teeth, as they appear here, are in very poor shape, and we would probably want to extract the bad ones. Ten days would be a minimum time for healing and we would like the therapist to wait three weeks, if possible. If we found that the teeth were in fairly good shape, we would restore those that need it, get rid of all periodontal calcium deposits, and instruct the individual regarding all the precautions about irradiated tissues. We would also teach him to apply sodium fluoride to his teeth.

Dr. Byers: Just as a hypothetical question, suppose this man had mandibular tori, Dr. Daly?

Dr. Daly: We have had some bad experiences with tori. If we remove them, a minimum of four weeks is required for healing, and if the patients received radiation before this time, we had some problems. Several of these patients developed necrosis and had to have a mandibular resection.

Dr. Jesse: If tori are to be in the field of irradiation, or if radium needles are placed against them, the problems are such that a primary surgical approach may be advocated.

Dr. Lindberg: Amen. The mandibular tori make the use of radium needles mechanically very difficult. You might as well do the surgical procedure and remove the tori at the same time. The surgeon should take out the tori with the cancer. If there is any reason to give postoperative radiation therapy, the tori are then not present to give you future problems.

Dr. Byers: This patient's neck was clinically N_1, the chest X-ray films and those of the mandibles were negative and biopsy showed squamous carcinoma. His treatment consisted of cobalt 60, 5,000 rads external to the primary and the entire neck bilaterally. Following this, a modified volume implant delivered 3,000 rads of radiation (Fig. 2B). Dr. Lindberg, would you care to comment?

Dr. Lindberg: The upper fields are opposed portals. An anterior field is employed for the lower part of the neck. We use a midline split, shielding the larynx when the lower portion of the neck is clinically free of metastases.

Dr. Byers: Figure 2C is an artist's schematic representation of the lesion. On the right you can see the volume implant in the floor of the mouth. The node in the preglandular area did not completely disappear. A left radical neck dissection was performed two months after completion of the radiation therapy. The specimen showed no cancer in 36 nodes. Does the panel consider the amount of radiation given this patient sufficient to sterilize the neck?

Dr. Lindberg: The dose of radiation to the node would probably be around 5,500 rads from the external beam plus a slight contribution from the radium. I do not consider this dose adequate enough to sterilize a 1.5 cm. clinically positive node.

Dr. Jesse: He had less than 6,000 rads to the neck. We would automatically do the neck dissection whether the node goes away or not. I probably would not have waited eight weeks to do it. We would have performed it between four to six weeks after radiation therapy.

Dr. Byers: Would you comment on the examination of the primary at the time of the planned neck dissection?

Dr. Jesse: Complete healing of an irradiated primary lesion may not occur before six weeks. You always have the problem of whether the primary is under control. If there is nothing to feel, I would leave it alone. If an ulcer is still present and you biopsy it at six weeks and the pathologist tells you that he sees malignant cells, you are immediately faced with the decision of whether these cells will grow. Any pathologist in the world can see the cancer cells in the biopsy specimen, but he cannot tell you whether they are viable and I do not think he can even guess well. If you get a positive interpretation at this point, then you are forced to resect the primary tumor as well as performing the neck dissection. I would, therefore, wait to perform the neck dissection until I was relatively sure of the status of the primary lesion. This is one reason we like doses of 5,000 rads or more as a preoperative dose to the nodes. The fact that the node was negative at 5,500 rads tells me I can wait awhile to see what the primary will do.

Dr. Byers: Are there any other comments from the panel or questions from the audience?

Question from Audience: Dr. Strong, if you will forgive me for using the term "leukoplakia," how would you manage these areas? Would you just continue to observe them? Would you excise them if any changes occurred?

Dr. Strong: I would refer back to what I said a little earlier about experience. If you look at enough mouths, in a high percentage of patients you can recognize which of these white patches are going to be significant and which are not. The area of hyperkeratosis along the occlusal margins of both cheeks which we frequently see is seldom significant. I would not treat these patches unless I was suspicious of them. Any that become ulcerated obviously should be biopsied.

Dr. Kent Westbrook, University of Arkansas, Little Rock, Arkansas: Why do a classical radical neck dissection after 5,000 rads?

Dr. Jesse: To be honest with you, I might not, nowadays. I hate to say that in an audience like this because when I say I do less than a classical radical neck dissection, it is often misinterpreted and the surgeon with little or moderate experience tries it and the patient has recurrence in the neck. You immediately have to understand that I am talking about a real team approach where everybody knows exactly what everybody else is doing. If you have a single node in the first echelon and you have no other nodes and if the whole neck has received 5,000 rads in five weeks or better, you do not have to perform a classical radical neck dissection. Now, I do not want everyone to do partial neck dissections, because I know what happens in the institutions in which there is not utmost cooperation between radiotherapists and surgeons. Too often, the radiotherapist and the surgeon do not communicate well or do not communicate often enough. If the therapist does not give the whole neck at least 5,000 rads of irradiation, then your patient has had it. Therefore, it is safest for most surgeons to do a classical radical neck dissection.

Dr. Strong: May I be the devil's advocate and state that if you are not going to do a classical radical neck dissection, why dissect it at all? Why not boost the dose of radiotherapy to the nodes in question?

Dr. Lindberg: Let me answer that. We have given 5,000 rads to the neck and have implanted radium needles and now you ask that additional radiotherapy be given over this area. We would prefer to have the neck node removed surgically rather than boost the dose up to the level where the node is surely sterile. To feel safe, I would have to give the node at least 7,000 rads, and this would greatly increase the patient's morbidity.

Question from Audience: Could you not get that kind of a dose reasonably well with an interstitial implant to the neck?

Dr. Lindberg: You could, but I think your complications and your sequelae, both functionally and cosmetically, are probably worse than would result with a modified or even a classical radical neck dissection.

Question from Audience: You said that the man's teeth were in poor condition. He is a chronic alcoholic and you said it was very difficult to ask these men to give up or limit adverse habits. Why don't you consider doing a surgical procedure which would include a coronal or marginal resection of the mandible, a resection of the floor of mouth, perform a left neck dissection, and subsequently treat the right side of the neck with radiation?

Dr. Strong: I would.

Dr. Byers: Dr. Strong pleads not guilty to that. Dr. Jesse is the one to whom you should direct your question.

Dr. Jesse: I did not say I could not do it. That is a very good way to do it. However, if radiation therapy succeeds without complications, the functional result is better than with the surgical procedure you outline.

Dr. Byers: Are there any other questions?

Dr. Drane: In his follow-up period, this patient certainly should be cautioned against having any dental surgery. The combination of radium and external radiation multiplies the chances of his having both soft and hard tissue breakdown. We would be aware of this and advise him not to have any extractions done in his hometown unless his dentist was aware of his therapy and had consulted with us regarding the proposed dental procedures.

CASE 3.—This is a 22-year-old woman with a small ulcer on the left side of her tongue which was cauterized with silver nitrate by her dentist when it continued to enlarge. An excisional biopsy was done. The margins of the specimen were equivocal for cancer cells. What is the role of the oral surgeon in dealing with this kind of lesion?

Dr. Pleasants: I do not think the cauterization should have been done. If the lesion does not go away after a short period of conservative therapy, a biopsy is certainly indicated. If expert head and neck surgeons are near, I think it is silly for anybody to excise a lesion except the man who is going to do the entire treatment. If you are in a small community, some miles from an expert, an incisional biopsy is certainly the procedure of choice, never an excisional biopsy.

Dr. Byers: When do you not advocate an excisional biopsy?

Dr. Pleasants: If the oral surgeon decides to do an excisional biopsy, he must have complete rapport with a pathologist so that the adequacy of the margins of excision are certain. Too often, such as in the case of the patient presented here, the margins of the biopsy are suspect. The treatment team is forced to perform extensive procedures, because they do not know whether the excision was adequate.

Dr. Strong: I do not think, except under the rarest of circumstances, that there is any more to be gained in making a diagnosis with excisional as opposed to incisional biopsy. I suspect the excision was thought to be therapeutic, and much to the surprise of the individual involved, the diagnosis came back "cancer." To his credit, he sent the specimen for its analysis. In my experience, this is one of the most difficult patients to handle because you have not the slightest idea as to what the extent of the original lesion was in spite of what rapport one may have with the referring physician because he rarely, if ever, can give you any specific information concerning its exact location, its exact size, and its exact infiltration. I do not think there is any place for an excisional biopsy unless, as has already been vividly pointed out, the excision can be done by the individual who is going to treat the patient definitively.

Dr. Byers: In this patient, the area of the primary showed a recent biopsy site with the black silk sutures still in place (Fig. 3A). The patient's mouth was extremely sore to palpation. The patient's neck had a small 1.5 cm. freely movable subdigastric node of doubtful clinical significance. The pathologist's diagnosis was squamous carcinoma, Grade II. Dr. Strong, how would you proceed?

FIG. 3.—*A*, excisional biopsy of squamous cell carcinoma of the tongue—margins of excision are probably positive for cancer. *B*, external 18 MEV photons—2,000 rads in five treatments. *C*, two-plane radium needle implant, 4,700 rads. *D*, floor of the mouth one year after radiation therapy.

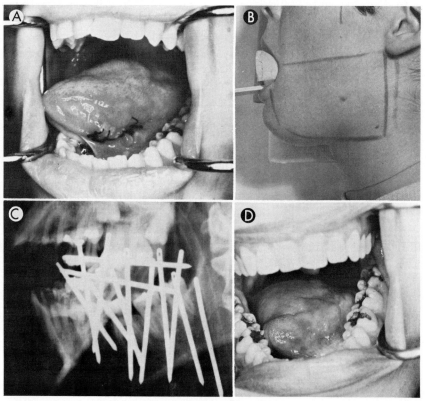

Dr. Strong: It is difficult to treat because I think we often overtreat such patients. I would put the patient on an intensive course of antibiotics and oral irrigations, waiting until the wound was in such a state that I could look at it again a week later and try to determine whether the induration persisted. I think if the induration was the result of a tumor, which I would doubt in view of that rather small incision, the treatment is going to be radically different than if it is not. Although you described a node, you did not tell me whether you thought that node was involved.

Dr. Byers: Clinically, it was thought to be negative.

Dr. Strong: I would do a wide local excision if the induration decreased the way I would think it would, and I would probably close the wound primarily fully expecting the specimen to show no residual tumor.

Dr. Byers: Would you ask the radiotherapist to see this patient?

Dr. Strong: I would have no objection to his seeing the patient. I think he is going to have the same problems I am in trying to determine what areas he would treat.

Dr. Lindberg: Well, I agree with Dr. Strong up to a point. I think he has made a very significant point in that three-dimensional removal is necessary. He is worried about the amount of induration which came to the midline, or possibly across the midline, from what appears to be a rather small biopsy site. We believe that all palpable induration must either be removed surgically or radiated. In our evaluation, you would have to do a hemiglossectomy if you did surgery, assuming, even if this is postsurgical hematoma, the residual cancer cells could migrate to the same areas where the blood did. Rather than subject the patient to a hemiglossectomy, we would prefer to irradiate the area. We may well be overtreating the patient, but I think we can cover a larger area with less loss of function than can a hemiglossectomy. Now, I am bringing up the subject of hemiglossectomy; I do not know if you would do that on this patient.

Dr. Strong: I would certainly hope that I would not have to do a hemiglossectomy, and this is why I would wait to see what happened to the induration. I could not agree with you more. You, obviously, can cover a much wider area with much less functional disability by using radiation than I can by surgery if you are going to insist that all that original induration be treated.

Dr. Byers: Dr. Daly, I am sure you were involved with this patient. Can I have some of your comments concerning this patient's dental care?

Dr. Daly: I do remember her quite well. We did a complete dental examination and took a panorex X-ray film; she had extremely high bone height. We have found that the more bone that is present around the teeth, the more difficult extractions are. Since there is a direct correlation between the difficulty of extractions and subsequent necrosis, we left all of her teeth in and put her on a preventive program with fluoride.

Dr. Byers: The patient was treated with an 18 MEV photon beam to the primary and subdigastric node—2,000 rads in one week followed immediately by a radium implant in two planes delivering 4,700 rads (Figs. 3B and 3C). Dr. Lindberg, could you give us a brief discussion as to why you used the 18 MEV photon beam as the external source?

Dr. Lindberg: Well, one advantage of using the single lateral 18 MEV over the Cobalt 60 unit is that you do not get significant radiation to the contralateral side of the mouth and neck. The 2,000 rads in one week is radiobiologically equal to about 3,400 in 3½ weeks. Then, we follow this with a double plane radium implant which actually covers all the area of the palpable induration.

Dr. Byers: Dr. Drane, would you comment on how you fashion various dental appliances for patients who are undergoing this type of radiation?

Dr. Drane: Yes. If we were to use the intraoral cone for this type of lesion, we would, of course, make a stent into the form that would help the therapist locate the cone in a repetitive position daily and move the other tissues out of the field as much as possible. The stent also moves the maxillary structures out of the beam by opening the mouth.

Dr. Byers: Figure 3D shows the primary site after the treatment. Dr. Daly, would you still continue the fluoride treatments?

Dr. Daly: We used to think that you would not get the postradiation caries unless you had doses of 5,000, 6,000, and 7,000 rads. However, in our study we found radiation caries after radiation doses as low as 2,000 in one week. Now, if a patient receives more than 2,000 rads, we put them on a preventive program.

Dr. Lindberg: For how long?

Dr. Daly: Indefinitely. We find that as long as they wear the fluoride they have no tooth sensitivity and postradiation caries are prevented. If they stop, they begin to develop caries.

Dr. Strong: Did this patient have any functional impairment of her tongue?

Dr. Byers: Practically none.

Dr. Jesse: I think any functional impairment was from the original biopsy.

Question from Audience: The panel was really concerned with the induration and this caused a great deal of concern as to how to treat the patient. Wasn't the original biopsy specimen available for examination? That is, if the tumor was grossly transected in all directions, that would have led to one approach. If indeed it was a small lesion and had free margins, I think the approach could have been something else.

Dr. Byers: Dr. Jesse?

Dr. Jesse: My experience is that most dental surgeons do not have a good rapport with the pathologists in their area; not because they do not like each other, but because they do not talk to each other much. The oral surgeon does an excisional biopsy and does not prepare it for the pathologist. He sends it over to the pathologist with little or no information other than where it came from. The surgeon may not have even suspected that this was a cancer. The result is a poor interpretation as to the adequacy of the margins. I think this is the reason why Dr. Pleasants decried the excisional in favor of the incisional biopsy. With the incisional biopsy, you still have the tumor there. The margins are still in place for examination.

Question from Audience: I was curious about the patient's smoking habits. I did not see any tobacco stains, and I wondered if she was a smoker and if so, what date she started.

Dr. Jesse: She is a nonsmoker.

Question from Audience: Could she have been treated just as well by external radiation?

Dr. Lindberg: Just as well? No, I do not think so. If you can treat this with external beam alone, that means you are crossfiring the entire mandible; the entire area receives a minimum of 5,000 rads, and I think radiation complications would be much higher. The great advantage of radium needles is that you put the radiation exactly where you need it. I do not think this could have been accomplished with an intraoral cone.

Question from Audience: Did the age of your patient have anything to do with your decision?

Dr. Lindberg: Well, the younger the patients, the less we like to radiate them. But when the alternative would be a fairly extensive surgical procedure, we believe radiation is the lesser of two evils.

Question from Audience: I notice that the treatment fields did include the upper part of the neck. Was this done intentionally?

Dr. Lindberg: For years, many of the early tongue and floor of mouth lesions were treated only by radium needles. Some patients developed mechanical implantation of cancer cells in the submental and submaxillary areas by pushing cells ahead of the needle. Nowadays, we give some external radiation first to kill or hurt the cancer cells so that we do not implant them with the radium needles. Remember that the end of a radium needle does not have any radium in it.

Dr. John MacFarlane, Montreal, Quebec, Canada: I would like to ask Dr.

Lindberg if the needling produces any less or more dryness in the mouth than treatment by external radiation.

Dr. Lindberg: One major advantage of the implant is that the salivary glands do not receive much irradiation. The dryness is only in the minor salivary glands in the implant area. Therefore, the dryness is a very local phenomenon.

Question from Audience: I would like to ask Dr. Jesse a question. It disturbs me that this young lady is going to have a long-time morbidity from the X-ray treatment. I mean for the rest of her life. What would be wrong, just to be the devil's advocate, with watching this and not treating it until you see the recurrence, maybe at a later date. How is that going to change the prognosis?

Dr. Jesse: Our statistics will show that if there is recurrent tumor, the chances of salvaging the patient by any modality are decreased a good deal. We admittedly overtreat, but this is better for the patient than to risk a recurrence with its poor prognosis.

CASE 4.—This patient is a 49-year-old man with an ulcerated sore of two months' duration on the tongue. He chewed tobacco for approximately 15 years. His teeth are in good condition. The primary tumor was an ulcerated, infiltrating 5×2.5 cm., T_3 lesion of the lateral oral tongue with some extension into the floor of the mouth (Fig. 4A). The tumor did not reach the anterior tonsillar pillar. The mobility of the tongue was normal. The patient had no nodes in the neck. The biopsy revealed a squamous carcinoma, Grade II. X-ray studies of the chest and mandible were negative. Dr. Lindberg, how would you prefer to handle this problem?

Dr. Lindberg: This particular patient presents a problem in that he has a fair-sized lesion infiltrating deeply into the floor of the mouth. This can be treated with a combination of external beam and radium needling. I think it is very significant that the patient's neck was negative. Biologically, the lesion is probably not aggressive. But if we elected to radiate him, we would treat the entire neck.

Dr. Byers: Bilaterally?

Dr. Lindberg: Yes.

Dr. Byers: Would you treat with external beam only, or would you boost this with an implant?

Dr. Lindberg: We would go at least to 5,000 rads externally. He should have a considerable amount of regression after the 5,000 rads and then we would have to reevaluate him to see if needles are feasible; I think they would be.

Dr. Byers: Dr. Strong, would you be interested in treating this patient surgically?

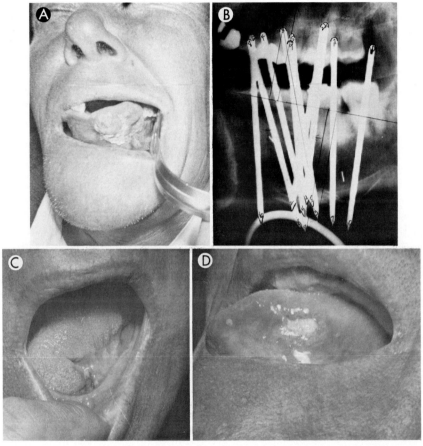

Fig. 4.—*A*, T₃N₀ squamous cell carcinoma of lateral oral tongue with infiltration into floor of the mouth. *B*, squamous cell carcinoma of the tongue treated by double plane radium implant. *C*, tongue six months after treatment by irradiation. *D*, recurrence in the tongue eight months later.

Dr. Strong: Yes, he has a big lesion. With the high propensity for subsequent nodal metastatic disease, any treatment of necessity must include the neck as well, since it falls within the definition of what I described to be a high-risk area. I would give him preoperative radiotherapy and then follow it with a neck dissection and a resection of the tongue. I would try to avoid resecting the mandible if I could possibly do so.

Dr. Byers: You would do a pull-through type procedure, then?

Dr. Strong: Yes. We have a limited number of patients in whom we have done a discontinuous procedure with success. I am not advocating that, but I am merely saying that it can be done.

Dr. Byers: Would you comment on the rationale for not doing pull-throughs? Suppose this tumor was right up to the margin of the mandible but there was a tumor-free margin?

Dr. Strong: Dr. Frank C. Marchetta at Roswell Park demonstrated that cancer which is not adherent to the bone seldom invades the bone and, therefore, one can reasonably leave bone behind. Often the osseous resection is for the convenience of the surgeon to help close the wound rather than to eradicate the tumor. If it is stripped of its periosteum, it has to be covered, but I do not think the bone of necessity has to be resected. If the tumor were densely adherent to it, I would do a marginal resection if I were reasonably convinced that the cortical bone was not involved. If careful examination of the specimen in the operating room did document that it was eroded, I possibly would go ahead and take out a segment of the mandible because I recognize my inability and that of my pathologist to judge, on frozen section, the amount of bone invasion.

Dr. Byers: Suppose after 4,000 rads in four weeks this tumor is practically gone. Could you still make a decision in the operating room as to whether you were going to take out more or less? Could you cheat, or would you cheat?

Dr. Strong: I would not dare. I would plan my operation based on what I saw at the initial evaluation.

Dr. Byers: Would you tattoo the periphery of this lesion, or how would you make sure that you were taking out the same amount of tissue?

Dr. Strong: I think that we could tattoo it. We simply place the dye beneath the mucosa with a needle. Do not inject the dye because the dye diffuses throughout the area and the tattoo becomes meaningless. I think that if one is meticulous in the graphic representation of these tumors with the aid of diagrams, he can be reasonably accurate in his description at the time of the original evaluation.

Dr. Byers: Let's move on to the treatment. The therapy consisted of 2,500 rads of 18 MEV external irradiation to the submental port in five days followed by double plane needle implant delivering 4,000 rads (Fig. 4B). The result at four months is shown in Figure 4C. The patient developed a recurrence in the tongue eight months later (Fig. 4D). Dr. Lindberg, would you comment on the possible explanation of why this patient's primary recurred?

Dr. Lindberg: The way he would be treated now is not what was done originally. We used the submental electron beam field delivering a rather low dose of 2,500 rads and then he had a 4,000 rad radium needle implant.

The neck was not treated. Today we would give more of the radiation by external beam and less with the radium in such a big lesion. We would also give the entire neck 5,000 rads of irradiation, because this patient is at high risk of developing nodes, as Dr. Strong has stated.

Dr. Byers: Dr. Jesse, how would you handle this recurrence?

Dr. Jesse: I think we would have to do a combined resection. After that amount of irradiation, I would be afraid not to resect the mandible. I would resect half the tongue, the floor of the mouth, and the left half of the mandible, and then repair the defect either primarily or with a forehead pedicle.

Dr. Byers: In other words, you would not cheat any on this as far as the amount of resection you would do now as opposed to what you have done originally?

Dr. Jesse: We now have an instance of recurrent disease and I would do a combined resection with a wide margin at this point. I do not know how big the recurrence is, but I would assume that it is more than just superficial.

Dr. Byers: It is difficult to say from reading the clinical chart. The recurrence appeared eight months following the completion of the patient's radiation therapy. There were no nodes palpable in the neck at the time. A partial glossectomy with pull-through and radical neck dissection were performed. The specimen showed no nodes positive. The patient is free of disease at five years. The mandible was covered with primary intraoral tissue.

Panel Discussion: Cancer of the Oropharynx and Hypopharynx

MODERATOR: RICHARD H. JESSE, M.D.

Chief, Section of Head and Neck Surgery, The University of Texas System Cancer Center, M. D. Anderson Hospital and Tumor Institute, Houston, Texas

Dr. Jesse: At this time I shall present the case report.

CASE 1.—This patient smokes two packs of cigarettes a day, drinks six beers a day, and works regularly. There is a 3.5 cm. squamous cell carcinoma in the retromolar trigone fixed to the periosteum of the mandible. The cancer is superficial in the soft palate and on the floor of the mouth. There is slight trismus. There is a 3 cm. subdigastric movable node (Fig. 1A). X-ray films of the mandible show a questionable break in the medial ascending ramus. (A film made after postoperative radiotherapy is shown in Figure 1B.)

Dr. Alfred S. Ketcham, National Cancer Institute, Bethesda, Maryland: Needless to say, this is a miserable lesion. Because it is such a miserable lesion, we would choose not to be conventional. We would place this man on a protocol study which we now have under way, giving him methotrexate in moderately high dosage. We would expect that he will achieve a rather remarkable remission of his tumor. At the end of two weeks we use citrovorum retrieval and do a conventional surgical procedure. Our conventional surgery would include a wide excision of the area, ipsilateral neck dissection, and a mandibular resection. We would take mandible because of fixation of tumor to bone, because of the better exposure, and because the closure is made easier. Patients in this protocol study having positive lymph nodes stay on methotrexate for six months; however, if the nodes are negative in the specimen, then we do not give methotrexate postoperatively.

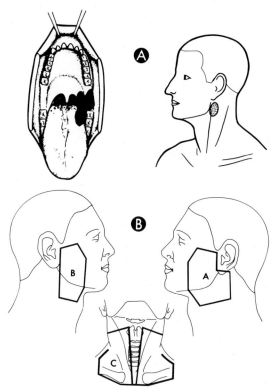

Fig. 1.—*A*, 3.5 cm. squamous lesion attached to periosteum of retromolar area—one 3 cm. movable ipsilateral node. *B*, postoperative radiation therapy—6,000 rads to the upper fields and 5,000 rads given to the lower anterior portal.

Dr. Jesse: Dr. Gottlieb, have you had any experience with this regimen of methotrexate?

Dr. Jeffrey A. Gottlieb, M. D. Anderson Hospital, Houston, Texas: This is far from conventional methotrexate therapy. Dr. Ketcham's doses are extremely high. This and the timing of the citrovorum factor rescue are quite critical here and not the type of thing to be undertaken without a great deal of experience.

Dr. Ketcham: If we were not doing the protocol study, we would do the surgical procedure I mentioned earlier and we would not use postoperative radiation.

Dr. Jesse: Dr. Bakamjian, Dr. Ketcham is going to resect the primary tumor with a 2 cm. margin, remove the mandible, and dissect the neck.

I assume at that point he will ask you to repair the defect. How would you handle it?

Dr. Vahram Y. Bakamjian, Roswell Park Memorial Institute, Buffalo, New York: With this size of resection I would do it with a deltopectoral flap; however, I do have other alternatives. We can use the forehead flap, cervical flaps in women, and, in small lesions, tongue flaps.

Dr. Jesse: Dr. Ballantyne, what would you do with this patient?

Dr. A. J. Ballantyne, The University of Texas System Cancer Center, M. D. Anderson Hospital and Tumor Institute, Houston, Texas: I think I would just treat this patient surgically with a neck dissection, resection of the ascending ramus of the mandible, and repair intraorally with a split thickness skin graft.

Dr. Jesse: Can you use a split skin graft when you clean out the pterygoid area?

Dr. Ballantyne: Yes, you can use a split graft almost anywhere in the mouth. I do not see any great advantage of big flaps over a split thickness skin graft in nonradiated areas.

Dr. Jesse: Dr. Perez, would you be interested in any radiation pre- or postoperatively or as the only modality of treatment?

Dr. Carlos A. Perez, Washington University School of Medicine, St. Louis, Missouri: We should distinguish this large, fixed lesion from the early tumors of the retromolar trigone and the anterior tonsillar pillar which do very well when treated only by radiation therapy. In this instance, because of the fixation of the lesion to the mandible and because of the extent of the lesion, we would prefer to treat the primary area and ipsilateral neck of the patient with 5,000 rads of preoperative radiation. If the patient had a surgical procedure as the initial treatment, I would not routinely give radiation after surgery unless there was a reason, such as multiple positive nodes or inadequate resection margins.

Dr. Jesse: Dr. Goepfert, if you were asked to operate on this patient after Dr. Perez gave him 5,000 rads, would you do exactly the same procedure you would have done had the patient not been irradiated?

Dr. Helmuth Goepfert, Baylor College of Medicine and The University of Texas System Cancer Center, M. D. Anderson Hospital and Tumor Institute, Houston, Texas: I would not change the extent of the resection. The original size of the lesion would have to be encompassed by the resection. The difficult problem really is after the patient has received the full dose of irradiation since then, the closure is difficult. You have to get some tissue to separate the carotid artery from the internal suture line.

Dr. Jesse: So you would like Dr. Bakamjian to use one of his pedicles?

Dr. Goepfert: Either the Bakamjian type of pedicle or a forehead flap if the patient would let me do it.

Dr. Jesse: Dr. Fletcher, would you want to give this patient postoperative radiation therapy?

Dr. Gilbert H. Fletcher, The University of Texas System Cancer Center, M. D. Anderson Hospital and Tumor Institute, Houston, Texas: Here is a man with a good-sized lesion, and there is a definite likelihood of a local recurrence. He has a good-sized node; the risk of a recurrence in the radically dissected neck is, I think, over 25 per cent. He also has a definite risk of contralateral metastasis. We must look at those odds and plan our strategy accordingly. This patient should have surgery first and then comprehensive postoperative radiation therapy which includes treating the opposite side of the neck. One could use the irradiation preoperatively if you wanted, but I think it would make repair more complex.

Dr. Jesse: What kinds of fields and what kind of dose would you use?

Dr. Fletcher: The whole left neck is at risk; therefore, we would use comprehensive treatment.

Dr. Jesse: You would treat the A and B fields shown on Figure 1B to 6,000 rads?

Dr. Fletcher: We would use the electron beam and give from 5,000 to 6,000 rads over the area of surgical resection where the remaining cancer cells may be relatively anoxic.

Dr. Jesse: So you would make a bigger field on the side of the lesion and a smaller field on the opposite side?

Dr. Fletcher: When you treat the opposite side, you always include the subdigastric area but do not have to treat the posterior chain. To prevent recurrence in the radically dissected neck, you have to include every bit of the surgical scar.

Dr. Jesse: This particular patient had successful treatment, utilizing a surgical resection and postoperative radiation. Let us take a hypothetical situation where we have used both radiation and surgical therapy and then get a recurrence. Dr. Gottlieb, what is your experience with bleomycin?

Dr. Gottlieb: It is important that we become familiar with this agent because we are going to hear more about it in the next two years. It is a new drug and it comes from Japan. It will be commercially available very shortly as Blenoxane. It comes in a 15 mg. vial. The usual dose is 7.5 mg. twice weekly or 15 mg. every week. There is a twofold reason why it is important for us to know about bleomycin. First, the drug is capable of causing regression of recurrent cancer in a patient who has been previously treated with the more conventional drugs such as methotrexate. Second, it is a drug that does not produce myelotoxicity of any significant degree—

an advantage which it has over methotrexate. Bleomycin is an unusual drug in that it concentrates in squamous tissue and particularly in that in the head and neck. Unfortunately, the regression time is usually of short duration. I think it is also important that we know some of the side effects. The gastroenteric effects are relatively mild and it produces a moderate alopecia. The patient commonly complains about changes in the skin, the occasional fever, and the sore mouth. Pulmonary toxicity has been the side effect that has had the most controversy because of the fear of inducing a fatal pulmonary fibrosis in patients treated with this drug. However, pulmonary toxicity seems to be something that can be avoided by keeping the dose low. As the dose increases above 250-300 mg., one starts to increase the risk of this type of toxicity, particularly in older patients. At 300 mg., 30 per cent of patients can be expected to have fairly good tumor regression. The action of this drug can apparently be potentiated by other agents. Kinetic studies show that bleomycin almost exclusively kills cells that are in the process of mitosis. By giving vincristine approximately 6 hours before bleomycin, we can increase to 10 times the number of cells in mitosis. This triples the efficacy of bleomycin, thus extending some remissions to six months or longer. It also permits us to use a lower dose of bleomycin and, therefore, to achieve a longer duration of therapy without producing pulmonary toxicity. I think that it is studies such as these that offer at least some hope for the future. Palliation is the role that chemotherapy has had and it was a sorry role, but I think that we are at least working on trying to make it a more effective weapon for the head and neck surgeon.

Dr. Jesse: Thank you. Does anybody have any comment related to this case?

Dr. Perez: I would like to make a couple of points. When you talk about replacing radiation therapy with chemotherapy as a preoperative modality, I think that one has to remember that (1) radiation has a much higher level of cell kill than does chemotherapy and (2) the drug produces more systemic morbidity than does radiation therapy. So far, no one has proved that one prevents distant metastasis in patients with squamous cancer by giving chemotherapy postradiation therapy or postoperatively.

Dr. Fletcher: Dr. Jesse, what about that national study of methotrexate? What did that show?

Dr. Jesse: The National Methotrexate Study will show that there is little if any benefit in patients undergoing radiation therapy randomized as to whether or not they receive methotrexate. The dose level was very low at 25 mg. every third day for five doses before irradiation.

Dr. Winchokowski, Washington, D.C.: I would like to ask Dr. Ketcham about a patient who is found to have 14 positive nodes in the neck dissection specimen. How many of these patients would he expect to have recurrence in the neck, and what would the salvage rate be at that point with radiation therapy?

Dr. Ketcham: If a patient has 14 nodes in the neck, that patient is likely to have occult systemic cancer so I do not think it matters what you do. We would give him immediate postoperative radiation to prevent regional recurrence. If the patient had one node positive in the neck, we would not electively use postoperative radiation to the ipsilateral side of the neck. We have not experienced a manifestation of cancer in the untreated contralateral side of the neck as great as 33 per cent. We would follow the contralateral side of the neck extremely closely but would not irradiate it.

Dr. Lane Hamilton, Ontario, Canada: In some of these patients who had both x-ray treatment and a surgical procedure, particularly if the mandible is left in place, one of the problems seems to be a severe degree of trismus. I would like to ask the panel how this can be obviated and if you do get trismus, what you do about it?

Dr. Ballantyne: There is not very much you can do. You can have the dentist give them the bite opener and try to open the bite, but if the trismus is progressive, then eventually you will have to resect a portion of the mandible so that the patient can open his mouth enough to clean it and eat satisfactorily.

Dr. Jesse: Do you ever just take out the condyle?

Dr. Ballantyne: I have taken out the condyles. I usually go a little further than that because with radiation and surgical treatment, the mandible tends to drift farther up and you will still get some trismus.

CASE 2.—This is a 58-year-old male with a lesion of the base of the tongue. His general condition is good but he smokes two packs of cigarettes a day and does not drink. There is a 3 cm. midline lesion in the base of the tongue. The glossopalatine sulcus was negative and the mobility of the tongue was good (Fig. 2A). There is a right subdigastric movable node 3 × 1.5 cm. and on the left there are three nodes in the mid and lower jugular, the largest being 2 cm. The pathology report is squamous cell carcinoma, Grade III.

Dr. Jesse: Dr. Goepfert, what would you do with this patient?

Dr. Goepfert: I would invite the radiotherapist to examine the mouth of this gentleman. I think that it is very important that we both determine where this lesion is, and how wide and deep the infiltrative component is. The important fact in the case of this patient is that one side of the neck is at least an N_1 and the other side is an N_2. It is a midline lesion so we have to treat both sides of the neck separately. I would ask the radiothera-

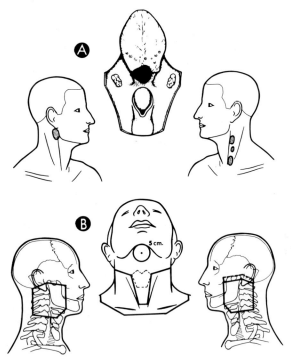

Fig. 2.—*A*, 3 cm. squamous cell carcinoma of the base of the tongue with clinically positive nodes as diagrammed. *B*, 5,000 rads ^{60}Co opposed lateral upper fields; 5,000 rads ^{60}Co given anterior lower field; 1,700 rads anterior electron beam field.

pist to treat the primary for cure and at the same time give radiation to both sides of the neck preoperatively. In four to six weeks, I would dissect the side of the neck with greatest involvement and four weeks after that, I would dissect the opposite side of the neck.

Dr. Jesse: Dr. Ketcham, how would you treat this man?

Dr. Ketcham: Our results with these lesions have been terrible. We have a study going with high dose bleomycin and irradiation which I am not enthusiastic about but which I think is very interesting. If that study were not going on and I did not feel obligated to enter a few patients into it, I would give this patient definitive radiation for cure, as has already been noted, and at the six-week or probably ten-week period, I would do simultaneous bilateral neck dissections. I would not touch the primary unless there was some indication that it is not controlled. If we wait ten weeks before the surgical procedure, we should have a good indication regarding control of the primary. I would start on the side with only one node and try to leave the jugular vein. Now, I do not advise anyone who does one neck dissection a month to do less than a conventional neck dissection. If you are going to save the jugular vein you have got to have some experience, because in my own case, this takes me another half hour or so of surgical time. Now I would like to mention another thing. I think it is mandatory that these patients have a complete cancer work-up, not just a head and neck work-up. A tongue cancer metastasizing to level 3 nodes may well have metastasized to the lung. We would do pulmonary tomography because the reports on clinical studies of patients with head and neck disease going to autopsy show that 55 per cent of them have disease below the clavicle, and in 99 per cent of those, the disease will be pulmonary.

Dr. Jesse: In 10 weeks, you would do the bilateral neck. Would you do any biopsy of the primary site?

Dr. Ketcham: I use the fibro-optic bronchoscope which is now available. We would take a very good look at the primary site. I would not be hesitant to perform a biopsy if there was any indication to do it, but I would not do it without reason because the biopsy site does not heal too well.

Dr. Jesse: What is your experience with the mortality of simultaneous bilateral neck dissection versus staged procedures?

Dr. Ketcham: We have had extremely satisfactory results with our bilateral neck dissections, and I would choose to do the procedures simultaneously rather than staged unless there was a reason to wait. We have had no mortalities in 30 simultaneous bilateral neck dissections. The morbidity is cut way down if you can leave one jugular vein.

Dr. Jesse: Dr. Strong, don't I remember Dr. Oliver Moore writing an article on the mortality of simultaneous bilateral neck dissection at your institution?

Dr. Elliot W. Strong, Memorial Hospital, New York, N.Y.: The operative mortality of bilateral simultaneous neck dissections, if I remember correctly, is 14 per cent. This encompasses both internal jugular veins, and in many patients includes resection of the primary lesion. This is, therefore, not the same operation that Dr. Ketcham is talking about.

Dr. Jesse: Dr. Fletcher, how would you treat this patient?

Dr. Fletcher: The way this lesion would be treated is shown in Figure 2B. It would be fair to say that we are quite revolutionary in the general planning for these patients. Because this was a midline lesion, we would give part of the radiation dose through a submental electron beam field. The lateral upper neck fields received 5,000 rads with the ^{60}Co unit with 1,700 rads being given by electron beam. The anterior lower field received a given dose of 5,000 rads. If the lesion is more laterally placed on the base of the tongue, you have to use a lateral ^{60}Co beam entirely and give a tumor dose of 7,000 rads. The method of treatment to the primary affects the way the nodes are treated. If the submental electron beam field is used, the nodes receive only 5,000 rads which is not enough to sterilize them. They either have to be boosted or, as we prefer, the surgeon must remove them. If the entire treatment to the primary is by lateral field, the nodes in the field receive 7,000 rads. This would probably sterilize a 3 cm. node if it disappears, but probably not a node which is much bigger. We do sterilize some clinically positive nodes at 7,000 rads, you know.

On the side with the multiple level nodes, the lower ones would not receive 7,000 rads and should be removed. Because we think that 5,000 rads will control subclinical deposits of cancer in lymphatics, our surgeons would probably "cheat" and not do a complete radical neck dissection but only remove the nodes or nodal chains which were originally clinically positive. They do cheat all the time, although Dr. Jesse will not admit it publicly; but the cheating is good. Radical neck dissection has reached a point of being a religious ritual. In the light of what we now know about the effective uses of radiotherapy in evidently subclinical disease, some changes are necessary in regard to some of the classical surgical procedures. Now we would not do a radical or bilateral radical neck dissection but rather a modified neck dissection.

Dr. Jesse: Dr. Ballantyne, would you be interested in doing anything different with this patient?

Dr. Ballantyne: The only thing I would add to the preoperative work-up is a lateral soft tissue film of the neck. If this is an excavating lesion on the base of the tongue and it goes down to the hyoid bone, then I do not think radiation therapy would be appropriate. This patient has an exophytic lesion and I think it can be adequately controlled by radiation. I do not hesitate to do a bilateral modified neck dissection, rather than a classical radical neck dissection, after 5,000 rads of irradiation.

Dr. Jesse: What do you mean by modified?

Dr. Ballantyne: I leave both sternocleidomastoid muscles and both veins, and remove the nodes. I would not, however, advocate this for everybody. I think you have to have good radiotherapists. You have to know how much radiation has been given and the exact fields employed, and you have to have some experience in doing modified neck dissections before you can do them routinely.

Dr. Ketcham: I have convinced myself that modified neck dissections can be done. I have found, however, that if I am going to leave the muscle and the vessel, it requires another hour of anesthesia time. I think we are all saying the same thing here. An individual is going to get in trouble if he is not doing them regularly, because it is difficult to clean out underneath the parotid and the submastoid angle with the muscle still in place.

Dr. Fletcher: But you leave the patient in better shape, and I think that is worth an extra hour, Dr. Ketcham.

Dr. Jesse: Are there any questions from the audience regarding this patient?

Dr. Ted Young, Toronto, Canada: Mr. Chairman, I wonder if I could direct a question to Dr. Ketcham and ask him if, on his complete work-up of this patient, he discovered a solitary 2 cm. node in the right upper lobe of the lung, or a small cancer in the sigmoid colon, how he would change his treatment of this patient.

Dr. Jesse: May I enlarge your question? I was going to ask him whether he did routine barium work-ups on all patients without a positive history of colonic trouble, or does he just do a digital rectal examination and sigmoidoscopy?

Dr. Ketcham: It is easier for me to speak when I am in an institution where economics are not a factor. What I would do if I were you, I do not know, but I can tell you what we have developed at the National Cancer Institute. Our routine on all patients with neck nodes includes an intravenous pyelogram, because we have examined more than one patient whose nodes are from the kidney instead of an unknown primary in the head and neck area. Now, to answer the question about what we do for a patient with suspected metastatic disease in the lung. If the patient were a nonsmoker, we would do his lung first. If this was found to be metastatic disease, or was highly suspicious of metastatic disease, we would be less apt to do a mutilating procedure in the head and neck area. If we found that this was a second primary in the lung, we would do the same procedure in the head and neck as we would ordinarily do. If we found the lung lesion postoperatively, whether it was one week or one year later, we would explore it.

Dr. Robert M. Byers, M. D. Anderson Hospital, Houston, Texas: I would like to bring up the point that patients having a surgical procedure following irradiation are often in negative nitrogen balance. Dr. Ballantyne, would you comment on this?

Dr. Ballantyne: You do not operate on these people until they start to gain weight. That is about the best way I know to insure that they are in positive nitrogen balance unless you want to do some complicated metabolic studies.

CASE 3.—The next patient is a 66-year-old man who smokes 12 cigars a day and also drinks a fifth of whiskey a day. The lesion is on the pharyngeal wall from the tip of the uvula above, crosses the posterior pillar on the right, invades the junction of the right posterior and lateral walls down to the level of the arytenoid. It is not on the left lateral wall; there are no nodes (Fig. 3A). The lesion involves less of the left side, but it is truly a bilateral lesion.

Dr. Jesse: Dr. Ketcham, what would you do with this one?

Dr. Ketcham: I think you have asked this question because of the nodes of Rauvier. The real problem here is the retropharyngeal dissemination of this tumor. I have a great deal of difficulty in surgically encompassing these nodes. We would put this patient into our protocol on bleomycin and radiation. Our conventional treatment is a pharyngectomy followed by irradiation. We try to do a primary closure. I would be worried about this man's rehabilitation because in order to do a resection, I would have to take his glossopharyngeal and superior laryngeal nerves and he may aspirate and have trouble swallowing. If we left his larynx I think he would have a 50 per cent chance of having to have it removed later. I would like to have this man have irradiation just as soon postoperatively as possible.

Fig. 3.—*A,* squamous cell carcinoma of the posterior pharyngeal wall of the oropharynx (T_3N_0). *B,* opposed portals for T_3N_0 lesion of posterior oropharyngeal wall.

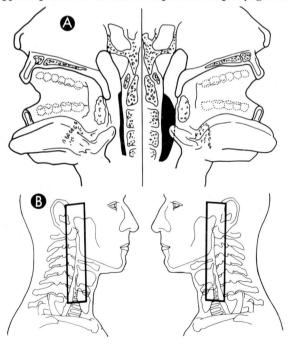

Dr. Jesse: Dr. Ballantyne, what would you do with it?

Dr. Ballantyne: If this were a woman, I would irradiate her without any question, presuming this were an exophytic lesion. Women do better than men. These pharyngeal wall cancers spread to the retropharyngeal nodes. The inferior group or the medial group of retropharyngeal nodes are positive in about 40 per cent of patients with pharyngeal wall cancers and also positive in about 40 per cent of patients with pyriform sinus cancers which invade the lateral pharyngeal wall. If you do have a patient with a pharyngeal wall cancer with positive posterior cervical nodes, you can be almost 100 per cent certain that he has positive retropharyngeal nodes.

Dr. Jesse: If you decided to operate on this patient, how would you approach it?

Dr. Ballantyne: I think most of these lesions can be approached through an infrahyoid incision. You excise the lesion and then you raise up the pharynx and do your bilateral retropharyngeal node dissection and then you repair the pharynx, usually with a skin graft. I do not think it is safe to save the larynx in people who have emphysema or chronic pulmonary disease, since the risk of aspiration is high.

Dr. Jesse: How do you tell if this lesion is exophytic?

Dr. Ballantyne: It is usually not difficult. If you can push on the tumor and move it over the vertebral fascia, then it is an exophytic lesion.

Dr. Jesse: Did you ever see one of these lesions attach itself to the prevertebral fascia?

Dr. Ballantyne: They practically never invade the prevertebral fascia. Once in a great while they do invade it, but for some reason they tend to spread along the muscle planes. If you can move the tumor relatively free over the underlying structures, then it is an exophytic tumor and will probably respond satisfactorily to radiation.

Dr. Jesse: All right, Dr. Fletcher, would you accept this patient for radiation?

Dr. Fletcher: The exophytic lesion will do quite well when treated with radiation therapy. If it is an excavating deep lesion, it does very poorly when radiated. In the latter type of lesion, using the concept of getting rid of subclinical disease by radiotherapy, I personally would like to see the surgeon excise and graft the lesion without taking too great a margin; then we would give radiotherapy as soon as possible.

Dr. Jesse: If you were treating this exophytic lesion primarily, are these the fields you would use (Fig. 3B)?

Dr. Fletcher: Many of these patients do not have lateral nodes on admission. The fields we would use in patients without nodes go inferiorly to the mouth of the esophagus to treat lymphatics in the submucosa; 7,000 rads of ^{60}Co irradiation would be delivered in seven weeks.

Dr. Perez: This lesion is primarily exophytic but it is going to have some infiltrative component. We would treat this patient with radiation therapy. We would use essentially the ports that Dr. Fletcher has shown in Figure 3B. Perhaps we would be a little more generous toward the base of the skull and include a little more of the lateral neck. We give 6,000 to 7,000 rads to the primary lesion in the midline and about 6,000 rads to the nodes. If, when the patient has received 5,000 rads, the lesion has not had good regression and a significant amount of infiltrating disease remains, we would then refer the patient for a surgical resection.

Dr. Ketcham: Some of the patients' photos shown here today showed nasogastric tubes. Often the patient has worn them for weeks or months. There is an alternative and I do not understand why people don't use it more often. We use a feeding esophagostomy which can be done very easily. We make a low incision, pull the trachea medially and encounter the vertebral fascia. The esophagus is just above and medial to it. We make a nick in it and drop the feeding tube in. These can be left in indefinitely. In our entire experience, we only have two patients in whom we had to close the fistula. After five to seven days, the patients change the tube as necessary.

Tumors of the Head and Neck: Clinicopathologic Discussion of Cases Illustrating Interaction of Diagnosis and Choice of Therapy

MODERATOR: WILLIAM O. RUSSELL, M.D.

Arranged by the Department of Pathology, The University of Texas System Cancer Center, M. D. Anderson Hospital and Tumor Institute, Houston, Texas and Co-sponsored by Texas Society of Pathologists

The panel included the following M. D. Anderson Hospital staff members in addition to Dr. Russell: A. J. Ballantyne, M.D., Surgeon; Howard T. Barkley, Jr., M.D., Radiotherapist; Barnett J. Finkelstein, M.D., Radiologist; Mario A. Luna, M.D., Pathologist; Victor Matalon, D.D.S., Surgeon (Prosthodontics); and W. W. Sutow, M.D., Pediatrician. Summary of panel discussion was prepared by Mary L. McCrackan, M.Sc. and reviewed by M. A. Luna, M.D.

THE ANNUAL SPECIAL PATHOLOGY PROGRAM consisted of an informal panel discussion of six case histories including patients with tumors of the jaws, soft tissues, and salivary glands, as well as odontogenic neoplasias. Discussions emphasized the full clinical correlation of the radiologic, pathologic, radiotherapeutic, chemotherapeutic, and surgical aspects of each case. The session was moderated by William O. Russell, M.D., Head, Department of Pathology and Professor of Pathology, M. D. Anderson Hospital. The introductory speaker was Elwood Baird, M.D., President of Texas Society of Pathologists and Associate Director of Clinical Laboratories, Professor of Pathology, The University of Texas Medical Branch at Galveston.

Case 1.—Benign Mixed Tumor of Deep Lobe of Parotid Gland

THERAPEUTIC APPROACH TO A DEEPLY LOCATED TUMOR.—This 60-year-old Caucasian woman was admitted to M. D. Anderson Hospital on August 3, 1971, with a history of a mass in the left tonsillar region and left parotid area of 22 years' duration. The patient had a tonsillectomy in 1948 following which she was told that she had a hemangioma. She received radiotherapy to the tonsillar region in another institution in 1953. The patient reported that the radiation slowed the growth, but it had recently increased in size before her referral to M. D. Anderson Hospital.

Physical examination was not remarkable except for a submucosal mass involving the left tonsillar fossa, the anterior tonsillar pillar, and the lateral portion of the left soft palate. External swelling was observed behind the ascending ramus of the left mandible. The mass was palpable between the mouth and the posterior mandibular area. The cervical lymph nodes were negative. The right parotid was unremarkable.

Nasopharyngeal tumor survey revealed asymmetry of the oropharyngeal shadow. On the base view, the soft tissue shadow was blunted, suggesting a lesion on the left side. A left carotid arteriogram showed a relatively avascular mass in the region of the left parotid.

DISCUSSION

DIAGNOSTIC RADIOLOGY.—Angiography is indicated for tumors of the head and neck and is of greatest value in delineating vascular lesions such as hemangioma, which this patient had been told she had. However, with parotid tumors, the diagnostic radiologists contribute less than with other types of neoplasms. With this patient, even using the subtraction technique which eliminates the bone so that the vasculature is more evident, only a vague outline of tumor was seen. All the angiogram demonstrated was that the tumor probably was not a hemangioma. The lesions which are most successfully outlined by angiography are the juvenile angiofibromas and the various chemodectomas. The angiogram is not used to provide a specific diagnosis for head and neck tumors. As with angiography in other anatomic sites, the primary purpose is to outline the tumor and delineate the blood supply. This preoperative information can be very significant for patients with tumors such as cavernous hemangioma which may have several different sources of blood. The surgeon may need to ligate some vessels. Also, the angiogram becomes very valuable in repeat surgery.

PATHOLOGY.—This patient had a benign mixed tumor of the parotid gland. The important gross features of mixed tumors are multilobulated masses with many nodules protruding out of the main tumor (Fig. 1A). These are connected to the main tumor and if any of these small nodules are left by the surgeon, the recurrence rate is very high. The benign mixed tumor is encased by a capsule which may vary from being thin and incomplete in some areas to well-developed and thick in other places. Mixed tumors contain epithelial elements and a mesenchymal like component which usually is cartilage or myxoid stroma (Fig. 1B). The epithelial component may be glandular; or the cells may be tall, cylindrical, and eosinophilic; or it may have squamous features. The prognosis of the benign mixed tumor does not depend on the histologic characteristics, but rather

Fig. 1.—Mixed tumor. *A*, whole organ section showing a multilobulated mass encased by the capsule (H and E, × 5). *B*, cartilage, myxoid tissue, and epithelial cells in a section (H and E, × 100).

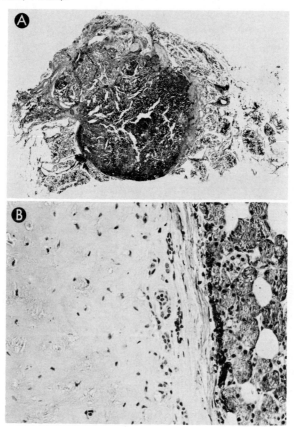

on the type of treatment given. In contrast with the benign mixed tumor, the malignant mixed tumor has a carcinomatous element which invades and destroys the normal capsule. In the M. D. Anderson Hospital series of malignant mixed tumors of the parotid gland, perineural invasion occurred in 50 per cent of patients. The differential diagnosis of malignant mixed tumors usually is easy. In borderline cases, necrosis, calcification, extensive fibrosis, and atypical mitoses may indicate malignant disease.

Surgery.—The ballottement test, in which one finger is placed on the mass in the mouth and another behind the ascending ramus of the mandible to detect an impulse behind the ramus, is an almost 100 per cent certain method of determining presence of a tumor in the deep lobe of the parotid gland. Tumors presenting submucosally in this region are almost certain to be parotid tumors. Most tumors of the deep lobe will not produce external swelling in the parotid region. The patient's external and internal swelling was caused by the very large size of the tumor. Pathologists receiving biopsy specimens from inside the mouth, in such situations, should think of a tumor of the deep lobe of the parotid gland. Actually, when the diagnosis is obvious from the ballottement test, no form of biopsy is indicated, and the physician should proceed with parotidectomy as the treatment of choice. In tumors of the deep lobe of the parotid which have been present for many years—this patient had known of her tumor for 17 years—the facial nerve may be displaced and almost subcutaneous in position. In this patient, the facial nerve was notably displaced, but was preserved. Tumors of this type also may extend up to the base of the skull, and if the pterygoid veins are involved some bleeding may occur, but this is not difficult to control.

About a year after the tumor was removed from the left side, the patient noted swelling on the right side. A second tumor was diagnosed, also in the deep lobe of the parotid gland. Parotidectomy was performed on the right side, with removal of the deep lobe and the upper jugular nodes. The tumor was a very well-circumscribed low grade mucoepidermoid carcinoma. The patient is now well, with no evidence of further disease.

Comment.—Bilateral tumors of the parotid gland are rare. In a series of about 2,100 major salivary gland tumors at Memorial Hospital, 45 patients had multiple separate tumors. Parotidectomy is the treatment of choice for tumors of this gland and with adequate surgical treatment, if the tumor is the benign mixed type, the local recurrence rate should be zero. In the M. D. Anderson Hospital series, only one recurrence of primary benign mixed tumor has been seen and a needle biopsy had been performed in that patient at another institution. About 10 per cent of parotid gland tumors occur in the deep lobe of the gland.

REFERENCE

Krolls, S. O., and Boyer, R. C.: Mixed tumor of salivary glands. *Cancer*, 30:276-281, July 1972.

Case 2.—Adenoid Cystic Carcinoma of Left Maxillary Antrum

Necessity for recognizing and determining the extent of cranial nerve involvement. This 70-year-old Caucasian woman had history of pain and swelling of the left side of the palate of six weeks' duration when admitted to M. D. Anderson Hospital on November 29, 1968. In September 1968, the patient noticed discomfort over the left palate causing her to remove her dentures which she had worn for about 35 years. Her dentist referred her to an oral surgeon who operated on the area and subsequently submitted a biopsy. Pathologic examination established the lesion as adenoid cystic carcinoma.

On physical examination, a smooth cystic swelling was found in the left upper gingivobuccal sulcus. The mucosa was intact. No tumor was palpable along the floor of the orbit. Extraocular movements were normal. Cervical lymph nodes were not palpable.

Sinus tumor survey showed a mass occupying most of the left antrum, and involving the left half of the nose, the left ethmoid sinus, and possibly the medial wall of the orbit. The sphenoid sinus on the left was cloudy; however, whether this was the result of sinusitis or tumor invasion could not be determined.

Discussion

Diagnostic radiology.—The sinus tumor survey consists of routine films of the paranasal sinuses and a set of anterior-posterior tomograms of the sinuses. Complete opacification of the left maxillary sinus was demonstrated with an obvious density in the left nasal fossa. The left frontal sinuses were somewhat clouded. The left maxillary sinus was dense and a portion of the posterior wall of the sinuses was destroyed. The tomograms showed the mass extended almost to the midline of the nasal fossa. Tumor was seen in the ethmoids, and the floor of the orbit showed evidence of destruction. The left pterygoid plates had densities between them, as well as sclerosis. The left foramen rotundum was much less well defined than the right. These were considered highly suspicious findings, but, again, the sinus tumor survey is performed primarily to determine the anatomic extent of disease for the surgeon or the radiotherapist. The changes in the foramen rotundum might indicate perineural metastasis. The primary radiologic evidence is change such as widening or destruction of the mandibular canal.

PATHOLOGY.—Adenoid cystic carcinoma is the most frequently occurring malignant tumor of the submaxillary and the minor salivary glands. In the M. D. Anderson Hospital experience, through 1970, in 120 patients, 85 tumors were located in the minor salivary glands, mainly in the oral cavity, palate, and tongue; 28 were in the nasal and paranasal sinuses, and 16 were in locations such as hypopharynx, nasopharynx, and other head and neck sites, while 21 were in the submaxillary and 14 in the parotid glands. The characteristic histologic pattern is composed of small cells with very dark nuclei. They form a glandular pattern surrounding the cystic structures in the typical cribriform pattern (Fig. 2). The tumors may be solid in some areas. Adenoid cystic carcinoma has a strong tendency to invade the perineural spaces. In the M. D. Anderson Hospital series, 70 per cent of the tumors showed significant perineural invasion. Margins were free of tumor but the tumor extended to the external palatine fossa, and the infraorbital nerve was invaded. There was extensive tumor involvement in the foramen rotundum and the perineural spaces.

SURGERY.—The difficulty in treating adenoid cystic carcinomas is created by their peculiar tendency to grow along nerves. Pain may suggest that the nerve is involved, but the only certain indication is numbness. The surgical

FIG. 2.—Adenoid cystic carcinoma showing typical cribriform pattern (H and E, × 50).

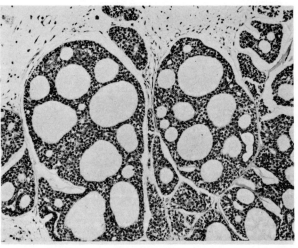

procedure for this patient was a maxillary resection with preservation of the orbit. The infraorbital nerve and the sphenopalatine ganglion were removed. When the second division of the fifth nerve was traced back to the foramen rotundum, biopsies still showed tumor. This meant one of two alternatives: to proceed with irradiation therapy or to have neurosurgeons remove the gasserian ganglion. Because of the extent of this patient's tumor, postoperative radiotherapy was judged preferable.

MAXILLOFACIAL PROSTHETICS.—Surgical removal of this tumor created an extensive defect which necessitated use of an obturator to permit the patient to eat. However, this now has had to be simplified because of trismus which has diminished the capacity of the oral cavity. The Maxillofacial Service continues to assist such patients regardless of prognosis.

RADIOTHERAPY.—A tumor dose of 6,000 rads was administered in six weeks through a pair of 60-degree wedge filters, anterior and lateral. The gasserian ganglion was included since the foramen rotundum was involved. No attempt was made to spare the eye. In order to avoid dosimetric alterations produced by the air cavity, it was packed with moistened gauze sponge. Sometimes such treatments are given with the obturator in place. This patient developed interstitial keratitis which was not amenable to therapy, and the irradiated eye was enucleated. However, the patient has remained relatively well for four and a half years. Just as eye complications may occur when the gasserian ganglion is surgically removed, including the eye in the radiation field will produce changes. Keratinization of the conjunctiva, iridocyclitis, cataract formation, and such complications can be expected, depending on the total dose. The problem apparently is caused by the obliteration of the fine vasculature which supplies the nerve, apart from the massive doses which produce acute destruction of neural tissue. In an earlier series of patients with adenoid cystic carcinoma studied at M. D. Anderson Hospital, among patients who initially were thought to be candidates only for palliation, one third lived for five years.

COMMENT.—With patients seen early enough to completely excise the tumor and control the perineural extensions, the risk of local recurrence or distant metastasis is greatly reduced. Patients with adenoid cystic carcinoma should be followed for 10 years or more because the tumor grows slowly and kills slowly.

Even patients with multiple pulmonary nodules in both lung fields survive with good local control of the primary tumor. Such nodules are known to remain relatively quiescent for years. For a patient with a single pulmonary nodule, resection may be indicated. Postmortem studies also support the thesis that the major effort should be directed toward local control of the primary tumors.

Although the diagnostic radiologist reports sclerosis in the pterygoid process, the surgeon should not be deterred in efforts to achieve control.

REFERENCES

Eneroth, C. M., Hjertman, L., and Moberger, G.: Adenoid cystic carcinoma of the palate. *Acta Otolaryngologica,* 66:248-260, February 1968.
Ballantyne, A. J., and Ibanez, M. L.: The extension of cancer of the head and neck through peripheral nerves. *American Journal of Surgery,* 106:651-667, March 1963.

Case 3.—Embryonal Rhabdomyosarcoma of the Nasopharynx

THERAPEUTIC APPROACH TO AN EXTENSIVE INOPERABLE LESION.—This eight-year-old girl was admitted in August 1967, for treatment because of a large tumor of the nasopharynx. The mass obstructed both nostrils and extended into the right auditory canal. The hard palate was displaced downward on the right, and a pendulum of tumor growth was visualized behind the uvula. Roentgenograms of the skull showed destruction of bone in the right mastoid area. Tumor also involved the right sphenoid sinus and the right side of the floor of the posterior fossa.

The pathologic diagnosis of a biopsy from the tumor was embryonal rhabdomyosarcoma.

DISCUSSION

DIAGNOSTIC RADIOLOGY.—The radiologist seeing an eight-year-old girl with a mass in the nasopharynx might think of the diagnosis of rhabdomyosarcoma on the basis of sex and age. Another lesion which becomes huge and resembles this tumor is juvenile angiofibroma. However, these lesions usually occur in teenage males rather than younger females. On the tomograms of this patient, opacification of the sphenoid sinuses was evident and the floor appeared to be destroyed. One major problem is whether the tumor is in the sinuses or whether the radiologic changes represent obstruction and infection. The most obvious finding, comparing the external auditory canals, was that the tumor was growing up through the base of the skull into the ear. However, following a vigorous regimen of simultaneous chemotherapy and radiotherapy, with extended chemotherapy, follow-up films demonstrated dramatic regression of the lesion. At the present time, the huge mass is no longer present. Some sclerosis may be seen at the base of the skull but this may be secondary to initial infection. Some repair of bone is evident. However, the fields did include the eye, and in November 1971, she had to have a cataract operation. Subsequently, with contact lenses, the patient has no visual problems.

PATHOLOGY.—Rhabdomyosarcoma is the most frequently encountered soft tissue sarcoma of the head and neck region. Of 70 patients with sarcomas in the head and neck reviewed in 1962, 48 had rhabdomyosarcoma, 38 of the embryonal type and 10 of the alveolar type. These tumors have cellular pleomorphic areas and myxomatous stroma. The numerous pleomorphic cells are elongated and have an eosinophilic cytoplasm (Fig. 3). Some cells are round but the eosinophilic cytoplasm of the neoplastic cells still is obvious. The electron microscope has proved helpful in the differential diagnosis of the more pleomorphic undifferentiated tumors. The rhabdomyosarcoma contains a large amount of glycogen which is demonstrated by simple PAS stain. However, the most diagnostic feature of the ultrastructure is presence of myofilaments in the cytoplasm of the tumor cells.

RADIOTHERAPY.—A tumor dose of 5,000 rads was administered with the majority of treatment through a three-wedge distribution, 45 degrees anteriorly, 45 degrees on the left lateral, and 60 degrees on the right. In addition, another 500 rads were given in two boosts, one over the temporal bone and another over the ethmoid sinuses. The patient received chemotherapy during her treatment, developed severe mucositis and dysphagia,

FIG. 3.—Embryonal rhabdomyosarcoma composed of pleomorphic malignant cells with cross striations in the cytoplasm (H and E, × 400).

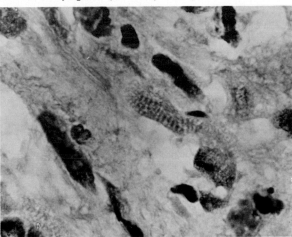

and lost considerable weight, despite maximum efforts by the pediatric staff. However, this child now exhibits none of the natural sequelae expected in heavily irradiated patients. A very important point is the preoperative or pretreatment evaluation of such patients to prevent interference with treatment by infection, abscessed teeth, or similar complications. The Maxillofacial Service now is evaluating all patients prior to chemotherapy so that treatment is not jeopardized by infection within the oral cavity. The importance of oral hygiene cannot be overemphasized as these rigorous treatment regimes are pursued successfully.

The possibility of this child developing thyroid carcinoma must be considered. However, from the Marshall Islands studies, it was learned that children who were exposed to irradiation under the age of ten had thyroid neoplasia, but none of the lesions have been malignant. Carcinoma of the thyroid has occurred in children treated for neuroblastoma of the head and neck; a child receiving mediastinal irradiation received sufficient scatter to develop carcinoma of the thyroid. Another child whose head was irradiated at the age of about one year returned with masses in the neck at age three. They were thought to be metastatic tumor, but biopsy proved the lesions to be papillary and follicular carcinoma of the thyroid gland. At age three years and six months the child had total thyroidectomy and modified bilateral neck dissection. It is postulated that because of the difficulty of positioning such a young child, she had received a significant amount of irradiation to the thyroid gland, which caused the carcinoma.

CHEMOTHERAPY.—Chemotherapy now is making very significant contributions to the control of childhood cancers. In 1967, when this patient was treated, staff members were just establishing the multimodal approach to treatment for tumors in children. Single cytotoxic agents had been used in metastatic lesions and it was thought that combination chemotherapy would be a good approach to rhabdomyosarcoma. This case demonstrates several points: combined radiotherapy and chemotherapy administered simultaneously; use of combinations of drugs; and prolonged chemotherapy (two years in this patient). While the child was receiving radiotherapy, actinomycin-D and vincristine were given. Cyclophosphamide and Cytoxan were not used in the initial phases of treatment because of the side effect of Cytoxan in producing bone marrow depression. Even the use of actinomycin-D and vincristine produced such severe toxicity in this child that the projected course of vincristine was reduced from 12 weekly doses to 10. The standard dosages are: Actinomycin-D, 15 mcg./kilo/day for five days or a total of 75 mcg./kilo/course. The aim was to take advantage of a possible synergism between actinomycin-D and radiotherapy. Vincristine dosage was 2 mg./meter^2/week for a projected 12 weeks. Eight doses were administered without too much difficulty, but the last two produced toxic reactions. Following radiotherapy, Cytoxan was begun in what was then the standard dose, 2.5 mg./kilo/day by mouth. This was continued for two years. This approach, known as VAC (vincristine, actinomycin-D, and Cytoxan) proved to be highly successful for this patient as well as a number of patients who subsequently received similar treatment.

REFERENCES

Bardwil, J. M., and MacComb, W. S.: Sarcoma of the head and neck. *American Journal of Surgery*, 108:476-479, October 1964.
Donaldson, S. S., Castro, J. R., Wilbur, J. R., and Jesse, R. H.: Rhabdomyosarcoma of head and neck in children, combination treatment by surgery, irradiation, and chemotherapy. *Cancer*, 31:26-35, January 1973.

Case 4.—Ewing's Tumor Located in the Mandible

MANAGEMENT OF AN IMPORTANT PEDIATRIC TUMOR IN A RARE SITE.—This 11-year-old Caucasian boy had a history of slightly painful swelling of the right mandible and parotid area, increasing rather rapidly within the month before admission to M. D. Anderson Hospital. In addition to the swelling, physical examination revealed some palpable nodes in the right upper neck. No other abnormalities were present. Roentgenograms of the mandible demonstrated multiple areas of punctate destruction. Skeletal survey was normal, as were the results of routine laboratory studies. Biopsy of the mandible revealed Ewing's tumor.

DISCUSSION

PATHOLOGY.—Ewing's sarcoma has distinct characteristics. The tumor cells are loculated by septa of connective tissue; darker cells are intermixed with cells having clear cytoplasms. The cells are very uniform in size, shape, and color at higher power, with no prominent nucleoli (Fig. 4), as is seen in histiocytic lymphoma. Nuclei are very prominent and more pleomorphic in histiocytic lymphoma, which is the usual differential diagnosis. Neuroblastoma is more frequently seen in the head and neck region than is Ewing's tumor, but in neuroblastoma neurofibers are usually seen. The most useful stain is demonstration of glycogen by PAS which stains it red, followed by digestion with diastase. Lymphomas and neuroblastomas are negative for glycogen. Electron microscopy is very useful in differentiation of small cell tumors. For example, neurofibers may not be evident with light microscopy in some neuroblastomas. With the electron microscope

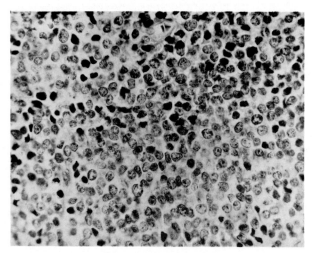

Fig. 4.—Uniform round cells with no prominent nucleoli in Ewing's tumor (H and E, × 300).

neurosecretory granules can be seen which are very characteristic of neuroblastoma. Both the rhabdomyosarcoma and Ewing's tumor are glycogen positive. The alveolar rhabdomyosarcoma cells are very similar to those of Ewing's tumor. However, the character of the nuclei will enable the pathologist to establish the differential diagnosis. In M. D. Anderson Hospital experience with Ewing's sarcoma of the mandible in young patients before 1966 only four patients were treated. Two of the tumors were in the body of the mandible and two were in the angle. All four patients received irradiation therapy. All tumors recurred and all four patients had the mandibles resected. These patients lived only 6 to 22 months. This is in contrast to the present case in which the multimodal approach with chemotherapy was applied.

RADIOTHERAPY.—From the viewpoint of the radiotherapists, Ewing's tumor has been considered a radiosensitive but not necessarily a curable lesion. The total M. D. Anderson Hospital experience before the time that this child was treated was marked by an approximately 40 per cent local recurrence rate. The tumor dose had been increased from 5,000 rads to 7,000 rads, but this had no effect on the recurrence rate. In this patient, the foramen ovale was considered to be at risk, so the entire mandible and the base of the skull were included in the fields. The mass was in excess of 6 cm. in thickness and measured 6 × 8 × 6 cm. Therefore, a cobalt field was used to deliver 1,000 rads tumor dose in the first week while additional dosimetry was calculated. The majority of radiotherapy was administered through a 45-degree wedge pair, anterior posterior, delivering 4,000 rads tumor dose. A boost was given to the field with 18 MEV electrons for a total of 6,000 rads.

Apparently most of the metastases from Ewing's tumor initially occur in the lungs. A national study is being formulated in which half of the children will receive prophylactic irradiation to the lungs. Earlier, similar thinking was applied to Wilms' tumor but it was found that children who received the prophylactic irradiation did eventually develop pulmonary metastases; whether Ewing's tumor will behave differently remains to be determined. Prophylactic whole body radiation has been suggested by some therapists.

CHEMOTHERAPY.—Ewing's tumor is considered to be less chemosensitive than rhabdomyosarcoma, but occasionally a child will respond to one of several agents. This patient was treated under a protocol developed by the departments of Pediatrics, Medicine, and Radiotherapy. Two drugs were used, vincristine and Cytoxan. In contrast to the daily doses given the previous patient with rhabdomyosarcoma, the approach had changed to administration of large doses of Cytoxan for a short time with rest periods between "pulses." The program requires approximately 32 weeks. Vincristine is given initially weekly for five doses and subsequently is administered on days 1 and 8 of each Cytoxan pulse. This is very rigorous therapy and produces bone marrow depression with leukopenia sometimes below 500, particularly during the phase when Cytoxan and radiotherapy are combined. But with close teamwork between the radiotherapists and pediatricians, most patients have been able to complete the course. Dosages are standard: 2 mg./meter^2, maximum of 2 mg./dose for vincristine and for Cytoxan approximately 10 mg./kilo orally or intravenously for 7 to 10 days. The Cytoxan pulse seldom is continued beyond the 10-day course.

This patient had tumor recurrence and the mandible was resected. Because of the history of irradiation and some difficulty in healing of the defect inside the mouth, his postoperative course of chemotherapy was one of the nitrosourea compounds, CCNU; the dosage was 130 mg./meter^2 every six weeks.

SURGERY.—When the tumor recurred, the mandible was resected from the mental foramen to the coronoid fossa. Along with disarticulation, a quantity of surrounding tissue, as well as masseter muscle and mucosa, was removed. Despite the fact that the resection was well around the radiological evidence of tumor, curettings of the bone marrow at the margins still showed tumor. Additional mandible was resected to within 1 cm. or 2 cm. of the midline. At that point, curettings were negative. Because of the histological findings, lack of skin, soft tissue, and mucosa, a prosthesis was not attempted. The mucosal defect was closed with a skin graft which took fairly well.

MAXILLOFACIAL PROSTHETICS.—With this type of tumor there usually is lack of tissue, preventing successful placement of a prosthesis. The most important rehabilitation factor is to have the patient initiate a series of exercises. These are designed to prevent deviation toward the defect side because of the heavy irradiation, chemotherapy, and surgery. A minor amount of effort will prevent problems in function and appearance. All growth has stopped because of the radiotherapy. The teeth developing at the time of initial surgery have remained the same. This is a typical reaction to such a dosage.

COMMENT. Only a few chemotherapeutic agents are effective for childhood tumors. Vincristine and Cytoxan are prominent. The chemotherapeutic combinations probably would be fairly similar regardless of the type of small cell malignancy. Alveolar rhabdomyosarcoma and embryonal rhabdomyosarcoma are treated identically. Embryonal rhabdomyosarcoma has a considerably better prognosis than does the alveolar type, however.

REFERENCES

Dahlin, D. C., Coventry, M. B., and Scanlon, P. W.: Ewing's sarcoma: Critical analysis of 165 cases. *Journal of Bone and Joint Surgery,* 43(A):185-192, March 1961.
Hustu, H. O., Pinkel, D., and Pratt, C. B.: Treatment of clinical localized Ewing's sarcoma with radiation therapy and combination chemotherapy. *Cancer,* 30: 1522-1527, December 1972.

Case 5.—Osteosarcoma of the Mandible

MANAGEMENT OF A PATIENT WITH PREVIOUS HISTORY OF EMBRYONAL RHABDOMYOSARCOMA TREATED WITH RADIOTHERAPY.—In May 1961 a three-year-old girl was first admitted to M. D. Anderson Hospital with history of recurrent embryonal rhabdomyosarcoma on the right nasolabial fold. The original lesion had been excised in another institution in August 1959, followed by 4,500 rads radiation therapy given in a small 2 × 2 inch field. On May 22, 1961, an excision of the right ala of the nose was performed with full thickness skin graft from the abdomen.

The patient was apparently free of disease and doing well until December 1971, when she noticed that the lower teeth in the midportion appeared to be pointing backward. She was seen by a dentist and an orthodontist. At that time x-ray films were taken. About the same time her mother died and her father was transferred to another city; this delayed any additional medical attention until May 1972, when a biopsy established the diagnosis of osteosarcoma. The patient was referred to M. D. Anderson Hospital for further therapy.

Physical examination showed a large mass in the chin, measuring 8 × 5 cm. The labial sulcus was distorted by what appeared to be a soft tissue mass. Radiological studies of the mandible demonstrated a mixed osteoblastic and osteolytic lesion in the symphysis of the mandible. This was associated with extensive spiculated periosteal reaction. No tumor activity was evident beyond the first bicuspid.

DISCUSSION

DIAGNOSTIC RADIOLOGY.—The lesion was located anteriorly and the Panorex film showed sclerosis and destruction along the alveolar margin. The occlusal view showed the lesion extended across the symphysis of the mandible. The large anterior soft tissue mass was spiculated. Mineralized tumor matrix in the soft tissues had a cloudlike appearance characteristic of osteosarcoma. Though the radiologic criteria are identical for the diagnosis of osteosarcoma of the mandible and osteosarcoma of the long bones, their biological behavior differs. Patients with the mandibular lesions usually are older, usually have local spread and recurrences but have longer survival. Patients with osteosarcoma of the long bones usually are younger, usually succumb to pulmonary metastases, and generally have poorer prognosis.

PATHOLOGY.—The original biopsy in 1959 showed a tumor composed of long, spindle-shaped, eosinophilic cells. Much of the stroma was myxoid. The cells had centrally located multiple nuclei and many could be seen with cross striations. The diagnosis was clearly rhabdomyosarcoma. In 1972, the biopsy of the mandible again showed sarcoma with many neoplastic cells with mitoses. The distinguishing characteristic was production of osteoid and bone. The histologic diagnosis of the second tumor was osteosarcoma (Fig. 5A). Excision of a portion of the mandible was performed.

The surgical specimen showed that the margins were free of tumor. The lesion was located primarily in the symphysis and invaded soft tissues (Fig. 5B). As these osteosarcomas distend the periosteum, trabeculae are left behind, giving the characteristic "sun ray" pattern on the roentgenograms. The histologic patterns of osteosarcomas are variable. Some obvious areas of chondrosarcoma with large neoplastic nuclei can be seen. Other areas contain definite neoplastic spindle cells with osteoblastic bone.

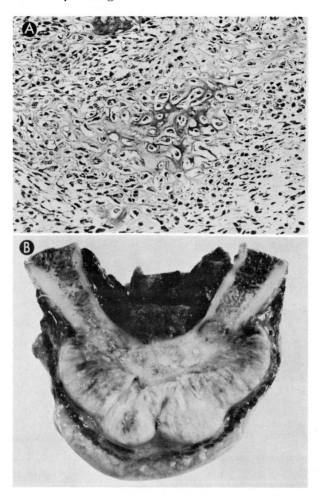

FIG. 5.—Osteosarcoma. *A*, section showing malignant spindle cells forming osteoid (H and E, × 80). *B*, whole section showing the lesion invading soft tissues.

Osteosarcomas of the mandible and the long bones are identical, histologically; however, mandibular lesions tend to be less anaplastic. The institutional experience with osteosarcoma of the maxilla and mandible was reviewed by Doctor Finkelstein in 1970. The series contained 12 cases in each site. These patients usually were older than those with osteosarcomas in the peripheral bones. Five of 10 patients with tumors of the mandible survived more than five years. The same tumors in the maxilla are more aggressive, primarily because of invasion of the brain.

Surgery.—When the rhabdomyosarcoma recurred in 1961, the patient had a wide local excision with skin graft. Any further reconstruction was inadvisable because the tissues were continuing to grow. Reconstruction will be postponed until full growth is achieved, resorting to a prosthesis for cosmetic purposes in the meantime. When the patient returned as a teenager in 1972, she had a large lesion involving the skin as well as the mandible. In contrast to tumors of the long bones, where the surgical procedure usually is resection of the entire bone, lesions in the mandible are approached differently. Only sufficient mandible is removed to excise the tumor. However, in this patient, the overlying skin had to be resected also. Curettings of both sides of the portion of the mandible excised showed that the margins were negative for tumor. A flap rotated up from the neck provided the soft tissue coverage. The forehead flap was preserved to repair the nose at some later date.

Maxillofacial prosthetics.—Because this patient still is growing, the result of any attempt to perform definitive repair by plastic surgery at this time would be grotesque at a later time. At the time of operation, an 18×8 inch stainless steel bar was inserted to maintain contour. A prosthesis was prepared, and at the present time the patient is quite presentable, though she returns approximately every 18 months for a new prosthesis because of the growth occurring. The stainless steel bar was selected as the simplest means of maintaining position. It is intended as a space-preserving expedient, not a final mandibular replacement which will be performed later, providing both lesions remain under control.

Chemotherapy.—This patient has been placed on an investigative regime of four-drug chemotherapy known as CONPADRI (Cytoxan; oncovin or vincristine; phenylalanine mustard or L-sarcolysin; and adriamycin). Presently, about 19 children are on this regime, but it was initiated too recently to show definite results. However, the survival rates appear to be improved over those for osteogenic sarcomas of all sites in children.

The question of second malignancies in children is being examined in great detail. Until recent advancements in the management of childhood malignant diseases, most children succumbed to the first tumor before a second lesion had time to develop. For example, in this patient there is a long survival period which gave the second tumor time to become evident.

Radiotherapy.—According to the established criteria for diagnosis of radiation-induced sarcoma, this patient's previous therapy in the nasolabial area could not have been responsible for the osteosarcoma of the mandible. As long as 24 years ago the following criteria were recognized: A histologically proven benign lesion or radiologically normal bone must be within the field of irradiation. The malignant change must be in the bone within the field of radiation and must be histologically proven to be a sarcoma. There should be a latent period of some years between the termination of radiation and the onset of the sarcoma. In retrospect, it appears almost impossible for the symphysis of the mandible to have been directly in the radiation field used for the nasolabial fold. The field of 5 cm. was moderately large for a child of three years, but it appears that it could not have been angled in such a manner to involve the symphysis. Hence, this patient's osteosarcoma was accepted as a second, spontaneous primary tumor.

However, in the review of the 24 patients with osteosarcoma, 12 in the mandible and 12 in the maxilla, several patients had tumors which met all the criteria for radiation-induced lesions. For example, one male patient received radiotherapy for a squamous cell lesion of the nasopharynx and later developed an osteosarcoma in the left maxilla. Another patient had received extremely high doses of irradiation for retinoblastoma in childhood and developed a tumor of the maxillary sinus. Furthermore, since osteosarcomas of the facial bones may appear as malignant degeneration of fibrous dysplasia, patients with fibrous dysplasia should be followed rather closely.

As for the role of irradiation in treatment of this patient's mandibular lesion, radiotherapists are not convinced it has a place either pre- or postoperatively. Large series of cases have been reported where preoperative irradiation was administered in doses as high as 12,000 rads but survival rates or length of survival were not improved.

REFERENCES

Finkelstein, G. V.: Osteosarcoma of jaw bones. *Radiologic Clinics of North America*, 8:425-443, December 1970.

Garrington, G. E.: Osteosarcoma of the jaws. Analysis of 56 cases. *Cancer*, 20: 337-391, March 1967.

Case 6.—Recurrent Ameloblastoma of Mandible

TREATMENT OF THIS IMPORTANT ODONTOGENIC TUMOR.—This 64-year-old Caucasian man was referred to M. D. Anderson Hospital in May 1969, with history of recurrent pain and increasing swelling of the right mandible of 5 months' duration. In 1951, he first noticed swelling of the right mandible which was diagnosed as ameloblastoma; curettement was performed. In 1959, he experienced a recurrence and a similar procedure was repeated.

On physical examination, swelling on the right side of the mandible extended from the first molar to the midline. No mucosal involvement was observed, but there was soft tissue swelling in the area of the mylohyoid and around the right mandible.

Radiological examination of the mandible by routine projections demonstrated a large multicystic lesion 6 × 4 cm. involving the anterior part of the body of the right hemimandible. It crossed the midline and extended almost to the mental foramen on the left. The cortex was expanded, especially in the inferior aspect of the lesion.

Discussion

Diagnostic radiology.—The Panorex film demonstrated sclerotic margins around a large lesion involving the right side of the mandible. Expansion of the bone was evident as was some break in the cortex. What might be described as a "soap-bubble" pattern was seen in some areas. Two curettements had been performed in the past. Radiologically, this multicystic lesion appeared to be of very low aggressiveness. It had none of the spiculation or anaplasia seen with osteosarcoma and Ewing's sarcoma. As many as 10 or 15 lesions might have almost identical radiographic features. A biopsy is necessary to arrive at the final diagnosis, but ameloblastoma would be one possibility. When a patient 64 years old presents with a lytic lesion in the mandible, it should be approached just as is a lesion of the long bone. First, any possibility of metastases or manifestation of myeloma should be ruled out. Metastases to the mandible occur from tumors of just about every anatomic site. Myeloma often involves the mandible but is not often recorded as the presenting complaint.

Pathology.—From the original biopsy, the lesion was recurrent ameloblastoma. Histologically, the tumor had very characteristic epithelial nests with connective tissue. Stellate reticulum formed the center of the nests with tall cuboidal cells on the periphery. In some areas, keratin metaplasia may be seen in the stellate reticulum; other areas may have granular cells. These variations have led to elaborate subclassifications which have no clinical application. The most important point is that the pathologist distinguish this lesion from other odontogenic tumors which behave differently. For example, two lesions which are most frequently seen in children and seldom recur after curettement are the adeno-ameloblastoma and the ameloblastic fibroma. The adeno-ameloblastoma is characterized by a glandular pattern and tubule formation with scattered calcification. The ameloblastic fibroma is composed of epithelial cells and neoplastic mesenchymal cells. Furthermore, the pathologist must distinguish the ameloblastoma from malignant tumors such as adenoid cystic carcinoma or squamous carcinoma which occasionally have necrosis or a pseudofollicular pattern.

When this particular surgical specimen was examined, the margins of resection were free (Fig. 6A). The tumor was destroying the body of the mandible and, in the wall of the specimen, numerous nodules occurred, representing the neoplastic cells (Fig. 6B). In some areas, the periosteum was very thin.

In the M. D. Anderson Hospital experience, solid ameloblastoma tends to recur more frequently than does the cystic type which this patient had. However, the most important factor is therapy, regardless of the histology of the tumor. No patients with metastatic ameloblastoma have been seen at M. D. Anderson Hospital. However, a few well-documented cases have been reported and the metastasis has been to the lungs after multiple recurrences and repeated surgical procedures. Many of the metastatic ameloblastomas were of the granular cell type. However, the histology is much less important than is the initial treatment for the first primary tumor.

SURGERY.—This case points up discussion of curettement versus surgical excision of the affected portion of the mandible. Occasionally, ameloblastoma occurs in children when the mandible or maxilla still is immature. These are essentially benign lesions and, in children, the mandible may be curetted if the procedure is done very thoroughly and carefully. If the lesion does recur, the mandible can be resected and a prosthesis used with good cosmetic results. However, in patients such as the one presented, whose mandible has matured, surgical resection and use of a prosthesis is

FIG. 6.—*A*, cystic ameloblastoma. *B*, ameloblastoma destroying mandible; notice epithelial cells arranged in follicles (H and E, × 20).

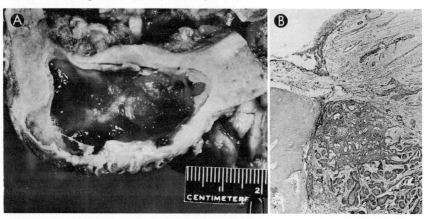

preferable. These tumors do not involve the mucosa. They rarely extend into the soft tissue or skin and the patient is left with all the requirements for insertion of a satisfactory prosthesis.

MAXILLOFACIAL PROSTHETICS.—A tantalum tray containing a marrow graft was used for this patient. In this procedure, the alignment is the critical factor. Therefore, an intra-oral stent was made prior to surgical treatment. At the time of placement of the tray, the entire prosthesis is held together as one rigid structure. Circum-mandibular wiring attached the mandible to the stent. Circum-zygomatic wiring completed the placement and the patient was maintained in this manner for seven weeks. Practically the full contour was achieved. When last seen the bone was well organized within the tantalum tray and the patient will be returning for surgery to remove the tray. The bone is sufficiently organized to function as a mandible.

A different approach was used in another male patient who had a large ameloblastoma involving the entire ascending ramus. Acrylic was used to reconstruct the ascending ramus and a stainless steel bar was inserted across. This type of prosthesis must be anchored to the remaining bone with an immovable fixture, so bolts were used. This patient's prosthesis now has been successfully in place for seven years.

REFERENCES

Gorlin, R. J.: Odontogenic tumors in man and animals: pathologic classification and clinical behavior. *Annals of the New York Academy of Sciences,* 108:722-771, May 1963.

Small, I. A., and Waldron, C. A.: Ameloblastoma of jaw. *Oral Surgery, Oral Medicine and Oral Pathology,* 8:281-297, April 1955.

Index

Cranial
  intracranial (*see* Intracranial)
  nerve involvement in adenoid cystic an-
    trum carcinoma, 379
Craniofacial exenteration, 199
Cutaneous hypersensitivity: to DNCB,
    214, 216
Cyclohexyl-chloroethyl-nitrosurea, 130
Cyclophosphamide: in rhabdomyosar-
    coma, in children, 283, 285
Cytosine arabinoside, 130

D

Daunorubicin: chemical structure of, 128
Death (*see* Mortality)
Deltopectoral flaps
  in oral defect repair, 241-247
  in pharyngeal reconstruction, 254-256
Dental care and radiotherapy, 225-231
  bone necrosis, 226-230
    cause of, 226-227
    extractions causing, 227-229
    management of, 229-230
  program, 225-226
    objectives of, 226
  tooth decay after therapy, 230-231
    prevention of, 230-231
Dentures: and oral cancer, 339-341
Diet (*see* Nutrition)
2,4-Dinitrochlorobenzene, 213
  delayed cutaneous hypersensitivity to,
    214, 216
DNCB, 213
  delayed cutaneous hypersensitivity to,
    214, 216
Dose
  cancerocidal, original concept of, 19
  preoperative, high vs. low, 49-50
  -response curve for subclinical disease,
    24-26
  tumor control, 26-27
  tumor size and, 27
Dressings: nursing care, 309
Droperidol, 117-118, 119
Dura: irradiation and surgery, 88

E

Energy requirements: daily, 327
Epiglottis: squamous cell carcinoma, 154-
    157
Epithelial tumors: radiosensitivity, 27-28
Esophagostomy: feeding through, 314

Esophagus
  (*See also* Tracheoesophageal)
  speech, comparison with normal and
    tracheoesophageal speech, 111
Ethmoid sinus
  carcinoma
    angiography, 161
    resection, 198
  fibrosarcoma, treatment, 198
  intracranial facial resection, surgical
    complications, 196
Ewing's tumor (*see* Mandible, Ewing's tu-
    mor in)
Extractions: teeth, causing bone necrosis,
    227-229
Extremities: soft tissue sarcomas of, irra-
    diation and surgery, 35
Eye
  lubricant, 317
  patch, for cosmetic palliation, 316

F

Face
  craniofacial exenteration, 199
  hemangioma, angiography, 172
  intracranial facial resection (*see* Intra-
    cranial facial resection)
  maxillofacial (*see* Maxillofacial)
Fast neutrons (*see* Radiotherapy, fast neu-
    tron)
Faucial arch
  cancer
    irradiation and surgery, 54
    surgical salvage for radiation failures,
      79
  carcinoma, subclinical disease, and irra-
    diation, 21, 22
Feeding
  through esophagostomy, 314
  jejunostomy and
    Mäydl, 315
    Witzel, 315
  tube (*see* Nasogastric tube feeding)
Fentanyl, 117-118, 119
Fibroma: nasopharynx angiofibroma, an-
    giography, 164-166
Fibrosarcoma: ethmoid sinus, treatment,
    198
Fistula: pharyngeal, after laryngectomy
    after radiation, 89
Flaps
  in oral defect repair, 237-249
    deltopectoral flaps, 241-247